Praise for Leslie Beck's Books

"Canada's nutrition guru has mapped out a plan that guarantees a new you. If you follow her 12-week plan, you will lose weight. Period." —*Calgary Herald*

"One of the most sensible 'diet books' out there." —*The Georgia Straight*

"Adolescence is a critical period for developing healthy eating and exercise habits, and the guidance provided in this book is invaluable."
—Chris Carmichael, personal coach to eight-time Tour de France champion Lance Armstrong and author of *Chris Carmichael's Food for Fitness*

"Teenagers are constantly confronted with fast food, poor cafeteria choices and eating on the go. *Healthy Eating for Teens and Preteens* provides them with straightforward, useable tools for making the right food choices."
—Dr. Marla Shapiro, medical consultant, CTV

"Leslie Beck offers indispensable advice for healthy living."
—James F. Balch, MD, co-author of *The Prescription for Nutritional Healing*

"If you'd like to eat more healthfully, Leslie Beck is a must-read."
—*Homemakers* magazine

"Leslie Beck, one of Canada's leading authorities on nutrition, has written another well researched, fabulously written and perfectly executed book, this time on boosting heart health. It's chock full of useful information and tips as well as scrumptious heart healthy recipes."
—Pauline Anderson, family health editor, *Canadian Living*

"[Beck's] book offers plenty of sound nutrition information and evidence-based diet strategies that can help protect you from coronary heart disease. It's all about implementing a sustainable, heart healthy lifestyle. The tools in this book will help you achieve this." —Dr. Rob Myers, Director of Cardiology, Medcan Clinic

"A comprehensive nutrition book aimed at teens that also includes terrific information for the whole family. It includes the most up-to-date information that will help your teen form a great foundation for a healthy lifestyle."
—Sally Brown, CEO, Heart and Stroke Foundation of Canada

"Parents and teens need all the help they can get, including nutrition advice. This book is so practical and thorough that I plan to share it with my daughter and son." —Linda Lewis, editor-in-chief, *Today's Parent*

"It is a relief to have Leslie Beck's well-researched, approachable and up-to-date guide to lifelong healthful eating." —Elizabeth Baird, *Canadian Living*

PENGUIN CANADA

THE COMPLETE NUTRITION GUIDE FOR WOMEN

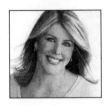

LESLIE BECK, a registered dietician, is a leading Canadian nutritionist and the bestselling author of nine nutrition books. Leslie writes a weekly nutrition column in *The Globe and Mail*, is a regular contributor to CTV's *Canada AM* and can be heard one morning a week on CFRB Radio's *The John Donabie Show* (Toronto) and CJAD Radio's *The Andrew Carter Show* (Montreal).

Leslie has worked with many of Canada's leading businesses and international food companies and runs a thriving private practice at the Medcan Clinic in Toronto. She also regularly delivers nutrition workshops to corporate groups across North America.

Visit Leslie Beck's website at **www.lesliebeck.com**.

Also by Leslie Beck

Leslie Beck's Nutrition Guide to Menopause

Leslie Beck's Nutrition Encyclopedia

Leslie Beck's Nutrition Guide for Women

10 Steps to Healthy Eating

Leslie Beck's Nutrition Guide to a Healthy Pregnancy

Healthy Eating for Preteens and Teens

The Complete Nutrition Guide to Menopause

The No-Fail Diet

Foods That Fight Disease

Heart Healthy Foods for Life

The Complete A–Z Nutrition Encyclopedia

THE COMPLETE NUTRITION GUIDE FOR WOMEN

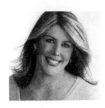

Staying Healthy with Diet, Nutrients and Supplements

Leslie Beck, RD

PENGUIN
CANADA

PENGUIN CANADA

Published by the Penguin Group

Penguin Group (Canada), 90 Eglinton Avenue East, Suite 700, Toronto, Ontario, Canada M4P 2Y3
(a division of Pearson Canada Inc.)

Penguin Group (USA) Inc., 375 Hudson Street, New York, New York 10014, U.S.A.
Penguin Books Ltd, 80 Strand, London WC2R 0RL, England
Penguin Ireland, 25 St Stephen's Green, Dublin 2, Ireland (a division of Penguin Books Ltd)
Penguin Group (Australia), 250 Camberwell Road, Camberwell, Victoria 3124, Australia
(a division of Pearson Australia Group Pty Ltd)
Penguin Books India Pvt Ltd, 11 Community Centre, Panchsheel Park, New Delhi – 110 017, India
Penguin Group (NZ), 67 Apollo Drive, Rosedale, North Shore 0745, Auckland, New Zealand
(a division of Pearson New Zealand Ltd)
Penguin Books (South Africa) (Pty) Ltd, 24 Sturdee Avenue, Rosebank, Johannesburg 2196, South Africa

Penguin Books Ltd, Registered Offices: 80 Strand, London WC2R 0RL, England

First published 2010

1 2 3 4 5 6 7 8 9 10 (WEB)

Copyright © Leslie Beck, 2010

All Health Canada information on pages 16, 20, 21, 24, 30, 67, 99, 203, and 206 is adapted and reproduced
with the permission of the Minister of Public Works and Government Services Canada, 2009.

LIBRARY AND ARCHIVES CANADA CATALOGUING IN PUBLICATION

Beck, Leslie (Leslie C.)
The complete nutrition guide for women : staying healthy with diet,
nutrients and supplements / Leslie Beck.

Includes index.
Previously published under title: Leslie Beck's nutrition
guide for women.
ISBN 978-0-14-316944-4

1. Women—Nutrition. 2. Vitamin therapy.
3. Minerals in nutrition. 4. Herbs—Therapeutic use.
I. Title. II. Series: Beck, Leslie (Leslie C.). Leslie Beck's nutrition guide for women.

RA778.B43 2010   613.2082   C2009-906074-4

Visit the Penguin Group (Canada) website at www.penguin.ca

Special and corporate bulk purchase rates available; please see
www.penguin.ca/corporatesales or call 1-800-810-3104, ext. 2477 or 2474

*This book is dedicated
to the memory of my grandmother, Dorothy Coulter;
to the women in my family;
and to the women I have worked with in my private practice.
I thank you for the incredible learning you motivate
and inspire me to achieve every single day.*

Contents

Acknowledgments

I would like to express a sincere thank-you to my researcher, Anne von Rosenbach, B.A., M.L.S., who so thoroughly and efficiently researched the many health conditions you will read about in this book—in 2000 and again in 2009. This book would not have been possible without Anne's support and research skills.

I am also appreciative of Emily Kennedy, M.Sc., a research assistant who has worked with me for the past three years, helping me research the many topics I discuss on *Canada AM* (CTV) and write about in my weekly *Globe and Mail* newspaper column. By updating the prevalence and incidence statistics on various health conditions, Emily was an asset in helping me write this edition of the book.

A heartfelt thank-you also goes out to Andrea Magyar, my editor at Penguin Canada, for her continued support of my work and for agreeing to the publication of this updated edition.

And finally, I am forever grateful to the many women I have counselled over the past twenty years in my private nutrition practice. Their questions about diet, nutrition and health have contributed to my learning and knowledge in the area of women's nutritional health. I am thankful to my clients for the ongoing opportunities to further develop my professional knowledge base and skills.

Introduction

More than 13 million adult women live in Canada today. And we can expect to live longer than did our grandmothers and great-grandmothers. A woman born in Canada in 1901 could expect to live, on average, until the age of 50, and a man until the age of 47. A century later, the situation has changed greatly. The average life expectancy for a woman in Canada today is almost 83 years, about five years longer than that of the average man.

The fact that women live longer is partly due to the fact that we practise better health than men. We're more apt to seek medical advice and we're more likely to report that we're making an effort to achieve a healthy weight, to eat better and to exercise more. Over the years, women have always been concerned about nutrition. Every day in my private practice I see women wanting dietary advice for themselves, their children and their partners. As caregivers for their families, women continue to be largely responsible for grocery shopping and meal preparation. At the same time, many women are looking after aging parents, as members of a phenomenon called the "sandwich generation." And as the female baby boomers consider retirement, there's a strong focus on living an active life, free of aches and pains. As women age, they want to fulfill their life goals with plenty of energy and in good health.

As a professional nutritionist (a Registered Dietitian), I have been giving women and men dietary and supplement advice for the past twenty years. When I see a client, I assess her diet, her supplement use, her personal and family medical history and her lifestyle, and then I make recommendations for change. Based on a woman's personal goals, I develop a customized nutrition and meal plan for her. My private practice is located in the heart of downtown Toronto, so many of my clients are professional, educated women who are taking charge of their health care.

The nutritional status of women

Despite our interest in nutrition and self-reported motivation to adopt a healthier diet, as women we experience more health problems and visit the doctor more often than men. And some of our nutrition habits receive a failing grade. Recent research suggests that Canadian women fall short of eating sufficient dairy products, fruit and vegetables—tendencies that are likely to limit your intake of important nutrients like folate, vitamins C and A, potassium, calcium, magnesium and dietary fibre.[1,2] And, although we're eating less fat than we did 30 years ago, we're getting heavier. It's estimated that slightly more than one-half (53.4 percent) of all Canadian women are overweight or obese; almost one-quarter (23 percent) are obese, having a body mass index of 30 or greater.[3,4] (To calculate your body mass index, see Chapter 2, page 37.)

Women have unique needs

It probably comes as no surprise that women have different nutrition needs than do men. The very biology of our bodies increases our need for many nutrients, such as calcium and iron. For instance, the hormonal fluctuations that women experience during their reproductive cycle have an impact on what nutrients we need and, often, what foods we eat. You'll also read how the subtle anatomical difference between the male and female urinary tract puts a woman at much greater risk for bladder infections. Pregnancy and breastfeeding are times when a woman needs to consume certain nutrients in greater amounts to nourish her growing baby. If careful attention is not given to diet, these nutrients are taken from a woman's body, leaving her depleted and at risk for health problems.

Women are also at unique risk for major nutrition-related health conditions, including heart disease, osteoporosis, breast cancer and weight-related problems. Some of these diseases are unique to women, whereas others affect women far more often than men. Risk factors for many of these diseases manifest differently for women than for men. For example, for women, having a low level of HDL (good) cholesterol is more predictive of heart disease than having a high level of LDL (bad) cholesterol. In men, high LDLs are more predictive of the disease. Being overweight puts women at risk for many health conditions, especially if excess body fat is stored around the middle.

And of course, women are much more vulnerable to societal pressures to be thin. Day after day we read in magazines and see on television that thin means beautiful, thin means successful. As a result, women are far more likely than men to be dieting, often in a quest to be underweight. The desire to be slim predisposes women to a pattern of losing and gaining weight repeatedly over the years, which can have consequences for long-term health. It also sets the stage for disordered eating, potentially leading to serious eating disorders.

How this book can help you

Fifteen years ago I was hard pressed to find good scientific information about how nutrition affected women's health. The fact was, women were less likely to be included in research studies, and the health conditions that afflict women were less likely to be studied. But that has all changed. Over the past two decades there has been an explosion in women's health issues. As findings from large trials involving women come to the forefront, scientists are unravelling the link between nutrition and women's health. This growing body of research has made writing this book possible.

Canadian women need nutrition advice that is easy to understand, relevant to their lifestyle and based on scientific evidence. Women don't need a new diet book that offers some far-fetched, unsustainable solution to losing weight. Instead women and girls need to know how food affects their weight, their energy levels and the health of their body. Canadian women need to know how to get more of the key nutrients that their health relies on. In this book, I translate current scientific research into practical food choices with defined serving sizes. When it comes to important nutrients like iron, calcium and folate, I tell you *how much* you need to be getting every day, *what foods* give you the most bang for your buck and, if you don't eat many of these foods, *how to supplement safely*.

This book is written for all women. It's for healthy women who want to stay well and lower their risk of disease. It's also for women who have a certain health condition and want to do whatever they can through diet and supplements to manage, or maybe even treat, their condition. This book is not only for adult women. It also has plenty of important information for younger women—girls and teens—who need to adopt eating habits that will lay the foundation for their future health.

How this book is organized

I've divided this book into seven parts. Parts 2 to 7 are dedicated to certain aspects of women's health—reproductive health, breast and bone health, emotional health and so on. I don't expect you to read this book cover to cover. Instead you should use it as a comprehensive reference guide to all aspects of your nutritional health care. You may be expecting your first baby and find my chapters on pregnancy and breastfeeding particularly relevant. Or you may be a woman in your late 40s experiencing hormonal ups and downs, who's more interested in my chapters on perimenopause, osteoporosis and heart disease. Finally, you may be afflicted with a particular condition, such as endometriosis or migraine headaches, and want to know how nutrition affects your health.

The first part of this book talks about the nutrition concerns of almost all women. Whatever your reason may be for picking up this book, be sure to read Chapter 1. In it, I give nutrition advice for *all* healthy women. You'll learn what nutrients are most important for optimal health, how much you need each day and how to get these nutrients in your diet. Chapter 2 deals with a topic that concerns many women: weight control. Here you'll find tools to assess your body weight and determine where you weigh in with respect to future health risks; there are also plenty of strategies that will help you successfully manage your weight over the years.

If you've read any of my other books, you're already familiar with my style. Here, too, I've tried to make the information very easy to read and easy to find. I begin each chapter with information you need to know— what causes the particular health condition, its symptoms, risk factors, conventional treatment and prevention strategies. In every chapter, I list my nutrition recommendations in four categories: dietary strategies; vitamins and minerals; herbal remedies; and other natural health products. And if you want a quick summary, just skip to the end of the chapter where I summarize my recommendations in "The Bottom Line."

I hope you and the other females in your family enjoy this book and find it a useful guide to better nutrition, improved energy and long-lasting health.

Leslie Beck, RD
Toronto, 2009

PART 1

NUTRITION ESSENTIALS FOR WOMEN

1

A healthy diet: nutrition advice for all women

As a nutritionist in private practice, I meet women every day who are concerned about their diet and nutrient intake. Many wonder if they're meeting their recommended daily intake for important vitamins and minerals. Too often, I see that their diets, like those of the average Canadian woman, are lacking in calcium, magnesium, folate, iron, zinc and fibre. Many women are also concerned about their body weight and want to take steps to ensure their weight isn't putting their health at risk. And others want to be proactive and do everything they can nutritionally to stay healthy and ease their transition into the menopausal years.

The information that follows in this chapter will help ensure your diet is providing what your body needs to stay healthy and reduce your risk of future health problems over the decades. The advice below will help you meet unique nutrient requirements that arise as women age. You'll also learn what foods and nutrients to limit in your diet to help reduce the risk of high cholesterol, high blood pressure, heart disease, diabetes, osteoporosis and certain cancers.

Every woman should strive to adhere to the following dietary guidelines. These healthy eating principles represent a common strategy to help prevent all chronic diseases that women face today.

15 Dietary guidelines

1. EMPHASIZE PLANT FOODS IN YOUR DAILY DIET.

Plan your meals around whole grains, fruit, vegetables, legumes and nuts—foods rich in fibre, vitamins, minerals and protective plant compounds called phytochemicals. When you do eat animal protein foods like meat or poultry, they should take up no more than one-quarter of your plate. Aim to eat a vegetarian meal with lentils, kidney beans, chickpeas, soybeans, tofu, soy products or tempeh three times per week. Snack on one serving—a small handful—of nuts five times per week. Studies have found that eating nuts on a regular basis can help lower high cholesterol and high blood pressure and reduce the risk of developing type 2 diabetes.

To increase your intake of these protein- and fibre-rich foods, try the following quick meal and snack ideas:

- Toss cooked legumes, like kidney beans or black beans, into leafy green and pasta salads. Add chickpeas to your favourite Greek salad recipe.
- Serve soup made from dried beans or peas. Try minestrone, split pea, black bean or lentil soup.
- Add cooked legumes or chopped firm tofu to commercial or homemade soups and stews.
- Add cooked chickpeas to grain dishes such as couscous or rice pilafs.
- Add black beans or pinto beans to tacos and burritos. Use half the amount of lean ground meat you normally would and make up the difference with beans.
- Sauté legumes, cubed tofu or tempeh with spinach and tomatoes and serve over cooked whole-wheat pasta.
- Add white kidney beans to a tomato-based pasta sauce for a Mediterranean-inspired meal.
- Add a handful of nuts to salads and stir-fries. Add chopped nuts to hot cereal and cookie and muffin batters.

2. INCLUDE AT LEAST 3 SERVINGS OF WHOLE-GRAIN FOOD IN YOUR DAILY DIET.

1 serving = 1 slice of bread, 1/2 cup (125 ml) cooked oatmeal, 1 oz (30 g) cold cereal, 1/2 cup (125 ml) cooked brown rice or whole-wheat pasta

Whole grains include whole-grain whole wheat, whole rye, whole spelt, brown rice, quinoa, millet, oats and flaxseed. These foods are naturally low in fat and good sources of vitamins, minerals, fibre, antioxidants and phytochemicals, all of which are thought to work together to guard against heart disease and type 2 diabetes.

Read labels and look for "100% whole grain" claims on food packages. The greater the percentage of whole grain, the greater the health benefit. Scan the ingredient list; choose products with a "whole" grain listed first (e.g., whole-grain whole wheat, whole rye, whole spelt, brown rice, oats, flaxseed). If a whole grain is listed second, you might be getting only a little whole grain, especially if there are only a few ingredients in the product. (Ingredients are listed by weight from most to least.)

3. INCLUDE 7 TO 10 SERVINGS OF FRUIT AND VEGETABLES IN YOUR DAILY DIET.

1 serving = 1 medium-sized fruit, 1/4 cup (60 ml) dried fruit, 1/2 cup (125 ml) cooked vegetables, 1 cup (250 ml) salad greens or 1/2 cup (125 ml) 100% pure juice

Fruit and vegetables are excellent sources of dietary fibre, potassium, vitamin C and folate, nutrients vital for maintaining good health and guarding against disease. A diet rich in colourful, nutrient-dense produce has been linked to lower rates of cancer, heart disease, stroke, cataracts, macular degeneration and type 2 diabetes. Adding fruit and vegetables to your diet can also help control blood pressure and cholesterol, decrease bone loss, promote weight loss and prevent a painful intestinal condition called diverticulitis.

To increase your intake of disease-fighting phytochemicals, choose a variety of coloured fruit and vegetables each day. To get more beta carotene, include one dark-green vegetable (e.g., spinach, kale, Swiss chard, rapini, broccoli) and one orange vegetable or fruit (e.g., carrots, sweet potato, winter squash, apricots, peaches, nectarines, mango, papaya) in your daily diet.

To help you increase your daily intake of fruit and vegetables, consider the following tips:

- Buy pre-chopped vegetables like baby carrots or broccoli and cauliflower florets. They're ready to throw in the microwave, steamer or salad bowl.

- Pick up fresh fruit or raw veggies from the salad bar at the local supermarket.
- Drink vegetable juice instead of diet drinks or coffee at lunch.
- Eat green or spinach salad for lunch. Use romaine and other dark-green lettuces in salad.
- Ask for tomatoes, cucumbers and lettuce in your sandwich. When making a sandwich yourself, reach for spinach leaves as a change from lettuce.
- Add quick-cooking greens like spinach, kale, rapini or Swiss chard to soups and pasta sauces.
- Fortify soups, pasta sauces and casseroles with grated zucchini and grated carrot.
- Bake (or microwave) a sweet potato for a change from white rice or pasta.
- Add slices of lemon, lime or orange to water for flavour and a little vitamin C.
- Top a bowl of breakfast cereal with fresh or frozen berries. Add berries to a breakfast smoothie made with low-fat milk or soy beverage.
- Top desserts such as sorbet, frozen yogurt or even chocolate cake with raspberries, blueberries or sliced strawberries.
- Out of season, reach for frozen fruit and vegetables.

4. EAT FISH, ESPECIALLY OILY FISH, TWICE PER WEEK.

Fatty fish like salmon, trout, sardines, mackerel, Arctic char and herring are particularly high in two omega-3 fats: DHA (docosahexanaenoic acid) and EPA (eicosapentaenoic acid). Eating fish at least twice per week may reduce the risk of heart attack, age-related macular degeneration (an eye disease that causes vision loss) and Alzheimer's disease.

Omega-3 fatty acids in fish are needed for the development and maintenance of the brain, eye and nervous tissue throughout life, beginning in the final trimester of pregnancy. An adequate supply of DHA is vital during the periods of rapid brain development in the womb, as well as during infancy and childhood. Since the amount of DHA a developing fetus or breastfed infant receives is dependent on a mother's diet, it's important for pregnant and breastfeeding women to include fish in their diet or take a fish oil supplement. (You'll learn more about omega-3 fatty acids in pregnancy in Chapter 16.) Fish rich in omega-3 fatty acids, such as salmon, trout and sardines, are also low in mercury.

5. CHOOSE FOODS LOWER IN SATURATED FAT.
AS MUCH AS POSSIBLE, AVOID TRANS FAT.

A high intake of saturated fat and trans fat is widely believed to contribute to the development and progression of coronary heart disease. A steady intake of these two fats increases the level of LDL (bad) cholesterol in the bloodstream, a major risk factor for heart disease. Worse, trans fat also lowers the level of HDL (good) cholesterol.

Saturated fat is found in all animal foods, including meat, poultry, eggs, milk, yogurt, cheese and butter. Choose animal foods that are lower in fat, such as lean cuts of meat (sirloin, tenderloin, flank steak, eye of round), skinless poultry breast, 1% or skim milk, 1% or non-fat yogurt, and part-skim or skim milk cheese. If you use butter, do so sparingly. In addition, many baked goods will contain high levels of saturated fat if they're made with butter.

Trans fats are formed during partial hydrogenation, a process used by the food industry to harden and stabilize liquid vegetable oils. You'll find trans fat in foods that list partially hydrogenated vegetable oil and/or vegetable shortening as ingredients. Roughly 90 percent of the trans fat in our food supply is found in commercially processed cookies, cakes, pastries, doughnuts, snack foods, fried fast foods and some brands of margarines. Read the Nutrition Facts box on foods you buy at the store and choose foods with little or no trans fat. Foods with a Daily Value (DV) for saturated plus trans fat of 5% or less are low in these so-called bad fats. Cut down on your consumption of processed foods such as crackers, cookies, snack foods and toaster pastries, since these foods supply most of the trans fat we consume. When buying margarine, choose one that is made from non-hydrogenated vegetable oil, as it will be trans fat free.

6. CHOOSE UNSATURATED COOKING OILS AND ADDED FATS.

Unsaturated fats include polyunsaturated and monounsaturated fats, both of which can help lower blood cholesterol when they are substituted for saturated fat. Health Canada advises all Canadians to consume 2 to 3 table-spoons (30 to 45 ml) of unsaturated fat per day to get essential fatty acids, compounds that our body can't make on its own.

Cooking oils high in polyunsaturated fat include sunflower, safflower, soybean, corn, grapeseed, hemp, flaxseed and walnut. Polyunsaturated oils provide essential fatty acids called linoleic acid and alpha-linolenic acid (ALA). Most of us already get plenty of linoleic acid, an omega-6 fatty acid that's widespread in processed foods made with soybean and corn oils. We don't, however, consume enough ALA, an omega-3 fatty acid found in flaxseed, walnut, canola and hemp oils.

Our excessive intake of omega-6 fats and our low intake of omega-3s is thought to play a role in the development of heart disease, cancer and autoimmune disease by promoting inflammation in the body. Studies suggest that higher intakes of ALA are protective from heart disease, especially if your diet lacks omega-3 fats from fish. Women require 1100 milligrams of ALA per day. One teaspoon (5 ml) of flaxseed oil delivers 2400 milligrams of ALA, a teaspoon of walnut oil has 470 milligrams and a teaspoon of canola oil has 419.

Excellent sources of monounsaturated fat include olive, canola, peanut, avocado and almond oils. Studies have shown that adding monounsaturated fat to your diet can help raise HDL (good) cholesterol and, among people with diabetes, improve how the body uses glucose.

Extra-virgin olive oil also contains phytochemicals that are thought to help dilate blood vessels, prevent blood clots and decrease inflammation in the body. (Extra-virgin and virgin olive oils are cold-pressed from olives, using minimal heat and no chemicals. As a result they retain the highest amount of phytochemicals and nutrients compared to pure olive oil, olive oil or light olive oil, which have been refined.)

7. LIMIT YOUR INTAKE OF REFINED (ADDED) SUGARS.

It's estimated that Canadian women consume, on average, 16 teaspoons (80 ml) of added sugar each day. And it's not just the usual culprits like soft drinks, cookies and candy that add sugar to your diet. Sugar also lurks in salad dressings, frozen dinners, pasta sauces, soy milk and even peanut butter and bread.

Eating too much sugar can increase your risk for heart disease by lowering HDL (good) cholesterol and raising blood triglycerides. A steady intake of sugary foods can also lead to overweight and obesity by adding a surplus of calories to your diet. In addition, a heavy intake of sugar-laden foods can increase your risk for insulin resistance, a condition in which the body cannot effectively remove sugar (glucose) from the bloodstream. Insulin resistance, in turn, ups your risk for developing type 2 diabetes.

To reduce your intake of refined sugars, replace soft drinks and fruit drinks with water, low-fat milk, unflavoured soy beverages, vegetable juice or tea. Choose fruit, yogurt or homemade smoothies over candy, cakes, cookies and pastries. Enjoy a small serving of dessert or other type of sweet once or twice per week at most.

Read the Nutrition Facts box when buying packaged baked goods. Compare products and choose a brand that has fewer grams of sugar per serving. Choose breakfast cereals that have no more than 8 grams of sugar per serving. (Cereals with dried fruit are an exception since the natural sugars in the fruit will increase the grams of sugar on the label.)

8. LIMIT FOODS WITH CHEMICAL ADDITIVES.

Read ingredient lists on foods. In general, foods that contain only a few— rather than many—ingredients will have fewer additives and preservatives. Wash fruit and vegetables under cool running water to remove pesticide residues. Or, if you prefer, buy organic produce.

9. REDUCE YOUR SODIUM INTAKE TO NO MORE THAN 2300 MILLIGRAMS PER DAY.

To help lower the risk of developing high blood pressure, reduce your intake of sodium. It's estimated that Canadian women, on average, consume as much as 2800 milligrams of sodium each day—two day's worth of sodium for woman over the age of 50. For sedentary Canadians aged 19 to 50, all it takes is 1500 milligrams of sodium to cover the body's requirement; older women need only 1300 milligrams per day. The daily upper limit—the maximum amount of sodium we should be consuming each day—is 2300 milligrams.

The following strategies will help you reduce your daily sodium intake:

- Read the Nutrition Facts box on packaged foods. Sodium levels vary widely across different brands of similar products. When checking sodium levels, focus on the number of milligrams listed for sodium in the Nutritional Facts table. This is the amount of sodium in milligrams per 1 serving of the food. You can also look at the % Daily Value (DV) of sodium to get a sense of whether 1 serving of food supplies a little or a lot of sodium. Foods with a DV of sodium of 5% or less are low in sodium. (The daily value for sodium on nutrition labels is set at 2400 milligrams, which is too high.)
- Pay attention to portion size. Sodium numbers on a nutrition label will underestimate your intake if you consume more than the serving size indicated.

- Limit your intake of processed meats such as bologna, ham, sausage, hot dogs, bacon, deli meats and smoked salmon.
- Limit your use of bouillon cubes, Worcestershire sauce, soy sauce and barbeque sauce.
- Rely less on convenience foods such as canned soups, frozen dinners and packaged rice and pasta mixes. Choose pre-made entrées or frozen dinners that contain no more than 200 milligrams of sodium per 100 calories.
- When possible, choose lower-sodium products. Many sodium-reduced brands contain 25 percent less sodium than the original version and some, like V8 juice, contain 75 percent less. If you can't find low-salt products in your supermarket, ask your grocer to stock them.
- Substitute other seasonings for salt when cooking—try garlic, lemon juice, salsa, onion, vinegar and combinations of herbs and spices.
- Remove the salt shaker from the table to break the habit of salting food at the table.

10. DRINK 9 CUPS (2.2 L) OF WATER EVERY DAY.

Water becomes the fluid in which all body functions occur. The fluid in your bloodstream transports nutrients and oxygen to your cells. The fluid in your urine removes waste products from your body. And the fluid in your sweat allows your muscles to release heat during exercise. If you drink too little fluid or lose too much through sweat, your body can't perform these tasks properly and you won't feel your best.

All beverages—with the exception of alcoholic beverages—count towards your daily water requirements. In addition to plain drinking water, fruit juice, milk, soy beverages, soft drinks, and even coffee and tea help keep you hydrated.

During exercise you do need to drink more water. Physical activity generates heat in your muscles, which your body releases through your skin as sweat. If you don't drink enough before, during and after exercise, your body can't properly release this heat. As a result your heart beats harder, your body temperature rises and ultimately your performance suffers. Drink 1/2 to 1 cup (125 to 250 ml) of water every 15 to 20 minutes during exercise.

11. LIMIT YOUR INTAKE OF CAFFEINE TO NO MORE THAN 450 MILLIGRAMS PER DAY.

Consuming too much caffeine can affect your ability to get a good night's sleep and, if you're not meeting your daily calcium requirements, can reduce bone density. Based on a review of the evidence, Health Canada contends that healthy adults are not at risk for adverse effects from caffeine, provided you limit your daily intake to 450 milligrams—the amount found in three 8 ounce (250 ml) cups of coffee or 10 cups (2.5 L) of tea. During pregnancy, women are advised to consume no more than 200 milligrams of caffeine per day. If you need to cut back on caffeine, start by avoiding caffeine in the afternoon. Choose caffeine-free or decaffeinated beverages like herbal tea, mineral water, fruit and vegetable juice or decaffeinated coffee.

Use the following list to help you stay within the recommended daily intake of no more than 450 milligrams of caffeine.

Caffeine Content of Common Beverages and Foods

Food	Caffeine (milligrams)
Coffee, brewed, 8 oz (250 ml)	100 mg
Coffee, instant, 8 oz (250 ml)	66 mg
Coffee, decaffeinated, 8 oz (250 ml)	3 mg
Espresso, 2 oz (60 ml)	54 mg
Starbucks coffee, venti, 20 oz (591 ml)	415 mg
Second Cup coffee, large, 20 oz (591 ml)	391 mg
Timothy's, large, 18 oz (532 ml)	245 mg
Tim Hortons, large, 20 oz (591 ml)	270 mg
Tea, black, 8 oz (250 ml)	45 mg
Tea, green, 8 oz (250 ml)	30 mg
Cola, 1 can, 355 ml	37 mg
Diet cola, 1 can, 355 ml	50 mg
Red Bull Energy Drink, 250 ml	80 mg
Mountain Dew AMP Energy Drink, 20 oz (591 ml)	91 mg
Snapple Diet Lemon Tea, 16 oz (473 ml)	42 mg
Dark chocolate, 1 oz (30 g)	20 mg

Keep in mind that the caffeine content of coffee can vary greatly based on the variety of coffee bean and the brewing equipment used.

12. AVOID—OR LIMIT—ALCOHOL.

Any type of alcoholic beverage—wine, beer or distilled spirits—adds excess calories to your diet and, more importantly, increases the risk of breast cancer. If you drink alcohol, consume no more than one drink a day, or seven per week. Replace alcoholic beverages with sparkling mineral water, Clamato or tomato juice or soda water with a splash of cranberry or pomegranate juice. Eliminate alcoholic beverages on evenings that you are not entertaining. Instead, save your glass of wine or cocktail for social occasions.

13. TAKE A MULTIVITAMIN AND MINERAL SUPPLEMENT EACH DAY.

There's clear evidence that taking a multivitamin with 400 micrograms (0.4 milligrams) of folic acid (a B vitamin) before and during pregnancy prevents neural tube defects, birth defects that affect the fetus' brain and spinal cord. And when it comes to iron, it's challenging—if not impossible—for menstruating women to meet their daily requirement (18 milligrams) from food alone. This is especially true for vegetarians and women who follow a low-calorie diet.

With age, we have more difficulty absorbing vitamin B12 from food. That's why the U.S. Institute of Medicine of the National Academies advises all adults over 50 to get their B12 from a supplement or from fortified foods such as soy beverages. Since B12 is found only in animal foods, strict vegetarians must also rely on a multivitamin to meet their daily needs. A multivitamin can provide a safety net if you don't get your full complement of nutrients from diet. And despite good intentions, most of us do not follow Canada's Food Guide to the letter. Stress, workplace demands and lack of time and energy are common barriers to eating healthfully.

Even so, it's important to eat a healthy diet first and then supplement with a multivitamin and mineral tablet. To help you choose foods brimming with vitamins and minerals, I've included a quick reference at the end of this chapter that outlines how much of each nutrient you need each day and which foods contain the most.

14. TAKE A 1000 IU (INTERNATIONAL UNITS)
VITAMIN D SUPPLEMENT EACH DAY.

Vitamin D is essential for prompting calcium absorption in the intestinal tract and maintaining calcium and phosphorus levels in the blood in order to build strong bones. In this way, vitamin D helps reduce the risk of osteoporosis. But mounting evidence suggests that this vitamin's benefits extend beyond bone health to the prevention of cancer, diabetes, coronary heart disease, multiple sclerosis and rheumatoid arthritis.

The majority of our vitamin D needs are met when sunlight strikes the skin, triggering vitamin D synthesis. When ultraviolet light hits the skin, it forms a pre–vitamin D. This compound then makes its way to the kidneys, where it's transformed into active vitamin D. But during our long winter in Canada, there isn't enough UVB radiation to produce any vitamin D in our skin. And in the summer, the sensible use of sunscreen blocks vitamin D production by more than 90 percent.

The fact that very few foods contain vitamin D (milk, oily fish, egg yolks and butter are among the few) and that our skin doesn't produce the vitamin in the fall and winter months makes it necessary to get vitamin D from a supplement. What's more, there's agreement among experts that the current "official" adequate intakes (AIs) for vitamin D are too low to reduce the risk of cancers. Evidence that taking a vitamin D supplement reduces cancer risk prompted the Canadian Cancer Society in 2007 to recommend adults consider taking 1000 international units (IU) of vitamin D each day throughout the fall and winter. Older adults, people with dark skin, those who don't go outdoors often and those who wear clothing that covers most of their skin should take the supplement year-round. The Canadian Cancer Society's vitamin D recommendation doesn't extend to children since, so far, research has focused only on adults.

It's prudent to supplement your diet with 1000 IU of vitamin D each day. (Add up how much you're already getting from your multivitamin and calcium supplements; the difference between that and the recommended 1000 IU is the dosage of vitamin D you need to buy.) Choose a vitamin D supplement that contains vitamin D3 instead of vitamin D2, which is less potent. Typically sold in 400 IU and 1000 IU doses, there's no need to be concerned if your intake exceeds 1000 IU slightly. The current safe upper limit—which vitamin D experts feel is far too low—is set at 2000 IU per day.

15. EXERCISE REGULARLY.

To control your weight and to reduce the risk of disease, aim to include aerobic, or cardiovascular, activities (brisk walking, jogging, stair climbing, cycling, swimming, cross-country skiing, aerobic classes, Spinning) and strength exercises (weights, push-ups, sit-ups) in your weekly routine. Aim to get at least four cardio workouts, 20 to 60 minutes in duration, each week and at least two strength training workouts.

As well, practise gentle reaching, bending and stretching to keep your joints flexible and your muscles relaxed. Yoga and pilates also help increase flexibility while strengthening your muscles. The more flexible you are, the less likely you'll get injured during exercise. If you get into the habit of doing flexibility exercises now, you'll be glad you did when you're older. Flexibility enhances the quality of life and independence for older adults.

Key nutrients for women across the decades

While the basics of healthy eating are essentially the same for women and men, unique nutritional needs arise for women as they age. The following strategies will help women eat healthfully and meet nutrient needs at every age.

IN YOUR 20S
Notable nutrients

Calcium	1000 milligrams per day
Folate	400 micrograms per day
Iron	18 milligrams per day

The main focus for women in their twenties should be building a strong nutrition foundation for the future. And that starts with calcium, folate and iron.

Calcium

Women continue to build bone density in their twenties. Peak bone mass—the maximum amount of bone a woman will have—is achieved by around the age of 25. Meeting daily calcium requirements—1000 milligrams—helps strengthen bones and lower the risk of osteoporosis. Research also suggests that a high-calcium diet might even ease PMS symptoms, including mood swings, fluid retention, food cravings and cramps. Use the table below to help you meet your daily calcium requirements.

Calcium Content of Selected Foods

Foods	Calcium (milligrams)
Dairy foods	
Milk, chocolate, 1 cup (250 ml)	285 mg
Milk, evaporated, 1/2 cup (125 ml)	350 mg
Milk, Lactaid, 1 cup (250 ml)	300 mg
Milk, Neilson TruTaste, 1 cup (250 ml)	360 mg
Milk, Neilson TruCalcium, 1 cup (250 ml)	420 mg
Milk powder, skim, dry, 3 tbsp (45 ml)	155 mg
Carnation Instant Breakfast Essentials drink, Nestlé, with 1 cup (250 ml) milk	540 mg
Cheese, cheddar, 1-1/2 oz (45 g)	300 mg
Cheese, cottage, 1/2 cup (125 ml)	75 mg
Cheese, mozzarella, 1-1/2 oz (45 g)	228 mg
Cheese, ricotta, 1/2 cup (125 ml)	255 mg
Cheese, Swiss or Gruyère, 1-1/2 oz (45 g)	480 mg
Sour cream, light, 1/4 cup (60 ml)	120 mg
Yogurt, plain, 3/4 cup (175 ml)	300 mg
Yogurt, fruit-flavoured, 3/4 cup (175 ml)	250 mg
Non-dairy foods	
Baked beans, 1 cup (250 ml)	150 mg
Black beans, 1 cup (250 ml)	102 mg
Kidney beans, cooked, 1 cup (250 ml)	69 mg
Lentils, cooked, 1 cup (250 ml)	37 mg
Soy beverage, fortified, 1 cup (250 ml)	330 mg
Soybeans, cooked, 1 cup (250 ml)	175 mg
Soybeans, roasted, 1/4 cup (60 ml)	60 mg
Tempeh, cooked, 1 cup (250 ml)	154 mg

Foods	Calcium (milligrams)
Tofu, raw, firm, with calcium sulphate, 4 oz (120 g)	260 mg
Tofu, raw, regular, with calcium sulphate, 4 oz (120 g)	130 mg
Sardines, 8 small (with bones)	165 mg
Salmon, drained, 1/2 can (with bones)	225 mg
Bok choy, cooked, 1 cup (250 ml)	158 mg
Broccoli, cooked, 1 cup (250 ml)	94 mg
Broccoli, raw, 1 cup (250 ml)	42 mg
Collard greens, cooked, 1 cup (250 ml)	357 mg
Kale, cooked, 1 cup (250 ml)	179 mg
Okra, cooked, 1 cup (250 ml)	176 mg
Rutabaga, cooked, 1/2 cup (125 ml)	57 mg
Swiss chard, cooked, 1 cup (250 ml)	102 mg
Swiss chard, raw, 1 cup (250 ml)	21 mg
Currants, 1/2 cup (125 ml)	60 mg
Figs, dried, 5 medium	135 mg
Orange, 1 medium	50 mg
Orange juice, calcium-fortified, 1 cup (250 ml)	300–360 mg
Almonds, 1/4 cup (60 ml)	100 mg
Brazil nuts, 1/4 cup (60 ml)	65 mg
Hazelnuts, 1/4 cup (60 ml)	65 mg
Molasses, blackstrap, 2 tbsp (30 ml)	288 mg
Molasses, fancy, 2 tbsp (30 ml)	70 mg

Source: Data adapted from the *Canadian Nutrient File*, Health Canada (2006). Available at: http://webprod.hc-sc.gc.ca/cnf-fce/index-eng.jsp.

CALCIUM SUPPLEMENTS. If you find it difficult to meet your daily calcium requirement from food alone, you'll need to reach for a supplement. You can't rely on a multivitamin and mineral supplement to provide enough calcium since most brands contain less than 200 milligrams of the mineral. Which calcium product you choose will depend on convenience, absorbability and tolerance.

- **Calcium carbonate and calcium citrate.** The most common compounds used in calcium supplements are carbonate and citrate. Calcium carbonate supplements are generally the least expensive and most widely used. They also contain twice as much elemental calcium—usually 500 or 600 milligrams per tablet—as supplements made from calcium citrate. Supplements made from calcium citrate generally have 250 to 350 milligrams of elemental calcium per tablet. Elemental calcium is the amount of calcium in a supplement that's available for your body to absorb; since your daily calcium requirements are based on the amount you need to absorb, this information is important. Most products list the amount of elemental calcium on the label, but some brands list only the total weight (milligrams) of the tablet, that is, the weight of the calcium plus that of the carbonate or citrate compound to which it's bound.

    If you have decreased stomach acid, or you're taking an acid-blocking medication, consider taking calcium citrate supplements. Calcium citrate is more readily absorbed in your intestine, so it can be taken any time of day, even on an empty stomach. Calcium carbonate requires extra stomach acid for absorption so it's best taken with food or immediately after eating.

- **Coral calcium.** These calcium supplements are made from marine coral beds off the coast of Okinawa, Japan. The U.S. Federal Trade Commission took legal action against companies making false and unsubstantiated health claims about coral calcium. Coral calcium is simply calcium carbonate. According to one U.S. study, some brands may contain high levels of lead, a naturally occurring heavy metal.

- **Other calcium supplements.** Calcium supplements made from unrefined oyster shell, bone meal and dolomite have fallen out of favour due to their higher levels of lead. Calcium citrate and refined calcium carbonate have the lowest lead content. Many experts say the exposure risk of lead in calcium supplements is relatively small and insignificant since the higher amounts of calcium present decrease intestinal absorption of lead.

Here are a few guidelines for taking calcium supplements:

- To determine how many calcium supplement tablets you need to take, know how much elemental calcium is in each. Read the ingredient list.

Spread out your calcium intake over the course of the day. Absorption from supplements is best in doses of 500 milligrams or less because the percentage of calcium your body absorbs decreases as the amount in the supplement increases. Therefore, if you need to take 1000 milligrams of calcium from supplements, you should take 500 milligrams twice a day instead of 1000 milligrams at one time.

- If you're averse to swallowing pills, try a chewable, liquid or effervescent calcium supplement. These supplements are well absorbed by the body since they're broken down before they enter the stomach.
- To prevent gas, bloating and constipation, ensure your diet provides adequate fluids and fibre. If this doesn't help, try another brand or form of calcium. Increase your calcium intake gradually—take 500 milligrams per day for one week, then add more calcium slowly.
- If you take medications, check with your pharmacist about possible interactions with calcium. Calcium can interfere with the body's ability to use certain drugs, including tetracycline, bisphosphonates (Fosamax, Actonel), hypothyroid medication (Synthroid) and iron supplements.
- Don't consume more than 2500 milligrams of calcium per day from food and supplements combined. Taking too much calcium can cause stomach upset, high blood-calcium levels, impaired kidney function and decreased absorption of other minerals.

Folate (folic acid)

In your 20s, it's also important to ensure that you are consuming the recommended amount of a B vitamin called folate, which is needed for healthy cell division and repair. (Folate refers to the B vitamin when it occurs naturally in foods; folic acid is the name of the synthetic version of the vitamin that's added to multivitamins and fortified foods.) It's well established that taking folic acid before and during the early weeks of pregnancy is vital to preventing neural tube defects (NTDs) in the developing fetus. NTDs are serious birth defects caused when development of the brain, spinal cord and/or their protective coverings, which occurs around the fourth week of pregnancy, is incomplete.

Since one-half of all pregnancies in Canada are unplanned, *all* women of childbearing age are urged to take a multivitamin providing 0.4 milligrams of folic acid. To reduce the risk of NTDs, the Society of Obstetricians and Gynaecologists of Canada advises healthy women to take a multivitamin with 0.4 to 1 milligrams of folic acid for at least two to three months before becoming pregnant and throughout pregnancy and breastfeeding.

Although a multivitamin will help women meet their daily folate requirements, you should also include folate-rich foods in your daily diet. Good food sources include lentils, black beans, cooked spinach, asparagus, broccoli, avocados and artichokes. The recommended dietary allowance (RDA) for folate for women of all ages is 400 micrograms. Meeting your folate requirements may also help reduce the risk of heart disease, breast cancer and cervical dysplasia. A deficiency of this important vitamin can increase your risk for these health conditions and can also cause anemia.

The best food sources of folate include cooked spinach, lentils, asparagus, artichokes, avocados and orange juice. In Canada, white flour, white pasta and refined cornmeal must be fortified with folic acid. It's estimated that fortified foods add 100 to 200 micrograms (0.1 to 0.2 milligrams) of folic acid to one's daily intake. Here's a list of selected foods and their folate content.

Folate Content of Selected Foods

Food	Folate (micrograms)
Chicken liver, 3.5 oz (100 g)	770 mcg
Black beans, cooked, 1/2 cup (125 ml)	135 mcg
Chickpeas, cooked, 1/2 cup (125 ml)	85 mcg
Kidney beans, cooked, 1/2 cup (125 ml)	120 mcg
Lentils, cooked, 1/2 cup (125 ml)	189 mcg
Peanuts, 1/2 cup (125 ml)	96 mcg
Sunflower seeds, 1/3 cup (75 ml)	96 mcg
Artichoke, 1 medium	64 mcg
Asparagus, 5 spears	110 mcg
Avocado, California, 1/2 medium	113 mcg
Avocado, Florida, 1/2 medium	81 mcg
Bean sprouts, 1 cup (250 ml)	91 mcg
Beets, 1/2 cup (125 ml)	72 mcg
Brussels sprouts, 1/2 cup (125 ml)	83 mcg

Food	Folate (micrograms)
Romaine lettuce, 1 cup (250 ml)	80 mcg
Spinach, raw, 1 cup (250 ml)	115 mcg
Spinach, cooked, 1/2 cup (125 ml)	139 mcg
Orange, 1 medium	40 mcg
Orange juice, freshly squeezed, 1 cup (250 ml)	79 mcg
Orange juice, frozen, reconstituted, 1 cup (250 ml)	115 mcg

Source: Data adapted from the *Canadian Nutrient File*, Health Canada (2006). Available at: http://webprod.hc-sc.gc.ca/cnf-fce/index-eng.jsp.

FOLIC ACID SUPPLEMENTS. As I advised above, all women of child-bearing age—those who could become pregnant, who are pregnant or who are breastfeeding—should take a multivitamin that supplies 400 micrograms (0.4 milligrams) of folic acid. If you're advised by your health care provider to take a folic acid supplement, be sure to choose one with vitamin B12 added. Supplementing with folic acid alone can mask a vitamin B12 deficiency, which could lead to irreversible nerve damage. Do not exceed 1000 micrograms of folic acid per day.

Iron

Iron is one of the most common nutrient deficiencies among women. Women who diet to lose weight, shy away from red meat and animal foods or engage in heavy exercise are all at risk for missing out on this important mineral. Women need more iron than men because they lose an average of 15 to 20 milligrams each month during their menstrual period. A woman's iron needs also increase during pregnancy. The consequences of iron deficiency are low energy, fatigue, listlessness, hair loss, pale skin, poor motivation to exercise and difficulty concentrating.

Menstruating women need 18 milligrams of iron per day. Vegetarian women need an extra 14 milligrams each day, for a total of 32 milligrams of iron, to account for reduced iron absorption from plant foods.

Good sources of iron include red meat, enriched breakfast cereals, whole-grain breads, dried fruit, legumes, tofu and nuts. A daily multivitamin with minerals will also help women meet daily iron needs. Use the following list to help increase your daily iron intake.

Iron Content of Selected Foods

Food	Iron (milligrams)
Beef, lean, cooked, 3 oz (90 g)	3.0 mg
Beans in tomato sauce, 1 cup (250 ml)	5.0 mg
Kidney beans, cooked, 1/2 cup (125 ml)	2.5 mg
Apricots, dried, 6	2.8 mg
Prune juice, 1/2 cup (125 ml)	5.0 mg
Spinach, cooked, 1 cup (250 ml)	4.0 mg
All-Bran Original, Kellogg's, 1/2 cup (125 ml)	4.7 mg
All-Bran Buds, Kellogg's, 1/2 cup (125 ml)	5.9 mg
Bran flakes, 3/4 cup (175 ml)	5.0 mg
Just Right, Kellogg's, 1 cup (250 ml)	6.0 mg
Raisin Bran, Kellogg's, 3/4 cup (175 ml)	5.5 mg
Shreddies, Post, 3/4 cup (175 ml)	5.9 mg
Cream of Wheat, 1/2 cup (125 ml)	8.0 mg
Oatmeal, instant, 1 pouch	3.8 mg
Wheat germ, 1 tbsp (15 ml)	2.5 mg
Molasses, blackstrap, 1 tbsp (15 ml)	3.2 mg

Source: Data adapted from the *Canadian Nutrient File*, Health Canada (2006). Available at: http://webprod.hc-sc.gc.ca/cnf-fce/index-eng.jsp.

The richest sources of iron are beef, pork, lamb, poultry and fish. These foods provide *heme* iron, the type that can be absorbed and utilized the most efficiently by your body. Sources of heme iron supply about 10 percent of the iron we consume each day. Even though heme iron accounts for such a small proportion of our intake, it is so well absorbed that it actually contributes a significant amount of iron.

The rest of our iron comes from plant foods such as dried fruit, whole grains, leafy green vegetables, nuts, seeds and legumes. These are sources of *nonheme* iron. The body is much less efficient in absorbing and using this type of iron. Vegetarians may have difficulty maintaining healthy iron stores because their diet relies exclusively on nonheme sources. The rate at which your body is able to absorb nonheme iron is strongly influenced by other factors in your diet. Practise the following to enhance your body's absorption of nonheme iron:

- Add a little animal food to your meal if you're not vegetarian. Meat, poultry and fish contain MFP factor, a special component that promotes the absorption of nonheme iron from plant foods.
- Add a source of vitamin C. Including some vitamin C in your plant-based meal can enhance the body's absorption of nonheme iron fourfold. The acidity of the vitamin converts iron to the ferrous form for ready absorption (your stomach acid enhances iron absorption in the same way). Here are some winning combinations:
  - whole-wheat pasta with tomato sauce
  - brown rice stir-fry with broccoli and red pepper
  - whole-grain breakfast cereal topped with strawberries
  - whole-grain toast with a small glass of orange juice
  - spinach salad tossed with orange or grapefruit segments
- Don't take your calcium supplements with an iron-rich meal, since these two minerals compete with each other for absorption.
- Drink tea between rather than during meals—tea contains tannins, compounds that inhibit iron absorption. Or add a little milk or lemon to your tea, since both inactivate its iron-binding properties.
- Cook your vegetables. Phytic acid (phytate), found in plant foods, can attach to iron and hamper its absorption. Cooking vegetables like spinach releases some of the iron that's bound to phytates.

IRON SUPPLEMENTS. To help you meet your daily iron requirements, a multivitamin and mineral supplement is a wise idea, especially for vegetarians and menstruating women. Most regular formulas provide 10 milligrams, but you can find multivitamins that provide up to 18 milligrams of the mineral.

If you're diagnosed with depleted iron stores or iron-deficiency anemia, your dietitian or doctor will prescribe single iron pills. Depending on the extent of your iron deficiency, you'll take one to three iron tablets (each containing 50 to 100 milligrams of elemental iron) per day. And depending on how much iron you take each day, a supplementation period of twelve weeks to six months is usually sufficient to treat anemia and restore your body's iron reserves. Your doctor will perform occasional blood tests to ensure that your iron supply has increased to an adequate level. Once your iron levels improve, discontinue the iron pills but continue taking a multivitamin and mineral supplement.

Too much iron may cause indigestion and constipation, though supplements of ferrous fumarate (e.g., Palafer, EuroFer) tend to be well tolerated. Excessive doses of iron can be toxic, causing damage to your liver and intestines. An iron overload can even result in death. To avoid these problems, don't take single iron supplements without having a blood test to confirm that you have an iron deficiency. (See Chapter 3, Anemia, for information on safe iron supplementation.)

IN YOUR 30S

Notable nutrients

Calcium	1000 milligrams per day
Folate	400 micrograms per day
Iron	18 milligrams per day
Magnesium	320 milligrams per day

In your 30s, your daily nutrient requirements remain unchanged, with the exception of magnesium. (Of course, if you become pregnant your daily requirements for certain vitamins and minerals do increase. See Chapter 16, Pregnancy, and Chapter 17, Breastfeeding, for specific advice related to these times.)

Magnesium

Magnesium requirements increase in the early 30s to help the body maintain enough of the mineral. An adequate intake of magnesium helps maintain strong bones and healthy blood pressure, and guards against type 2 diabetes and heart disease. Studies even suggest that magnesium may prevent migraine headaches, reduce high blood pressure and ease the symptoms of premenstrual syndrome.

The best sources of magnesium include legumes, nuts and seeds, whole grains and vegetables. Green vegetables are particularly good sources of magnesium because the centre of the chlorophyll molecule—the compound that gives green vegetables their colour—contains magnesium. Use the following list to help boost the magnesium content of your diet.

Magnesium Content of Selected Foods

Food	Magnesium (milligrams)
Wheat bran, 2 tbsp (30 ml)	46 mg
Wheat germ, 1/4 cup (60 ml)	91 mg
Almonds, 1 oz (23 nuts)	84 mg
Brazil nuts, 1 oz (8 nuts)	64 mg
Peanuts, 1 oz (35 nuts)	51 mg
Sunflower seeds, 1 oz (30 g)	100 mg
Black beans, cooked, 1 cup (250 ml)	121 mg
Chickpeas, cooked, 1 cup (250 ml)	78 mg
Kidney beans, cooked, 1 cup (250 ml)	80 mg
Lentils, cooked, 1 cup (250 ml)	71 mg
Navy beans, cooked, 1 cup (250 ml)	107 mg
Soybeans, cooked, 1/2 cup (125 ml)	131 mg
Tofu, raw, firm, 1/2 cup (125 ml)	118 mg
Dates, dried, 10	29 mg
Figs, dried, 10	111 mg
Green peas, cooked, 1/2 cup (125 ml)	31 mg
Spinach, cooked, 1/2 cup (125 ml)	81 mg
Swiss chard, cooked, 1/2 cup (125 ml)	76 mg
Halibut, 3 oz (90 g)	90 mg

Source: Data adapted from the *Canadian Nutrient File*, Health Canada (2006). Available at: http://webprod.hc-sc.gc.ca/cnf-fce/index-eng.jsp.

MAGNESIUM SUPPLEMENTS. If a blood test indicates that you have very low magnesium stores, a daily magnesium supplement will be necessary. As well, due to a condition or age, some people may benefit from a daily magnesium supplement. Certain diuretics used to treat high blood pressure (e.g., Lasix, hydrochlorothiazide) cause magnesium to be excreted in the urine. Individuals with poorly controlled diabetes may also benefit from a magnesium supplement since increased magnesium loss in the urine is associated with elevated blood sugar. (Older women are at risk for magnesium deficiency because they tend to consume less in their diets than younger adults and magnesium absorption decreases with age.)

Even if you don't fall into one of the above categories, you may feel your magnesium intake is below par despite your best efforts to eat magnesium-rich foods, and so you might consider taking a magnesium supplement. But keep in mind, when it comes to reducing high blood pressure, studies show that magnesium-rich foods do the trick, not supplements. These foods also supply other nutrients and antioxidants linked to better health. Although magnesium supplements may be helpful in boosting your daily intake, be sure to include magnesium-rich foods in your daily diet.

Magnesium supplements combine magnesium with another substance. You'll find supplements made of magnesium oxide, magnesium citrate, magnesium carbonate, magnesium fumarate and magnesium sulphate. It's the amount of elemental magnesium in a supplement (listed on the label) and its bioavailability that influence the mineral's effectiveness. Bioavailability refers to how much magnesium is absorbed in the intestines and is ultimately available to be used by your body's cells and tissues. Research suggests that magnesium oxide has a lower bioavailability than other forms of magnesium.

Magnesium supplements are typically sold in 200 or 250 milligram doses. Unless you have been diagnosed with a magnesium deficiency, you shouldn't need more than this amount if you're also including magnesium-rich foods in your diet.

If you take calcium supplements, a simple way to boost your intake of magnesium is to buy calcium pills with magnesium added. Calcium/ Magnesium supplements are sold in a 2:1 or 1:1 ratio of calcium to magnesium. A 2:1 Cal/Mag supplement will usually supply 300 milligrams of calcium and 150 milligrams of magnesium. If you need to take such a supplement twice daily to meet your calcium needs, you'll be consuming 300 milligrams of magnesium, close to the recommended daily intake. Supplement manufacturers often promote a 2:1 ratio as being ideal for absorption despite the fact there is no credible research to support this.

Magnesium supplements can cause diarrhea and abdominal cramping if taken in high doses. Don't exceed the safe upper limit of 350 milligrams of supplemental magnesium per day.

Weight control

It's during the 30s that many women complain they can't manage their weight as easily as they could in their 20s. Women often find that reversing a small weight gain takes more effort that it used to when they were younger. That's because a woman's metabolism starts to slow down in her 30s due to age-related muscle loss. To prevent weight gain in your 30s, you need to eat less and exercise more to keep your weight steady.

For every year after 30, women need to reduce their intake by 7 calories per day. In other words, by the age of 40, a woman should be eating 70 fewer calories per day than she did at age 30. The first step: Reduce your calorie intake by cutting unnecessary calories from sweets, sugary drinks and refined starchy foods while still emphasizing foods rich in folate, calcium and iron.

To make small calorie cuts, identify two or three areas in your diet where you can trim calories each day, such as replacing cream in your coffee with milk, using a smaller plate at dinner or opting for water instead of a sugary beverage. Replace your glass of orange juice with an orange at breakfast to save 50 calories. Substitute a teaspoonful of mustard for a tablespoonful of mayonnaise on your sandwich to save 100 calories. Swapping your side of rice at dinner with a serving of vegetables will also cut at least 100 calories. Of course, bigger calorie savings can be had by switching from a bagel with cream cheese to an English muffin with reduced-fat cream cheese (save 300 calories). Or forgoing the mid-morning muffin at Starbucks for a piece of fruit (save 370 calories).

Determine how you can burn off an extra 100 calories each day. Use a pedometer to track your daily steps. Aim to increase your daily total by 2000 steps to burn off an extra 100 calories. For weight loss, aim for 12,000 to 15,000 steps per day.

IN YOUR 40S
Notable nutrients

Calcium	1000 milligrams per day
Folate	400 micrograms per day
Iron	18 milligrams per day
Magnesium	320 milligrams per day
Soy foods	Once or twice daily
Saturated and trans fat	Limit to 20 grams per day
Sodium	1500 milligrams per day

During this decade, women begin the transition into perimenopause, the five- to ten-year period before the onset of menopause. (Menopause occurs when twelve months have passed since a woman's last menstrual period; a woman then begins her post-menopausal years.) Although vitamin and mineral requirements remain unchanged, women in their 40s should concentrate on choosing nutritious foods to minimize perimenopausal symptoms such as hot flashes and insomnia and maximize health.

Now is the time to fine-tune your diet to reduce saturated (animal) fat, refined sugars and sodium. Incorporate more whole grains, oily fish, legumes, fruit and vegetables. Consume no more than seven alcoholic beverages per week. Limit caffeine to 450 milligrams per day, or much less if you suffer sleep disturbances. Look for ways to reduce your sodium intake to no more than 2300 milligrams per day. (See earlier sections in this chapter for more detailed information on elements of a healthy diet.)

Soy isoflavones

Adding foods such as tofu, soy beverages, soy burgers and soy nuts to the diet may help some women ease hot flashes. Soybeans contain natural plant compounds called isoflavones, which have a similar structure to the hormone estrogen and, as a result, have a weak estrogenic effect in the body. Even though isoflavones in soy are about 50 times less potent than estrogen, they still offer a source of estrogen. When a woman's estrogen levels are low during perimenopause, a regular intake of foods like roasted soy nuts, soy beverages and tofu can help reduce hot flashes. (See Chapter 19, Perimenopause, for detailed information on soy and hot flashes.)

The following tips will help you incorporate soy foods in your daily diet:

- Pour an unflavoured soy beverage on breakfast cereals or in a smoothie; use it in cooking and baking (soups, casseroles, muffins, pancake batters).
- Cube firm tofu and add it to soups—canned (lower sodium) or homemade.
- Grill firm tofu on the barbecue. Brush tofu and vegetable kebabs with hoisin sauce or marinate them in teriyaki sauce.
- Substitute firm tofu for ricotta cheese in recipes.
- Use soft tofu in creamy salad dressing or dip recipes.
- Throw canned soybeans, drained and rinsed, in a salad, soup or chili.

- Replace up to one-half of all-purpose flour in a recipe with soy flour.
- Enjoy 1/4 cup (60 ml) of roasted soy nuts as a midday snack or added to a green salad.
- Replace ground beef with soy ground round in chili, pasta sauce and tacos.
- Try veggie burgers (made from soy protein) and veggie dogs on the grill.

IN YOUR 50S AND BEYOND
Notable nutrients

Calcium	1500 milligrams per day
Iron	8 milligrams per day
Sodium	1300 milligrams per day
Vitamin D	1000 IU per day year-round
Vitamin B12	2.4 micrograms per day from a supplement
Fibre	21 grams per day

In Canada, most women reach menopause around the age of 51 and then enter post-menopause, the phase of life when osteoporosis, heart disease and breast cancer risks increase. It's now, more than ever, that women need to be proactive about their nutritional health and adopt healthy habits that help them stay healthy into their 60s, 70s and beyond.

Calcium
At age 50, a woman's calcium requirements increase to 1500 milligrams daily. In most cases, women need to rely on calcium supplements to ensure an adequate intake.

Iron
Not all nutrient requirements increase at age 50—your body needs less of some nutrients. Once a woman stops menstruating, she needs only 8 milligrams of iron per day. (Vegetarian women still require 1.8 times more iron at this age; they need 14 milligrams daily from food and a multivitamin.)

Vitamin D
After the age of 50, women (and men) have a reduced capacity to produce vitamin D in the skin through sun exposure. For this reason, you need to

take your daily 1000 IU vitamin D supplement year-round, not only during the fall and winter months.

Vitamin B12

Aging also affects the status of vitamin B12, a nutrient needed for healthy nerve and blood cells and the production of DNA. Vitamin B12 is found exclusively in animal foods, including meat, poultry, fish, eggs and dairy products. Studies suggest that up to 30 percent of people over the age of 50 may not produce enough stomach acid to absorb B12 from foods.

To meet the recommended daily intake of 2.4 micrograms, beginning at age 50, women are encouraged to take a multivitamin supplement or eat fortified foods such as soy, rice or almond beverages, and soy products if you're not already doing so.

Fibre

Daily fibre requirements also decrease slightly after age 50, from 25 grams to 21 grams per day. The recommended daily intake of fibre is tied closely to your daily calorie requirements. As women age and require fewer calories, they also require a little less fibre each day. This doesn't mean you should stop adding fibre-rich foods to your daily diet. Quite the contrary. Even 21 grams of fibre can be challenging to consume each day unless you're carefully choosing high-fibre foods. Getting enough fibre is an important strategy to keep blood cholesterol and blood-sugar levels in the healthy range and to keep your bowels regular. It's estimated that Canadians get at most 14 grams of fibre each day, only one-half of what's recommended. Use the list below to help you meet your daily fibre needs.

Fibre Content of Selected Foods

Food	Fibre (grams)
Cereals & Grains	
100% bran cereal, 1/2 cup (125 ml)	12.0 g
All-Bran Buds, Kellogg's, 1/3 cup (75 ml)	12.0 g
Bran flakes, 3/4 cup (175 ml)	6.3 g
Corn Bran, Quaker, 1 cup (250 ml)	6.3 g
Oat bran, cooked, 1 cup (250 ml)	4.5 g
Oatmeal, cooked, 1 cup (250 ml)	3.6 g

Food	Fibre (grams)
Pita pocket, whole wheat, 1	4.8 g
Whole-wheat bread, 100%, 2 slices	4.0 g
Spaghetti, whole wheat, cooked, 1 cup (250 ml)	4.8 g
Rice, brown, cooked, 1 cup (250 ml)	3.1 g
Flaxseed, ground, 2 tbsp (30 ml)	4.0 g
Wheat bran, 2 tbsp (30 ml)	3.0 g
Legumes	
Beans and tomato sauce, 1/2 cup (125 ml)	10.0 g
Black beans, cooked, 1/2 cup (125 ml)	6.0 g
Lentils, cooked, 1/2 cup (125 ml)	4.5 g
Almonds, 1/4 cup (60 ml)	4.0 g
Peanuts, 1/4 cup (60 ml)	3.5 g
Fruit & Vegetables	
Figs, dried, 5	8.5 g
Pear, with skin, 1 medium	5.1 g
Strawberries, 1 cup (250 ml)	3.8 g
Prunes, dried, 3	3.0 g
Raisins, seedless, 1/2 cup (125 ml)	2.8 g
Apple, with skin, 1 medium	2.6 g
Apricots, dried, 1/4 cup (60 ml)	2.6 g
Orange, 1 medium	2.4 g
Blueberries, 1/2 cup (125 ml)	2.0 g
Potato, baked with skin, 1 medium	5.0 g
Sweet potato, mashed, 1/2 cup (125 ml)	3.9 g
Green peas, 1/2 cup (125 ml)	3.7 g
Brussels sprouts, 1/2 cup (125 ml)	2.6 g
Corn, 1/2 cup (125 ml)	2.3 g
Carrots, 1/2 cup (125 ml)	2.2 g
Broccoli, 1/2 cup (125 ml)	2.0 g

Source: Data adapted from the *Canadian Nutrient File*, Health Canada (2006). Available at: http://webprod.hc-sc.gc.ca/cnf-fce/index-eng.jsp.

Sodium

Now is the time to become vigilant about sodium, especially if you didn't pay attention to your sodium intake when you were younger. That's because at age 50 daily sodium requirements decrease from 1500 to 1300 milligrams. Consuming excess sodium can contribute to high blood pressure, a major risk factor for coronary heart disease. Although heart disease was once considered a man's disease, after menopause, women are just as likely to suffer a heart attack as men. (See page 9 for strategies to reduce your sodium intake.)

Before menopause, the naturally occurring hormone estrogen provides built-in protection from heart disease. Estrogen reduces the body's total cholesterol level by regulating the amount of cholesterol produced by the liver and helping cells clear LDL (bad) cholesterol from the bloodstream. This helps raise a woman's HDL (good) cholesterol and lower her LDL cholesterol. Estrogen may also help keep blood vessels more flexible. With menopause and the loss of estrogen, the reverse happens: a woman's LDL cholesterol level rises and her HDL cholesterol level falls. By the time a woman is 65 years old, her risk of heart attack equals a man's because she no longer produces estrogen. (It's important to note that estrogen doesn't protect all women from heart disease. Premenopausal women who have diabetes have the same risk of heart attack as men of the same age.)

A primer on vitamins and minerals for women

Dietary surveys suggest that many women don't consume enough calcium, magnesium, iron and zinc—key nutrients for health. To help you—and your family—increase your intake of key vitamins and minerals, use the following guide to choose nutrient-packed foods. You'll also learn how much of each nutrient you need each day—the recommended dietary allowance (RDA). I'll often refer you to this table in the chapters that follow.

Vitamin and Mineral RDA Guide and Best Food Sources

Key vitamins	RDAs for women (mcg = micrograms mg = milligrams)	Best food sources
Vitamin A	700 mcg	Liver, oily fish, milk, cheese, eggs
	Pregnancy: 770 mcg	Beta carotene: carrots, sweet potato, winter squash, broccoli, kale, spinach, apricots, peaches, mango
	Breastfeeding: 1300 mcg	
Vitamin B1 (thiamin)	1.1 mg	Pork, liver, fish, whole grains, wheat germ, enriched breakfast cereals and breads, legumes, nuts
	Pregnancy: 1.4 mg	
	Breastfeeding: 1.4 mg	
Vitamin B2 (riboflavin)	1.1 mg	Milk, yogurt, cheese, fortified soy and rice milk, meat, eggs, legumes, nuts, whole grains
	Pregnancy: 1.4 mg	
	Breastfeeding: 1.6 mg	
Vitamin B3 (niacin)	14 mg	Red meat, poultry, fish, liver, eggs, dairy products, peanuts, almonds, enriched breakfast cereals, wheat bran
	Pregnancy: 18 mg	
	Breastfeeding: 17 mg	
Vitamin B6	Age 19–50: 1.3 mg	Red meat, poultry, fish, liver, eggs, legumes, nuts, seeds, whole grains, green leafy vegetables, bananas, potatoes, avocados
	Age 50+: 1.5 mg	
	Pregnancy: 1.9 mg	
	Breastfeeding: 2 mg	

Key vitamins	RDAs for women (mcg = micrograms mg = milligrams)	Best food sources
Vitamin B12	2.4 mcg	Meat, poultry, fish, eggs, dairy products, fortified soy and rice milk
	Pregnancy: 2.6 mcg	
	Breastfeeding: 2.8 mcg	
Folate	400 mcg	Lentils, legumes, seeds, cooked spinach, asparagus, artichokes, orange juice
	Pregnancy: 600 mcg	
	Breastfeeding: 500 mcg	
Vitamin C	75 mg (110 mg for smokers)	Citrus fruit and juices, kiwi, cantaloupe, strawberries, broccoli, cauliflower, cabbage, tomato juice, bell peppers
	Pregnancy: 85 mg	
	Breastfeeding: 120 mg	
Vitamin D	1000 IU*	Fluid milk, egg yolks, oily fish, fortified soy and rice milk
	Pregnancy: 2000 IU*	
	Breastfeeding: 2000 IU*	
Vitamin E	15 mg	Vegetable oils, nuts, seeds, soybeans, whole grains, wheat germ, avocado, leafy green vegetables
	Pregnancy: 15 mg	
	Breastfeeding: 19 mg	
Vitamin K	90 mcg	Green peas, broccoli, leafy green vegetables, cabbage, liver
	Pregnancy: 90 mcg	
	Breastfeeding: 90 mcg	

*Represents the current recommended dietary intake to reduce cancer risk. This amount is above the official RDA, which is now considered too low.

Key minerals	RDAs for women (mcg = micrograms mg = milligrams)	Best food sources
Calcium	Age 9–18: 1300 mg	Dairy products, fortified soy and rice milk, broccoli, leafy green vegetables, almonds, legumes, tofu, canned salmon (with bones), sardines, fortified fruit juice
	Age 19–50: 1000 mg	
	Age 50+: 1500 mg	
	Pregnancy: 1000 mg	
	Breastfeeding: 1000 mg	
Iron	Age 9–13: 8 mg	Red meat, poultry, tuna, salmon, eggs, enriched breakfast cereals, whole grains, baked beans, lentils, blackstrap molasses, raisins
	Age 14–18: 15 mg	
	Age 19–50: 18 mg	
	Age 50+: 8 mg	
	Pregnancy: 27 mg	
	Breastfeeding: 9 mg	
Magnesium	Age 9–13: 240 mg	Whole grains, almonds, Brazil nuts, sunflower seeds, legumes, tofu, leafy green vegetables, prunes, figs, dates
	Age 14–18: 360 mg	
	Age 19–30: 310 mg	
	Age 30+: 320 mg	
	Pregnancy: 350–360 mg	
	Breastfeeding: 310–320 mg	
Potassium	4700 mg	Bananas, oranges, orange juice, cantaloupe, peaches, avocados, broccoli, Brussels sprouts, spinach, tomato juice, lima beans, peas

Key minerals	RDAs for women (mcg = micrograms mg = milligrams)	Best food sources
	Pregnancy: 4700 mg	
	Breastfeeding: 5100 mg	
Selenium	55 mcg	Brazil nuts, shrimp, salmon, halibut, crab, fish, pork, organ meats, wheat bran, whole-wheat bread, brown rice, onion, garlic, mushrooms
	Pregnancy: 60 mcg	
	Breastfeeding: 70 mcg	
Zinc	8 mg	Beef, pork, lamb, yogurt, milk, wheat bran, wheat germ, whole grains, enriched breakfast cereals, legumes, pumpkin seeds, cashews
	Pregnancy: 11 mg	
	Breastfeeding: 12 mg	

2

Strategies for weight control

Now that you've read Chapter 1, you have a good idea of the key nutrients women need for an overall healthy diet. The rest of the book deals with certain conditions and the role nutrition plays in preventing and managing them. But a large and growing number of women have nutrition concerns apart from, or in addition to, specific health conditions. In this chapter, I'll address one topic that concerns many women: managing their weight.

Women and weight control

For many women (myself included), weight control has always been top of mind. Since I was a teenager I've had to watch what I eat and exercise regularly in order to maintain a healthy weight. Some women find that staying trim comes naturally and they don't have to work very hard at it (oh, how I envy them!). But as women get older, many find that it becomes more difficult to take off a few unwanted pounds. Many of my perimenopausal clients complain about a "softening around the middle" despite their best efforts at weight control. But carrying excess weight is not just a matter of appearance. There's compelling evidence that being overweight puts you at risk for a number of health problems, including breast cancer, ovarian cancer, type 2 diabetes, high blood pressure and heart disease. Indeed, many of my female clients are motivated to lose weight to stay healthy—not to fit into a certain sized pair of jeans.

Luckily, despite the age factor and the challenge of female hormones, weight management is possible through a healthy diet and regular exercise. Over the years, I've helped scores of women lose excess body fat with practical—and sustainable—diet advice.

HOW HEALTHY IS YOUR WEIGHT?

Most women rely on the bathroom scale to decide whether they're happy with their body weight. But to get a more accurate picture of your health, there are other numbers you need to consider—though I certainly don't advocate throwing out the scale. Weighing-in helps motivate people to stick to a weight-loss plan. And it's also a very important way to stay on top of small weight gains before they accumulate. Think about it—it's much easier to lose an extra 3 pounds than it is 10 or more. As useful as the scale may be, knowing your weight doesn't tell you everything you need to know about your health risk. Determining how much body fat you have—and where you carry it—is important not only for weight control but also for identifying your risk for disease.

BODY MASS INDEX (BMI)

If you're between the ages of 18 and 65, body mass index (BMI) is a height and weight formula that gives a pretty reliable snapshot of your body fat. Your BMI is calculated by dividing your weight (in kilograms) by your height (in metres squared). The easiest and quickest way to determine your BMI is to use an online calculator—you'll find one on my website (www.lesliebeck.com)—but you can also do the calculation yourself.

Calculate Your BMI

1. Determine your weight in kilograms (kg)
   (Divide your weight in pounds by 2.2) _____ Weight (kg)

2. Determine your height in centimetres (cm)
   (Multiply your height in inches by 2.54) _____ Height (cm)

3. Determine your height in metres (m)
   (Divide your height in centimetres by 100) _____ Height (m)

4. Square your height in metres (m²)
   (Multiply your height in metres by height in metres) _____ Height (m²)

5. Now, calculate your BMI
   (Divide #1, your weight [in kg], by #4, your height [in m²]) _____ BMI

Doctors and dietitians use the BMI to classify your body weight and assess your risk for disease as follows:

- BMI values less than 18.5 are considered underweight and increase a person's risk for conditions such as osteoporosis, nutrient deficiencies and eating disorders.
- BMI values from 18.5 to 24.9 are defined as healthy or normal weight and linked with a lower risk of health problems.
- If your BMI falls between 25 and 29.9, you're classified as overweight.
- A BMI of 30 or greater is considered obese. As your BMI goes up, so does your risk for certain cancers, type 2 diabetes, heart disease, high blood pressure and gallbladder disease.

Keep in mind, though, that sudden or considerable weight gains or weight losses may also indicate health risk, even if this occurs within the "normal" BMI category.

The BMI is not without drawbacks. For starters, it doesn't tell you where you're carrying your body fat, which is important in determining the risk of heart disease. It also doesn't distinguish between body fat weight and muscle weight. Because muscle weighs more than fat, heavily muscled people may have a high BMI but very little fat.

WAIST CIRCUMFERENCE

If you want to know where your body fat is located, and how that fat is affecting your health, you need to measure your waist. Simply take a measuring tape and measure your waist at the narrowest part of your trunk, about 1 inch (2.5 cm) above your belly button, without holding the tape too tightly or too loosely. (Resist the urge to suck in your stomach!)

Excess fat around the abdomen (apple shape) is associated with greater health risk than fat located on the hips and thighs (pear shape). When it comes to health, not all fat cells are alike. Whereas BMI measures overall fat, your waist circumference is a good measure of abdominal fat. The fat around your middle consists of subcutaneous fat, the fat just beneath the skin that you can pinch, and visceral fat, a type of deep fat that packs itself around your organs. It's visceral fat that's considered dangerous to your health because it secretes chemicals that increase the body's resistance to insulin and cause inflammation throughout the body.

A waist circumference of 31.5 inches (80 cm) or greater for women increases the likelihood of type 2 diabetes, high blood pressure, elevated cholesterol, heart attack, stroke, metabolic syndrome and some cancers. Lower thresholds for waist circumference are recommended for Asian women because studies suggest health risk increases among many Asian populations at lower levels of body weight than in Caucasian populations.

Your Waist Circumference and the Risk of Disease

For women	Risk of disease
<31.5 inches (<80 cm)	Lower
≥31.5 inches (≥80 cm)	Increased

WAIST-TO-HIP RATIO (WHR)

The waist-to-hip ratio is simply your waist circumference divided by your hip measurement. It's another index of body fat distribution used by doctors and researchers. However, some studies suggest it's less accurate than waist circumference at predicting health risk. Even so, it does a much better job of predicting the risk of heart disease in women and men than BMI alone.

Your Waist-to-Hip Ratio (WHR) and the Risk of Disease

For women	Risk of disease
≤0.8	Lower
>0.8	Increased

Winning strategies for weight loss

If you've determined you need to lose excess weight, there's no time like the present to get started. You're ready to embark on a weight-loss plan if you consider losing weight a long-term lifestyle change rather than a short-term quick fix. I can tell you right now that people who approach losing weight with a long-term attitude are far more successful. To increase your chances of success, I strongly recommend that you consult with a registered dietitian to help you lose weight safely and effectively. To find a private-practice dietitian in your community check out the website www.dietitians.ca. Working one-on-one with an expert means you'll get a meal plan that's customized to your schedule and food preferences. Regular follow-up visits allow you to monitor your progress, adjust your plan as needed and discuss ways to overcome challenges and potential obstacles to success.

While it's beyond the scope of this book to outline a weight-loss plan, I can share with you some key strategies that will help you shed excess pounds. They're the very strategies that I've given my clients for the past twenty years. They seem like common-sense tips, but trust me, they really work. They're strategies that you can live by today, tomorrow and years down the road. (You'll find four specific diet plans for weight loss in my book *The No-Fail Diet*.)

1. SET A REALISTIC, MEASURABLE GOAL.

If your body mass index (BMI) is over 25, determine what weight you need to be in order for it to fall in the healthy zone. Make your weight goal a 3 pound weight range rather than one single number. It's not realistic to always weigh in at the exact same weight on the scale. After all, you need a little wiggle room for holidays and entertaining.

Consider setting mini goals. Rather than keeping your eye on a long-term goal such as losing 25 pounds (11.3 kg) or more, set your sights on smaller goals to help you stay motivated and maintain momentum. Breaking your weight-loss goal into 5 to 10 pound (2 to 4.5 kg) blocks will allow you to experience success along the way. Mini goals don't have to be centred on weight loss. They can be daily, weekly or monthly goals that challenge you to exercise more, eat more vegetables, eat more fish or drink more water.

Aim to lose weight at a safe rate of 1 to 2 pounds (0.5 to 1 kg) each week. Rapid weight loss that results from following a very low-calorie diet actually makes it harder to maintain your weight loss. When you put your body through a period of starvation by drastically cutting calories, you burn muscle and trigger hormonal changes in your body that cause it to be more efficient at storing fat. When you inevitably abandon the diet, your metabolism is slower, making it easier to gain your weight back.

2. REDUCE CALORIES TO 1200–1600 CALORIES PER DAY.

A good general target for women is 1400 calories per day. If you're very active, start with 1600 calories. If you're unable to exercise, aim to get 1200 calories each day. Cut calories by eliminating sugary drinks and sweets as well as fatty, salty foods such as fast food meals, french fries and potato chips. Reduce portion sizes of meat and starchy foods like rice, pasta and potatoes. Instead, fill your plate with vegetables, which fill you up with fewer calories. Replace snacks of pretzels, crackers and muffins, which supply a lot of calories in even a small portion, with less energy-dense foods like fresh fruit and raw vegetables. If you're in the habit of snacking after dinner, replace those calories with a cup of tea, herbal tea or light hot chocolate. Before you embark on losing weight, keep a food diary for seven days to see where your extra calories are sneaking in.

3. PLAN YOUR MEALS AND SNACKS IN ADVANCE.

If you come home from work tired and hungry without a plan for dinner, chances are you'll order in. Or graze your way through the evening. On the weekend, plan a weekly menu of healthy meals and snacks. If planning a week's worth of meals seems too daunting, plan for the next day only. I have many of my clients keep their food journal one day in advance. This way it serves as a plan they're more likely to stick with. To ensure you keep to your plan, make time for grocery shopping (make a list in advance!) and batch cook on the weekend.

4. EAT AT REGULAR INTERVALS THROUGHOUT THE DAY.

Eating a meal or snack every three to four hours will help to boost your metabolism, improve your energy level and maintain a consistent blood-sugar level. Eating regularly also prevents you from becoming overly hungry and helps to eliminate mindless snacking and overeating at the next meal. If your meals are more than four hours apart, plan to have a snack. But here's my rule: *No snacking on starchy foods* like bagels, pretzels, low-fat cookies, low-fat crackers or fat-free muffins. Because these foods are quickly converted to blood glucose, they're more likely to lead to premature hunger and cravings for sweets. Healthier snacks include yogurt and fruit, dried apricot and almonds, a non-fat latte, a homemade fruit smoothie or a small energy bar. Choosing these snacks will also help get more fibre and calcium into your diet.

5. ASSESS YOUR PORTION SIZE.

I recommend that you measure your food portions during the first two weeks of following a weight-loss plan. Get to know what 1/2 cup (125 ml) or 1 cup (250 ml) of brown rice looks like on your plate, or what 3 ounces (90 g) of salmon looks like.

TIPS TO REDUCE PORTION SIZE

- **Buy small packages of food at the grocery store.** Economy-sized boxes of cookies, crackers, pretzels and potato chips encourage overeating. If you resist the "more for less" thinking, you'll end up eating less. If you're serving dessert for guests, buy (or make) only what you plan to serve. Lingering leftovers can tempt even the most dedicated dieter into overeating.

- **Serve smaller portions at mealtime.** If you sit down to a plate overflowing with food, the chances are good that you'll finish it. Most of us have a tendency to clear our plates, a habit that's rooted in childhood. If you don't serve yourself at dinner, instruct whoever does to put less food on your plate.

- **Use smaller plates.** This trick really works. Instead of filling a dinner plate with food, serve yourself less food on a luncheon plate (7 to 9 inches/2.8 to 3.5 cm in diameter). The plate looks full and you'll end up eating less food. I vividly remember one client telling me that the only thing she did differently to lose 10 pounds was to serve her dinner on a luncheon plate. Ditto for glasses. Reserve large glasses for water and use smaller ones for low-fat milk (1 cup/250 ml) and 100% fruit juice (1/2 cup/125 ml).

- **Plate your snacks.** Never, ever snack out of the bag. When you continually reach your hand into that bag of mini rice cakes or pretzels, you never really get a sense of how much you're eating. It just doesn't register. You end up eating far more that you should. Whether your snack is crackers and low-fat cheese, air-popped popcorn or apple slices, measure out your portion and put it on a plate. And then pay attention to the fact that you're eating!

6. EAT BREAKFAST, EVEN IF YOU'RE NOT HUNGRY.

Studies show that people who eat the morning meal do a better job of keeping their weight in check than those who go without. Eating breakfast kick-starts your metabolism and helps you consume fewer calories over the course of the day. People who eat breakfast are less likely to mindlessly snack in the morning and overeat at lunch and dinner. If you don't feel hungry in the morning, eat something small—a low-fat yogurt, a soy milk smoothie or even an apple. Pretty soon you'll wake up with an appetite for breakfast.

7. STOP EATING WHEN YOU FEEL SATISFIED, NOT FULL.

Think about your hunger level prior to eating and how full you felt after eating. Listening to your body can help prevent you from eating too many calories. Use the following scale to assess how you feel before you eat, halfway through a meal and after you finish eating. Your goal is to stop eating when you reach level 5 on the hunger scale.

Hunger Scale

1	You feel starving. You can't concentrate because you feel so empty. You need food now!
2	You feel hungry and know that your stomach needs food, but you could wait a few minutes before eating.
3	You feel slightly hungry. You could eat something, but you couldn't eat a large meal.
4	Your hunger has almost disappeared. You could eat another bite.
5	**You are no longer hungry. You feel satisfied, not full.**
6	You feel slightly full.
7	You feel overly full and uncomfortable. Your waistband is noticeably tighter.
8	You feel stuffed, bloated, even nauseous. Some people call this the "Thanksgiving Day" full.

If you eat too quickly, you're more likely to overeat and feel stuffed. To slow your pace—and eat less—put down your knife and fork after every bite and chew your food thoroughly. You'll also be less likely to overeat if you avoid distractions, such as watching television, checking email or reading, while eating. Reserve the kitchen or dining room table for meals to help you pay attention to what—and how much—you're eating.

8. KEEP A FOOD JOURNAL.

I recommend this strategy to all of my clients because, quite simply, it works. Many studies have shown that people who keep food diaries lose more weight and keep more pounds off in the long run. A recently published study of 1500 overweight and obese adults—one of the largest weight-loss studies ever—found that people who wrote down what they ate at least five days each week lost twice as much weight as those who didn't.[1]

For the first four weeks of following your meal plan, write down what you eat and how much you eat. Tracking every bite—for better or worse—that passes your lips forces you to see what you're really eating. It will highlight what needs tweaking in your diet and help keep you focused on your goals. You can also use your food diary to track your intake of healthy foods that you're trying to eat more of, such as fish, nuts (keep portion size small!), legumes, whole grains, fruit and vegetables.

9. WEIGH IN WEEKLY.

According to the National Weight Control Registry, a U.S. database of over 5000 people who have lost a significant amount of weight and kept if off, 75 percent of participants say their success comes from weighing themselves at least once per week.[2] Weighing in helps you measure your progress. Seeing your efforts reflected on the bathroom scale motivates you to stick to your plan. On the flip side, if the scale doesn't budge, or if the needle creeps up after the weekend, you'll more likely pay closer attention to following your plan. Avoiding the scale because you're afraid of what it might tell you is a surefire way to let small weight gains accumulate into big ones. The women I see in my practice who have a significant amount of weight to lose tend to be the ones who haven't stepped on a scale in years.

10. INDULGE ONCE PER WEEK.

Putting a food on a forbidden list makes it more desirable and can make you feel deprived. When you're stressed, angry or bored, you're more likely to crave what you can't have, a feeling that can lead to bingeing. Rather than eliminating the foods you love, plan a weekly splurge so you won't feel deprived. (I mean a single treat—a dessert, a chocolate bar, an order of french fries—not one day's worth of indulgences.)

While a weekly treat will help you stick to your weight-loss resolution, I don't advise that you keep treats in the house. Successful dieters in the

National Weight Control Registry say they stay on track by keeping high-fat foods out of the house and stocking their kitchen with healthy foods.[3]

11. DON'T BE DISCOURAGED BY WEIGHT-LOSS PLATEAUS.

When your weight loss has come to a halt without any change in diet, exercise or other lifestyle factors, this is called a weight-loss plateau. It can be frustrating, but trust me when I tell you that plateaus are a natural part of the weight-loss process. They often occur when you reach a weight that you have not been below for quite some time. As you lose weight, your body requires fewer calories and your rate of weight loss may temporarily slow down.

It takes persistence and consistency to break through a plateau. The key is to not give up. If you say to yourself it doesn't matter what you eat because your weight isn't budging, you'll never break through that number on the scale. Do *not* eat less food in order to speed up your weight loss! The best way to work through a plateau is to take your exercising up a notch to burn more calories. If you've been doing the same workout routine for months, it's time to challenge your body. Consider cross-training by adding different types of cardiovascular workouts to your weekly routine.

12. DEAL WITH MOMENTARY LAPSES.

We're all human. Whether you've had a busy social calendar or you've just returned from a three-week food-filled vacation, you're bound to have put on a few pounds. (That's why I advised you earlier to choose a weight *range* to stay within.) The key to long-term weight maintenance is nipping small gains in the bud, before that 3 or 5 pound gain becomes 10, that easily turns into 20 if you're not watching it. I'm sure many of you know just what I mean. I recommend monitoring your weight on a regular (i.e., weekly) basis. When you see a few pounds creep on, have a plan of action to take them off: Keep a food diary for a few weeks, add an extra workout each week for a month or give up your weekly treat until your weight is back down. Choose something that will work for you and remember: It's only natural to stray from your plan once in a while. It certainly doesn't mean you've ruined all your hard work. If you backslide, get right back on track. You'll be pleasantly surprised to learn that an occasional slip-up won't prevent you from achieving your goal.

13. START AN EXERCISE PROGRAM.

The majority of participants in the National Weight Control Registry say they exercise regularly to maintain their weight loss. Most combine walking with another type of planned exercise such as aerobics classes, biking or swimming. Regular exercise helps you stay trim by burning calories and increasing your metabolism. It also increases your motivation to eat a more healthful diet. If you've successfully lost weight, research suggests it takes close to one hour of moderate aerobic exercise five days per week to keep the pounds off.

Aim to get four cardiovascular workouts each week (brisk walking, jogging, stair climbing, swimming, cross-country skiing or aerobics classes). Gradually build up to a minimum of 30 minutes each session. When you're ready, add weight training two or three times a week. Studies have found that adding a weight workout to a weight-loss program speeds up weight loss.

Leslie's Meal Plan for Healthy Weight Loss

Your daily food servings
All serving sizes are measured after cooking. To make nutrient-packed food choices, follow the principles outlined in Chapter 1.

Protein foods	6 to 8 servings
1 serving =	1 oz (30 g) lean meat, poultry, fish
	1 oz (30 g) part-skim cheese
	1 whole egg or 2 egg whites
	1/4 cup (60 ml) cottage cheese
	1/3 cup (75 ml) cooked legumes (i.e., kidney beans, chickpeas, black beans)
	1/4 cup (60 ml) firm tofu, chopped
	1/2 small soy burger
	1/4 cup (60 ml) soy ground round
	2 tbsp (30 ml) roasted soy nuts

Your daily food servings

Starchy foods	*4 to 6 servings*
1 serving =	1 slice bread (70–90 calories)
	1/4 of a bagel
	1 small (6 inch/15 cm) soft tortilla
	1/2 cup (125 ml) pasta
	1/2 cup (125 ml) corn or 1/2 cob
	1/3 cup (75 ml) rice or quinoa
	1/2 cup (125 ml) hot cereal
	1/2 to 3/4 cup (125 to 175 ml) cold cereal
	1/2 cup (125 ml) 100% bran cereal
	1/3 cup (75 ml) Kellogg's All-Bran Buds with Psyllium
	1/2 medium potato or 1/2 cup (125 ml) sweet potato
	7 whole-wheat soda crackers or 2 rice cakes
Fruit	*2 to 3 servings*
1 serving =	6 oz (175 ml) unsweetened fruit juice
	1 medium-sized piece fruit
	1 cup (250 ml) berries or fruit salad
	4 small plums or apricots
	2 kiwi
	1 small grapefruit
	2 tbsp (30 ml) raisins or dried cranberries
Vegetables	*4+ servings*
1 serving =	1/2 cup (125 ml) cooked or raw vegetables
	1 cup (250 ml) leafy vegetables (e.g., salad)
	3/4 cup (175 ml) vegetable juice or tomato juice
	1/2 cup (125 ml) tomato sauce
Milk	*2 servings*
1 serving =	1 cup (250 ml) skim or 1% milk
	3/4 cup (175 ml) low-fat yogurt
	1 cup (250 ml) fortified soy beverage

Your daily food servings

Fats & Oils	4 servings
1 serving = 1 tsp (5 ml) vegetable oil, butter or margarine	
1 tsp (5 ml) mayonnaise	
2 tsp (10 ml) fat-reduced mayonnaise	
2 tsp (10 ml) salad dressing	
4 tsp (20 ml) fat-reduced salad dressing	
1 tbsp (15 ml) nuts/seeds	
1-1/2 tsp (7 ml) nut butter	
2 tbsp (30 ml) hummus	
1/8 avocado	
6 medium olives	
Water	9 cups (2.2 L)
Coffee, tea, herbal tea	
Milk, soy beverages and juice also count towards your daily water requirements.	

BREAKFAST PORTIONS AND MEAL IDEAS
Your Basic Breakfast: Portion Guide

1 Protein serving (Optional)
1 OR 2 Starchy Food servings
1 Fruit serving
1 Milk serving
Water (i.e., coffee, tea, herbal tea, if desired)

Choose one of the following breakfasts—or create your own meal:

1. 1/2 cup (125 ml) 100% bran cereal or 1 cup (250 ml) whole-grain cereal (choose a cereal with at least 5 grams of fibre and no more than 8 grams of sugar per serving)
   1 cup (250 ml) 1% or skim milk or fortified, unflavoured soy beverage

3/4 cup (175 ml) 100% fruit juice or 1 cup berries or 2 tbsp (30 ml) raisins

Water

2. 1 or 2 slices whole-grain toast with 2 tbsp (30 ml) sugar-reduced jam

   3/4 cup (175 ml) low-fat yogurt (flavoured is okay) or 1 medium-sized skim-milk latte

   3/4 cup (175 ml) 100% juice or 1 medium-sized fruit

   Water

3. 1 cup (250 ml) cooked oatmeal or Red River Hot Cereal (add ground flaxseed, salba or wheat germ)

   Top with 3/4 cup (175 ml) plain or vanilla-flavoured low-fat yogurt or 1 cup (250 ml) milk

   1 cup (250 ml) berries or 2 tbsp (30 ml) dried cranberries

4. Breakfast Blender Smoothie

   Blend together these ingredients:

   1 cup (250 ml) milk or calcium-fortified soy beverage

   1/2 medium-sized banana

   1/2 cup (125 ml) whole frozen berries or 1 whole orange, peeled

   Ice, if desired

   Enjoy with 1 slice of whole-grain toast with sugar-reduced jam

MID-MORNING SNACK

If lunch is more than four hours after breakfast, choose one of the following:

3/4 cup (175 ml) 1% MF yogurt; or

1 medium-sized fruit

LUNCH PORTIONS AND MEAL IDEAS

Your Basic Lunch: Portion Guide

3 Protein servings

1 OR 2 Starchy Food servings

2 Vegetable servings

2 Fat servings

2 cups (500 ml) water

Choose one of the following lunches—or create your own meal:

1. Sandwich on 2 slices of whole-grain rye, pumpernickel or whole-wheat bread, or a pita pocket made with 3 oz (90 g) lean protein (turkey, chicken breast, tuna or salmon)
   2 tsp (10 ml) mayonnaise or 4 tsp (20 ml) salad dressing, if desired
   2 vegetable servings (baby carrots, vegetable soup, green salad or vegetable juice)
   Water

2. 3 oz (90 g) grilled chicken breast or tuna or 3/4 cup (175 ml) 1% cottage cheese
   Large green salad
   4 tsp (20 ml) salad dressing or 2 tsp (10 ml) olive or flaxseed oil
   1 whole-grain roll or 1/2 whole-grain pita pocket
   Water

3. Veggie burger made with soy protein (not a "grain" burger)
   1 whole-wheat roll or a small whole-wheat pita pocket (about 160 calories)
   Add mustard, relish, sliced vegetables
   Green salad
   4 tsp (20 ml) salad dressing
   Water

4. 1 cup (250 ml) cooked pasta with tomato sauce with 3 oz (90 g) lean ground beef or chicken or 3/4 cup (175 ml) lentils
   Large green salad
   4 tsp (20 ml) salad dressing
   Water

MID-AFTERNOON SNACK

If dinner is more than four hours after lunch, choose one of the following:

1 piece of fruit and 3/4 cup (175 ml) low-fat yogurt; or
4 dried apricots and 10 plain, unsalted almonds; or
1 energy bar: Look for a bar with 7 to 15 grams of protein and no more than 200 calories. You'll find a wide selection in health food and sporting-goods stores (my favourites are Luna Bar and Elevate Me! bar); or

1 whole food bar (i.e., Lärabar, Source Salba Real Whole Food Bar); or 1/2 to 1 cup (125 to 250 ml) of raw vegetables and 1/4 cup (60 ml) of hummus

DINNER PORTIONS AND MEAL IDEAS
Your Basic Dinner: Portion Guide

5 Protein servings
0 Starchy Food servings
2 Vegetable servings (or more)
2 Fat servings
2 cups (500 ml) water

Or, if you want starch at this meal, use the portion guide outlined for lunch.

Choose one of the following dinners—or create your own meal:

1. Large green salad with one of the following:
   2 cups (500 ml) of greens plus raw vegetables; or
   5 ounces (150 g) of baked or grilled salmon or chicken breast
   4 tsp (20 ml) salad dressing
   Water
2. Egg white omelet (use 1 whole omega-3 egg and 1/2 carton of egg whites)
   Add chopped vegetables, 2 tbsp (30 ml) grated low-fat cheese, salsa if desired
   Steamed vegetables or large green salad
   4 tsp (20 ml) salad dressing
3. 5 oz (150 g) baked salmon fillet (wrap in foil with lemon juice and fresh chopped dill; bake at 450°F/230°C for 25 to 30 minutes)
   Steamed vegetables and/or green salad
   4 tsp (20 ml) salad dressing
   Water

4. 5 oz (150 g) roasted pork tenderloin (brush with hoisin sauce; bake at
   375°F/190°C for 25 to 30 minutes)
   Steamed vegetables and/or salad
   4 tsp (20 ml) salad dressing or 2 tsp (10 ml) oil
   Water
5. 5 oz (150 g) grilled sirloin or beef tenderloin steak*
   Large green salad and/or steamed vegetables
   4 tsp (20 ml) salad dressing or 2 tsp (10 ml) oil
   Water
   *Limit your intake of red meat to twice per week.
6. 5 oz (150 g) white fish; e.g., halibut, tilapia, sole (marinate with your
   favourite dressing or brush with hoisin sauce; bake at 450°F/230°C
   for 15 to 20 minutes)
   Steamed or stir-fried vegetables or salad
   Water

PART 2

LOW ENERGY LEVELS, FATIGUE AND PAIN

3
Anemia

Anemia literally means "too little blood." It's the most common disorder of the blood, and the most prevalent nutritional problem in the world today. Anemia is any condition in which too few red blood cells are present, or in which the red blood cells are too small or contain too little hemoglobin (the pigment that transports oxygen throughout your body).

Anemia lowers the oxygen-carrying capacity of the blood and starves tissues in your body of the energy they need to function properly. Anemia affects the whole body, causing fatigue, shortness of breath, lack of energy and many other complications.

There are several kinds of anemia, but the most common and severe type is iron-deficiency anemia. Women are especially at risk of developing iron-deficiency anemia throughout their reproductive years. In fact, iron deficiency is the most common nutrient deficiency in Canadian women. It's estimated that up to 84 percent of Canadian women don't meet their daily requirement for iron. In some studies, the prevalence of low iron stores has ranged from 25 to 39 percent.

Deficiencies of folate and vitamin B12 can also cause anemia. Shortchanging your body of these vitamins affects your red blood cells differently than a lack of iron. You'll read how to prevent these types of anemia later in this chapter.

Anemia is not a disease itself, but it can be a symptom of many different conditions, including nutrient deficiencies, bleeding, excessive red blood cell destruction and defective red blood cell formation. Anemia is treated by stopping the source of blood loss and/or rebuilding your body's nutrient stores through the use of supplements and diet.

What causes anemia?

Blood is essential to human life. It carries nutrients, oxygen, hormones, cellular waste and other substances to and from all parts of your body. Almost 50 percent of your blood is composed of red blood cells, which contain an essential oxygen-carrying protein called hemoglobin. To stay healthy, your body requires a steady supply of oxygen to nourish tissues and keep them functioning efficiently. The red blood cells circulate in your bloodstream, transporting oxygen from your lungs to the working muscle cells and tissues of your body.

Many nutrients are required for red blood cell production. Iron, vitamin B12 and folate are the most important nutrients, but small quantities of vitamin C, riboflavin and copper are also necessary, along with a specific balance of hormones. If your body doesn't have adequate amounts of these nutrients and hormones, red blood cell production slows down and eventually causes anemia.

Anemia develops when there is a reduction in the number and the size of red blood cells or when the amount of hemoglobin contained in the red blood cells is too low. Anemia limits the amount of oxygen your blood can deliver to your body. Essentially, your cells become starved for energy.

The most common type of anemia is iron-deficiency anemia. The mineral iron is essential for making hemoglobin, the main component of red blood cells. Your body uses its iron supply very efficiently: Iron from dead red blood cells is recycled to produce new ones. Consequently, the recommended dietary intake for iron is relatively low (you'll learn how much iron you need each day later in this chapter). A healthy, well-balanced diet provides some or all of the iron your body needs to ensure healthy red blood cell production. However, vegetarians, menstruating women and pregnant women often don't meet their daily iron requirements from diet alone.

Women are particularly vulnerable to iron-deficiency anemia, especially during their reproductive years. Because of the regular blood loss that occurs during menstruation, women have higher iron requirements than men. Pregnancy also depletes iron stores at a much faster rate than normal. The growing fetus and placenta require a higher blood volume and a larger supply of iron. Pregnant women need additional iron and are very likely to develop iron deficiency unless they supplement their dietary intake. A traumatic childbirth can also cause a sudden blood loss, which can lead to anemia, low blood pressure and other complications.

In adults, the main cause of iron deficiency is blood loss. Conditions that result in chronic or repeated bleeding, such as nosebleeds, hemorrhoids, certain cancers, ulcers or other gastrointestinal problems, will deplete iron stores and may eventually lead to anemia. The condition can also develop because of a sudden blood loss due to an injury or surgery.

Although excessive blood loss is the main cause of iron-deficiency anemia, your dietary intake of iron is extremely important for maintaining your body's iron stores. A diet that chronically lacks the proper amount of iron will lead to iron deficiency, and ultimately anemia.

Diet may not be the only culprit behind a case of iron deficiency. You may be consuming enough iron every day, but your body may not be absorbing it properly. Poor iron absorption will have a negative effect on your iron stores and could easily lead to anemia. Certain factors in your diet can impair your body's ability to absorb iron from food, and that's discussed in the section below. Furthermore, thyroid hormones and certain drugs may interfere with your ability to utilize iron effectively.

Anemia is often a side effect of chronic disease, especially in the elderly. Health conditions such as infection, inflammation and cancer will suppress red blood cell production and deprive the developing cells of much-needed iron. In more rare instances, anemia can develop when the destruction of red blood cells exceeds the rate of production. This type of anemia can result from many conditions, including an enlarged spleen, various autoimmune disorders, red blood cell abnormalities and cancer. Elderly women with a chronic disease may also be taking medication that is known to destroy red blood cells prematurely.

In addition to iron deficiency, there are several other nutritional factors that can cause anemia. Deficiencies in vitamin B12, vitamin C or folate (folic acid) can cause abnormalities in red blood cell production. Impaired absorption of vitamin B12 can lead to *pernicious anemia*. If your diet lacks folate, another B vitamin, *megaloblastic anemia* can result.

Symptoms

Iron-deficiency anemia is a progressive condition. It usually develops in stages, so it can take months or even years before symptoms appear. The main symptoms of anemia include fatigue, weakness, loss of appetite, loss of energy, shortness of breath, cold hands and feet, difficulty concentrating, hair loss, pale skin, and increased susceptibility to infection. It's important to keep in mind that you may feel these symptoms even if you're not classified as "anemic." A marginal iron deficiency, measured by a low level of ferritin in the blood, can affect your energy levels, too, although not as severely. (Ferritin is one of the chief forms in which iron is stored in the body.)

Tongue irritation, cracks at the side of the mouth and spoon-like deformities in the fingernails also may result from iron deficiency. Some people with anemia develop pica, a craving for non-food substances such as ice, dirt or pure starch. In young children, iron deficiency may cause irreversible abnormalities in brain development, resulting in impaired attention span, cognitive function and learning ability. However, scientists don't know the severity of iron deficiency necessary to produce these developmental changes.

Anemia ranges from mild to severe, and the symptoms also vary accordingly. Mild anemia doesn't have any significant long-term consequences. It may simply result in dizziness, faintness, thirst, sweating or a rapid pulse. These symptoms usually disappear when iron supplies are restored. More severe cases of anemia may lead to medical problems involving the heart. Because anemia lowers the amount of oxygen in the bloodstream, the heart must beat faster and deliver more blood to the tissues. If the heart is unable to keep up with this increased demand, symptoms of heart failure may develop, including difficulty in breathing, swollen legs and angina.

The speed at which blood is lost will also affect the symptoms of anemia. When blood loss is sudden and occurs over several hours or less, the loss of only one-third of the body's blood volume causes death. If bleeding takes place over a longer period, such as days or weeks, the body can tolerate a loss of up to two-thirds of its blood volume, often without suffering anything more than a feeling of fatigue or weakness.

Who's at risk?

If you fall into any of the following categories, you're at risk for developing iron-deficiency anemia:

- You're female.
- You're pregnant.
- You engage in regular endurance exercise (e.g., long distance running, triathlons).
- You follow a low-calorie diet (less than 1200 calories per day).
- You're a vegetarian.
- You have an intestinal disorder that affects nutrient absorption in the small intestine (e.g., Crohn's disease, celiac disease).

All women of reproductive age are at risk of developing iron deficiency, and at even greater risk if their diet lacks iron-rich foods. Women who are pregnant or breastfeeding are also predisposed to anemia because of the additional demands of the growing baby and placenta. Female runners or triathletes lose iron through sweat and can become iron deficient, especially if their diet lacks iron. Any woman who reduces her calorie intake to lose weight or eats an unbalanced vegetarian diet is also at risk.

Teenage girls are another high-risk group due to the onset of menstruation, increased growth requirements and a diet that often has an inadequate intake of iron.

Infants are born with sufficient stores of iron, but this iron supply becomes depleted during the first few months of life. Exclusively breastfed babies and babies fed on whole cow's milk are especially at risk of developing iron deficiency. For this reason, pediatricians recommend that infants receive additional iron from iron-fortified cereals or formulas from the time that they are six months of age.

Surveys indicate that young children also fall into a high-risk category for iron deficiency. Children from low-income families or from ethnic groups such as Chinese and Aboriginal peoples may not eat sufficient quantities of iron-rich foods to maintain a healthy iron supply.

Diagnosis

Blood tests are used to diagnose anemia. Your doctor will look at the level of hemoglobin in your blood to determine the degree of iron deficiency. A simple blood test can also determine the amount of iron that's stored in your liver. On rare occasions it may be necessary to examine a sample of bone marrow to assess the iron content of your red blood cells.

Blood tests that identify the size, shape, colour and number of red blood cells are used to identify anemia that is caused by deficiencies in other vitamins, such as vitamin B12, vitamin C and folate (folic acid). Anemia that is a result of chronic disease or other physical disorders will normally be identified as part of the diagnosis of the underlying medical condition.

Conventional treatment

Excessive bleeding is often a primary cause of anemia, so the first step in treatment usually involves locating and stopping the source of the bleeding. In most cases, iron supplements are prescribed as a short-term therapy for iron deficiency (read more about this below).

When anemia is severe or the blood loss is rapid, you may need a blood transfusion to immediately replenish your iron supplies. If excessive menstrual bleeding or another uterine problem causes your anemia, your doctor may prescribe oral contraceptives to reduce your monthly blood flow.

The other types of vitamin-deficiency anemia are also treated with a daily regimen of vitamin supplements. People with vitamin B12 and folic acid deficiency must take supplements for their entire life. Anemia caused by medical disorders or chronic disease usually disappears once the underlying cause of the condition is addressed.

Preventing and treating iron-deficiency anemia

In most chapters in this book, I discuss food/dietary strategies first, then vitamins and minerals, and finally herbal remedies and other natural health products if applicable. In the case of anemia, I must start off with vitamins and minerals since they are key strategies to both preventing and treating the different types of anemia. Certain foods are important for enhancing the body's absorption of these nutrients, especially in the case of iron. So, let's begin with the mighty "micro" nutrients, the vitamins and minerals.

VITAMINS AND MINERALS
Iron

Most of the body's iron is found in two proteins: hemoglobin in red blood cells and myoglobin in muscle cells. As a component of these two proteins, iron helps carry oxygen throughout the body and release it to tissues where it's used for energy. To help prevent the signs and symptoms of an iron deficiency, it's critical that women consume adequate amounts of iron every day. Women aged 19 to 50 who are menstruating require 18 milligrams of iron each day; older women need 8 milligrams. Teenaged females need 15 milligrams. If you're a vegetarian, your daily iron requirements are increased by a factor of 1.8; that means if you're between the ages of 19 to 50, you must consume 32 milligrams of iron each day.

The richest sources of iron are beef, fish, poultry, pork and lamb. They supply heme iron, the type that can be absorbed and utilized the most efficiently by your body. Heme sources of iron make up about 10 percent of the iron we consume each day. Even though heme iron accounts for such a small proportion of our intake, it's so well absorbed that it actually contributes a significant amount of iron.

The rest of our iron comes from plant foods such as dried fruit, whole grains, leafy green vegetables, nuts, seeds and legumes. These are nonheme sources of iron, and the body is much less efficient in absorbing and using this type of iron. Vegetarians may have difficulty maintaining healthy iron stores because their diet relies exclusively on nonheme sources. (That's why the RDA for iron is higher for vegetarians.) The rate at which your body is able to absorb nonheme iron is strongly influenced by other factors in your diet, as you'll read in the sections that follow.

To boost your intake of iron, aim to include in your diet some of the foods from the Iron in Foods table in Chapter 1, page 21.

Over the years, our dietary preferences have changed considerably. Today, we eat more grains, fruit and vegetables and less meat than we did thirty years ago. This trend towards a plant-based diet has affected our overall intake of iron. In an attempt to lose weight or to watch their blood cholesterol level, women often restrict the amount of meat they eat. This can make it very difficult to achieve the recommended daily requirements for iron. Statistics indicate that adolescent girls also tend to limit their meat intake.

Enhancing absorption of nonheme iron

ANIMAL FOODS. Meat, poultry and fish contain the most bioavailable (most easily absorbed and utilized by the body) heme iron. These sources also contain a special component called MFP factor, which promotes the absorption of nonheme iron from other foods eaten with them. So, if you're wanting to absorb more iron from your brown rice stir-fry, throw in a little lean beef. This trick will work for those of you who don't follow a vegetarian diet.

VITAMIN C. If you're a vegetarian, here's a strategy worth noting: Including a little vitamin C in your plant-based meal can enhance the body's absorption of nonheme iron fourfold. In fact, vitamin C is the most potent promoter of nonheme iron absorption. The acidity of the vitamin converts iron to the ferrous form that's ready for absorption (your stomach acid enhances iron absorption in the same way). Here are some winning combinations:

- whole-wheat pasta with tomato sauce
- brown rice stir-fry with broccoli and red pepper
- whole-grain breakfast cereal topped with strawberries
- whole-grain toast with a small glass of orange juice
- spinach salad tossed with orange or grapefruit segments

CALCIUM. Chances are you've heard that calcium can interfere with iron absorption, especially when iron and calcium are taken simultaneously. It's true that these minerals (as well as magnesium and zinc) are absorbed the same way in the intestinal tract, so they can compete with one another for transport across the intestinal tract. But recent research has shown that taking a calcium supplement with meals for up to six months doesn't affect iron levels in healthy adults. However, if you're taking calcium supplements *and* iron pills to treat anemia, it's advisable to take them at separate times.

TEA. Natural compounds in tea called tannins can bind with iron and make it unavailable for absorption. Tannins are found in black tea and, to a lesser extent, in coffee, nuts and some fruit and vegetables. If you're a tea drinker, enjoy your cup of tea between meals. Or add a little milk or lemon to your tea, since both inactivate its iron-binding properties.

PHYTATE-RICH FOODS. Another compound in plant foods called phytic acid (phytate) can attach to iron and inhibit its absorption. These compounds are found in dietary fibre, nuts, spinach and other leafy vegetables. The recommended daily intake for dietary fibre (21 or 25 grams, depending on your age) isn't associated with impaired iron absorption. You'd have to be eating a diet that's extremely high in fibre (50 grams or more each day) before you'd interfere with the body's absorption of minerals.

Cooking vegetables such as spinach releases some of the iron that's bound to phytates. For this reason, cooked vegetables are always a better source of minerals than their raw counterparts.

Multivitamin/mineral and iron supplements

To help you meet your daily iron requirements, I do recommended a daily multivitamin and mineral supplement. Most formulas provide 10 milligrams of iron, but you can find multivitamins that provide up to 18 milligrams of the mineral. Menstruating women and vegetarians should choose a formula that supplies 10 to 18 milligrams of iron; men and post-menopausal women should look for 5 to 10 milligrams of iron in a multivitamin. During pregnancy, women are advised to take a prenatal formula that supplies 27 to 30 milligrams of iron.

If you're diagnosed with iron-deficiency anemia, your doctor will prescribe single iron pills. Depending on the extent of your iron deficiency, you may take one to three iron tablets (each containing 50 to 100 milligrams of elemental iron) per day. If you're advised to take an iron pill, take it on an empty stomach to enhance absorption. Taking your iron supplement with a vitamin C pill or a glass of orange juice can further enhance iron absorption. Many people find that taking their iron supplement before bed instead of during the day reduces stomach upset. Iron can be constipating, so I recommend you make a special effort to boost your fibre and water intake to prevent this side effect.

A supplementation period of three to six months is usually sufficient to treat your anemia. However, you may need to take the supplements for a longer period in order to completely restore your body's iron reserves. As your iron levels improve, your symptoms will gradually disappear.

While taking iron you may notice that your stools turn black. There's no need to worry—this is a normal and harmless side effect of the treatment. Your doctor will perform occasional blood tests to ensure that the bleeding has stopped or that your iron supply has increased to a healthy level.

When it comes to iron supplements, it's important to remember that more is *not* better. Your intestine can absorb only a limited amount of iron, so the benefits don't increase with larger doses. On the contrary, too much iron may cause indigestion and constipation. Excessive doses of iron can actually be quite toxic, causing damage to your liver and intestines. An iron overload can result in death. To avoid these problems, don't take iron supplements without first having a blood test to confirm that you're suffering from an iron deficiency.

Preventing and treating other types of anemia

VITAMINS AND MINERALS
Folate

An ongoing deficiency of this important B vitamin leads to what is known as megaloblastic or macrocytic anemia. Folate is needed to synthesize DNA, the genetic material that's required by all cells. When your body lacks folate as a result of poor diet, impaired absorption or an unusually high need for the vitamin, the DNA metabolism is harmed, especially in rapidly dividing cells like red blood cells.

The anemia of folate deficiency is characterized by large, immature red blood cells. Without folate, DNA production slows and red blood cells lose their ability to divide. These immature cells are enlarged and oval shaped. As such, they cannot carry oxygen or travel through the tiny blood vessels (capillaries) as efficiently as normal red blood cells.

To help prevent anemia associated with a folate deficiency, aim to meet your recommended daily allowance: 400 micrograms (0.4 milligrams). If you're pregnant, your folate requirement rises to 600 micrograms (0.6 milligrams) per day to cover the needs of rapidly multiplying cells.

The best food sources of folate include cooked spinach, lentils, asparagus, artichokes, avocados and orange juice. In Canada, white flour, white pasta and refined cornmeal must be fortified with folic acid. It's estimated that fortified foods add 100 to 200 micrograms (0.1 to

0.2 milligrams) of folic acid to one's daily intake. For a look at some of the best dietary folate sources, see the Folate in Foods table in Chapter 1, page 19. You'll notice that some of the best sources of folate are leafy green vegetables. In fact, the vitamin's name is derived from the word *foliage*. Foods deliver folate in a bound form; because your intestine prefers folate in its free form, special enzymes located on the surface of your intestine must first break down the bound folate. The free folate is then absorbed into your bloodstream and delivered to your body's cells.

Sounds fine so far. The problem is that this complicated system of handling folate from the diet is vulnerable to injuries in the intestinal tract. If your intestinal cells are harmed, then folate is lost from the body. Alcohol abuse and chronic use of aspirin and antacids can disrupt the absorption of folate. If you use the occasional aspirin to relieve a headache you need not be concerned, but if you rely heavily on these medications you are at risk of developing a folate deficiency. The medication Azulfidine (sulfasalazine), used to treat inflammatory bowel diseases such as Crohn's disease or ulcerative colitis, also interferes with folate absorption.

Other medications that can affect folate levels in the body include oral contraceptives, barbiturates, Metformin (a medication used for impaired fasting glucose and type 2 diabetes) and certain anticonvulsant drugs. If you take any of these prescription drugs, check with your pharmacist for possible nutrient interactions.

Folic acid supplements

Folate refers to the B vitamin in its natural form found in foods. Folic acid describes the synthetic vitamin found in vitamin supplements or fortified foods like white bread and white pasta. To meet your daily folate requirements, include in your diet at least two or three folate-rich foods from the table on page 19. And, of course, all women of childbearing age should take a multivitamin and mineral that provides 0.4 milligrams of folic acid. A B complex supplement that provides all eight B vitamins in one pill will also give you this amount of folic acid.

If you decide to take a folic acid supplement, make sure to buy one with vitamin B12, since these two nutrients work closely together. The body uses folic acid to activate B12 and vice versa. So a deficiency of one vitamin can eventually lead to a deficiency of the other. Supplementing with folic acid and neglecting to meet your B12 requirements can hide an underlying B12 deficiency. Folic acid supplementation will correct the anemia, and a blood test will find your red blood cells normal, but the nerve symptoms of a B12 deficiency can still progress.

Folic acid is well tolerated. It's generally recommended that you don't exceed the tolerable upper limit of 1000 micrograms per day. However, if you suffer from a malabsorption problem, higher doses can be safely used (be sure to take vitamin B12 too).

I don't recommend that you take a single supplement of folic acid unless you've been advised to do so by your doctor to treat a deficiency or if you're planning a pregnancy or are pregnant. (Women at high risk of giving birth to a baby with a neural tube defect are advised to take 5 milligrams of folic acid per day; you'll learn more about this B vitamin in Chapter 16, Pregnancy.) Recently, there has been concern that high doses of folic acid might do more harm than good. In a randomized controlled trial of 1021 men and women who previously had pre-cancerous polyps removed from their colon, those who took a folic acid supplement (1 milligram) got just as many new polyps as those who took placebo pills. People in the folic acid group had higher rates of advanced tumours and multiple tumours, although this could have been a chance finding (i.e., the evidence wasn't what researchers call statistically significant). This finding raised the possibility that if taken early, folic acid may prevent polyps from forming in the first place, but if taken once polyps have formed, large amounts of folic acid could accelerate their growth.[1] (Research also suggests that taking a high-dose folic acid supplement (1 milligram) could raise the risk of prostate cancer.[2] For these reasons, I advise people against taking high-dose folic acid supplements or B complex supplements that provide 1 milligram of folic acid. Get your folate from your diet and a multi-vitamin that provides 400 micrograms (0.4 milligrams).

Vitamin B12

Vitamin B12 and folate work very closely together in the body. Without enough B12, your body is unable to use folate, leading eventually to a folate deficiency and megaloblastic anemia (your blood test will show large, immature red blood cells). Alone, vitamin B12 maintains the protective covering of nerve fibres. Your bones also rely on this B vitamin for normal metabolism.

In addition to developing the anemia related to a folate deficiency, a lack of B12 can lead to pernicious anemia. This type of anemia is caused by impaired B12 absorption, not by poor dietary intake. After you consume

B12 from your diet, the acid in your stomach helps to release the vitamin from proteins in food. The vitamin then binds to an intrinsic factor that enables B12 to be absorbed into the bloodstream.

A vitamin B12 deficiency can occur for two reasons. Some people produce an insufficient amount of hydrochloric acid in their stomach. This condition, called atrophic gastritis, is common in older adults. Without enough stomach acid, B12 can't be released from food proteins and it won't be absorbed into the blood.

Some people inherit a defective gene for intrinsic factor. They don't produce this necessary factor that attaches to B12 and transports it into the bloodstream. A B12 deficiency caused by a lack of intrinsic factor leads to pernicious anemia. This anemia is characterized by a deficit of red blood cells, muscle weakness and nerve damage. Most doctors prefer to treat pernicious anemia with injections of vitamin B12, although oral supplements may also be effective. A recent study found that taking a B12 supplement dissolved under the tongue, twice daily, was as effective as shots in restoring B12 levels.[3]

Women of all ages need 2.4 micrograms of B12 each day. This vitamin is found exclusively in animal foods. If you eat meat, poultry, fish, eggs and dairy products on a regular basis you're probably not at risk for a B12 deficiency. The vitamin is also added to soy and rice beverages and some soy products like veggie burgers.

Vitamin B12 Content of Selected Foods

Food	Vitamin B12 (micrograms)
Beef, lean, 3 oz (90 g)	2.8 mcg
Mussels, shelled, 3 oz (90 g)	20 mcg
Salmon, sockeye, cooked, 3 oz (90 g)	4.9 mcg
Milk, 1 cup (250 ml)	1.0 mcg
Cheese, cottage, 1%, 1 cup (250 ml)	0.7 mcg
Cheese, cheddar, 1-1/2 oz (45 g)	0.4 mcg
Yogurt, 3/4 cup (175 ml)	1.0 mcg
Egg, 1 whole	0.6 mcg
Soy beverage, fortified, 1 cup (250 ml)	1.0 mcg

Source: Data adapted from the *Canadian Nutrient File*, Health Canada (2006). Available at: http://webprod.hc-sc.gc.ca/cnf-fce/index-eng.jsp.

B12 supplements

If you're a strict vegetarian who eats no animal products and you don't drink a fortified soy or rice beverage, I strongly recommend a B12 supplement. In fact, women (and men) over the age of 50 should be getting their B12 from a supplement or fortified foods. That's because the bodies of up to one-third of older adults produce inadequate amounts of stomach acid and are therefore inefficient at absorbing B12 from food.

 If you take certain medications you should consider taking extra B12 in the form of a supplement. If you suffer from reflux or ulcers and take acid blockers (e.g., Tagamet, Zantac, Pepcid), your body may not absorb enough B12 (as well as iron). Metformin, used to manage type 2 diabetes and polycystic ovary syndrome, can also deplete B12 levels. If you take these medications, your doctor should monitor your blood periodically for signs of anemia.

To get your B12, I recommend a good multivitamin and mineral supplement or a B complex supplement that contains the whole family of B vitamins. If you take a single B12 supplement, take 500 to 1000 micrograms once daily.

THE BOTTOM LINE...

Leslie's recommendations for preventing and managing anemia

1. To prevent iron-deficiency anemia, be sure to include iron-rich foods in your daily diet.
2. To maximize the absorption of nonheme iron (the type of iron predominant in grains, legumes, vegetables and fruit), include a source of vitamin C with each meal.
3. If you're not a vegetarian, include a little meat, poultry or fish with meals rich in nonheme iron.
4. If you're a tea drinker and you rely on nonheme sources of iron to meet your needs, enjoy your tea apart from your meals.
5. To ensure you're meeting your daily iron requirement, take a multivitamin and mineral supplement that contains 10 to 18 milligrams of iron. If you're no longer menstruating, there's no need to get more than 10 milligrams of iron in your supplement since your daily needs have declined.
6. If you're iron deficient or you have anemia, take 50 to 100 milligrams of elemental iron one to three times a day or as directed by your doctor.

Get your blood retested after twelve weeks of treatment. When your iron stores are replenished, stop taking iron supplements. High doses of iron are toxic when taken for a long period of time.

7. If you're taking supplemental iron pills and you already take calcium tablets each day, don't take these supplements at the same time. Take them at least two hours apart.

8. To prevent megaloblastic anemia, ensure you meet your daily requirement for folate. The best food sources include lentils, kidney beans, black beans, cooked spinach, asparagus and orange juice.

9. To help you reach your daily target of folate, choose a multivitamin and mineral pill that contains 0.4 milligrams of folic acid. Or, if you prefer, take a B complex supplement that provides this amount.

10. If you're advised to take a single folic acid supplement, be sure to buy one that has vitamin B12 added. That's because folic acid supplementation can mask a B12 deficiency.

11. To prevent anemia caused by a folate deficiency, make sure you're getting your daily vitamin B12 requirements. B12 is needed to activate folate.

12. If you're a strict vegetarian (vegan) who eats no animal products, be sure to include a B12-fortified soy beverage in your daily diet. Take a 500 or 1000 microgram B12 supplement.

13. If you're diagnosed with pernicious anemia, your doctor will likely prescribe monthly vitamin B12 injections. If shots aren't your thing, consider taking 1000 micrograms of sublingual (under the tongue) B12 twice daily.

4
Chronic fatigue syndrome (CFS)

Relentless fatigue ... punishing exhaustion ... limited energy. This daunting list represents only a few of the symptoms commonly associated with the disabling disease known as chronic fatigue syndrome (CFS). CFS is an enigma—a largely misunderstood illness that saps vitality and steals mental acuity. Very little is known about the causes of CFS and even less about the possible cures. We do know, however, that most cases of CFS occur in white, middle- to upper-class women.

CFS is a disease characterized by profound fatigue that's not improved with bed rest. People with CFS are easily exhausted by the slightest physical or mental activities. Because there's no cure, CFS can persist for years, dramatically altering the lives of women who suffer from it.

What causes CFS?

Chronic fatigue syndrome is a complicated disorder defined by symptoms of severe, debilitating fatigue. Over the years, doctors have diagnosed chronic tiredness under a variety of different names, including nervous exhaustion, Yuppie flu, Epstein-Barr virus disease or myalgic encephalo-myelitis. In 1988, a committee of experts studying the illness selected a new name, chronic fatigue syndrome, to represent the most noticeable and consistent symptom of the disease.[1] Since then, CFS has become an important social and public health issue and is currently the focus of intense research.

There doesn't seem to be one single cause for CFS. Instead, nearly twenty years of research indicates there are likely a number of different factors, working alone or in combination, that might cause CFS. Initially, it was thought a viral infection produced CFS. Scientific attention was focused on the Epstein-Barr virus, herpes-type viruses and infections that cause polio. But extensive studies were unable to establish a direct connection between CFS and these or any other infectious agents. Despite this, scientists still speculate that a virus may help trigger the disease.

Much of the ongoing research into the cause of CFS has focused on the roles of the immune, hormonal and nervous systems. CFS may be caused when an infection or virus attacks someone with a weakened immune system. Once the infection has passed, the immune system doesn't return to its normal state. Instead, it remains active, continuously producing excess immune-activating factors. As these factors circulate through the bloodstream, they may cause profound fatigue. Studies do find that many people with CFS have chronically over-active immune systems, with white blood cells that are less able to fight off viruses.

It's also thought that oxidative stress caused by free radicals in the body may play a role in the development and progression of CFS.

Often people with CFS have a history of allergies, which, for some unknown reason, seems to predispose them to the disease. There's also the possibility that a severe metabolic dysfunction may be the culprit behind CFS. Many CFS sufferers show evidence of extreme shifts in metabolism that limit heart and lung functions, making it difficult and even physically damaging to carry out normal activities. Research has also linked brain abnormalities with CFS, especially those associated with sleep-related disorders.

Certain malfunctions of the nervous system can produce racing heartbeats or sudden drops in blood pressure. These conditions seem to be associated with the development of CFS in ways that are not yet fully understood. As well, periods of physical or emotional stress have an impact on the nervous system. Stressful events stimulate the brain to produce cortisol and other stress hormones. Because stress may be a trigger for the development of CFS, it's possible that there's a connection between the disease and altered levels of stress hormones.

CFS isn't caused by depression, although the two illnesses often appear together. However, many people with CFS don't suffer from depression or other psychiatric disorders.

Symptoms

CFS is marked by extreme fatigue that has lasted at least six months and is not relieved by rest. It's a fatigue that goes far beyond the exhausted, overtired feelings that we all get from time to time—it's relentless and causes a substantial reduction in daily activities. In addition to fatigue, CFS includes the following characteristic symptoms:

- relapse of symptoms after physical or mental exertion
- sleep disturbances; unrefreshing sleep
- impaired thinking, forgetfulness, confusion, difficulty concentrating
- muscle pain and weakness
- joint pain, often in multiple joints
- headaches
- sore throat
- tender lymph nodes in the neck or armpits

Because the disease involves a faulty immune system, it's also common for people with CFS to experience food allergies, other fungal infections (e.g., yeast infections) and frequent bouts of the common cold.

CFS symptoms and their duration vary widely from individual to individual. Approximately 50 percent of people with CFS return to a fairly normal lifestyle within five years. The other half will still be dramatically ill even after ten years. Some people recover from the disease in two to three years, only to suffer a relapse at a later time. CFS can be cyclical, producing alternating periods of illness and relatively good health.

Who's at risk?

CFS is thought to affect 350,000 to 480,000 Canadians.[2] It can affect people of every age, gender, ethnicity and socioeconomic group. Despite this, the condition is most common in people in their 40s and 50s. Research also indicates that women report the condition four times more often than men, possibly because women are more willing to seek medical treatment for fatigue.[3]

Diagnosis

There are no diagnostic laboratory tests for CFS. Individuals who suffer from CFS must be carefully evaluated by a physician to rule out other treatable medical conditions that have similar symptoms, such as fibromyalgia, mononucleosis, Lyme disease, multiple sclerosis, hypothyroidism, cancer, depression and hormonal dysfunction.

To determine whether you have CFS, a thorough evaluation of your health will be necessary. This will include an examination of your medical history, a physical examination and a review of your mental state. Because CFS is diagnosed through a process of elimination, your doctor will order a series of laboratory and X-ray screening tests to rule out other possible causes of your chronic fatigue. Once these other medical conditions have been eliminated, your doctor will consider CFS if you meet the following criteria:

1. Unexplained, persistent or relapsing fatigue that lasts for at least six months; fatigue that isn't the result of ongoing exertion or other medical conditions; and
2. The presence of at least four of the following symptoms:
   * substantial impairment of short-term memory or concentration
   * sore throat
   * tender lymph nodes
   * muscle pain
   * multi-joint pain without swelling or redness
   * headaches of a new type, pattern or severity
   * unrefreshing sleep
   * post-exertion fatigue that lasts more than twenty-four hours

Conventional treatment

Medications prescribed for CFS are intended to provide relief of symptoms. They're not considered cures for the disease. Today, doctors use a combination of therapies and a gradual approach to rehabilitation in treating this disease.

Low-dose *tricyclic antidepressants* seem to have a positive effect on some people with CFS, possibly because they improve the quality of sleep. Another form of antidepressant, known as *SSRIs (serotonin reuptake inhibitors)*, has also provided treatment benefits. In some cases, benzodiazepines, a type of drug used to treat anxiety and sleep problems, will improve the quality of life for CFS sufferers. *NSAIDs* (non-steroidal anti-inflammatory drugs) will help fight the aches and pains, and *antihistamines* may relieve the allergy symptoms associated with the condition. You'll probably need to try more than one type of drug before you find the right combination for you.

Lifestyle changes such as prevention of overexertion, reduced stress, gentle stretching, yoga and physical therapy are also used to treat CFS. Learning to manage your fatigue will help you improve the ability to function. Behaviour therapy can help you find effective ways to plan daily activities so that you can take advantage of peak energy levels. Exercise is also important in the management of CFS. Although exercise may seem to aggravate the symptoms, it's essential to maintain some muscle strength and conditioning. Throughout the course of this disease, it's important to learn to pace yourself physically, emotionally and mentally, since extra stress can exacerbate symptoms.

Managing CFS

If you have CFS, nutrition plays an important role in your recovery to good health. As you'll read below, scientists have found that a number of vitamins and minerals are deficient in many people with CFS. This seems to be mostly due to the illness itself, rather than a poor diet. Even marginal nutrient deficiencies can contribute to your fatigue symptoms, and the lack of important nutrients can also delay your healing process.

DIETARY STRATEGIES

Follow a wholesome, healthy and well-balanced diet. The quality of the foods eaten seems to be most important in helping to restore energy levels. Some practitioners recommended a low-sugar, low-yeast diet; however, research hasn't shown this eating plan to be any more effective at improving energy levels and quality of life than an overall healthful diet.[4]

- **Emphasize plant foods** in your daily diet. Fill your plate with grains, fruit and vegetables. If you eat animal protein foods like meat or poultry, they should take up no more than one-quarter of your plate. Try vegetarian sources of protein like legumes and soy.
- **Choose foods and oils that are rich in essential fatty acids.** Fish, nuts, seeds, flaxseed and flaxseed oil, canola oil, omega-3 eggs, wheat germ and leafy green vegetables are examples.
- **Choose foods rich in vitamins, minerals and protective plant compounds.** Reach for whole grains as often as possible. Eat at least three different coloured fruits and four different coloured vegetables every day.
- **Eliminate sources of refined sugar** as often as possible: that means cookies, cakes, pastries, frozen desserts, soft drinks, sweetened fruit juices, fruit drinks, candy, etc.
- **Buy organic produce or wash fruit and vegetables** to remove pesticide residues.
- **Limit foods with chemical additives.**
- **Avoid caffeine** (this can worsen fatigue by interrupting sleep patterns).
- **Drink at least 9 cups (2.2 L) of water every day.**
- **Avoid alcohol.** If you drink alcohol, limit your intake. Women should consume no more than one drink a day, or seven per week.
- **Take a multivitamin and mineral supplement each day** to ensure you're meeting your needs for most nutrients. Buy a product that contains no artificial preservatives, colours, flavours or added sugar, starch, lactose or yeast. This should be declared in small print below the ingredients list. If you experience gastrointestinal upset when taking a multivitamin, try a "professional brand" supplement available at certain health food stores. These products contain no binding materials and are suitable for people with food sensitivities. However, they're expensive, and you have to take at least three to six capsules a day to meet your recommended intake levels. Brand names include Genestra and Thorne Research.

To help you follow these principles, reread my dietary guidelines in Chapter 1 to learn what foods you should be eating more often.

If you experience bloating, cramps, gas, diarrhea or skin rashes after eating, it's a good idea to be tested for food allergies. Ask your family doctor for a referral to an allergy specialist.

Because no single cause has been identified for CFS, there's no single diet or supplement program that can be said to cure the condition. However, there is research to suggest that the vitamins, minerals and herbs I discuss below can improve CFS symptoms. Since these supplements are all considered safe in the amounts indicated, it makes sense to try one or more of these for a trial period. You should always make an effort to boost your intake of these nutrients through your food choices too.

Omega-3 fatty acids

A number of studies have shown that patients with CFS have depressed levels of the omega-3 fatty acids DHA and EPA in their blood cells. Scientists also speculate that a persistent viral infection may impair the body's ability to synthesize omega-3 fatty acids. Since DHA and EPA are used to help regulate the immune system and reduce inflammation in the body, lower levels of these fats may contribute to the symptoms of CFS.

Researchers have reported symptom improvements in many patients treated with omega-3 fatty acid supplementation. Patients given high-dose EPA showed improvement within eight to twelve weeks.[5-7]

Aim to eat oily fish, rich in omega-3 fatty acids, twice per week. In addition, take a fish oil supplement that supplies both EPA and DHA. See Fish Oil Supplements later in this chapter.

VITAMINS AND MINERALS

Antioxidants

Since CFS is often accompanied by signs of oxidative stress and by decreased antioxidant levels in the body, individuals with the condition may benefit from increasing their intake of antioxidant nutrients. Start by adding the following antioxidant-rich foods to your daily diet.

VITAMIN C. The recommended daily intake is 75 milligrams per day for women. The best food sources include citrus fruit, citrus juices, kiwi, mango, cantaloupe, strawberries, broccoli, Brussels sprouts, red pepper and tomato juice.

VITAMIN E. The recommended daily intake for women is 15 milligrams of alpha-tocopherol, equivalent to 22 international units (IU) of natural source or 33 IU of synthetic vitamin E. The best food sources include vegetable oils, sunflower seeds, almonds, hazelnuts, peanuts and kale.

BETA CAROTENE. There's no recommended daily intake for beta carotene. Research suggests that consuming 3 to 6 milligrams daily will maintain blood levels of beta carotene in the range linked with disease prevention. The best food sources include carrots, winter squash, sweet potato, kale, spinach, turnip greens, collard greens, romaine lettuce, broccoli, apricots, cantaloupe, peaches, nectarines, mango and papaya.

SELENIUM. Adults need 55 micrograms of selenium per day. The best food sources include Brazil nuts, seafood, tuna, cod, beef, turkey breast and chicken breast.

B vitamins

Without B vitamins, our bodies would lack energy. These eight nutrients are indispensable for yielding energy compounds from the foods we eat. Many B vitamins serve as helpers to enzymes that release energy from fat, protein and carbohydrate. Compared with healthy people, patients with CFS often have lower levels of B vitamins in their blood.[8-11] One study also found that enzymes dependent on B vitamins were less active in people with CFS. No published studies have assessed the effect of vitamin B supplements on fatigue symptoms. The following table will help you choose foods rich in B vitamins.

Foods Rich in B Vitamins

B vitamin	RDA for women aged 19+ (mg = milligrams, mcg = micrograms)	Best food sources
Thiamin (B1)	1.1 mg	pork, ham, bacon, liver, whole-grain or enriched breads and cereals, dried peas, beans and lentils, nuts
Riboflavin (B2)	1.1 mg	milk, yogurt, cottage cheese, meat, leafy green vegetables, whole-grain or enriched breads and cereals
Niacin (B3)	14 mg	milk, eggs, poultry, fish, whole-grain or enriched breads and cereals, nuts, all protein-containing foods
B6	1.3 to 1.5 mg	whole grains, bananas, potatoes, legumes, fish, meat, poultry

B vitamin	RDA for women aged 19+ (mg = milligrams, mcg = micrograms)	Best food sources
Folate	400 mcg	spinach, orange juice, lentils, asparagus, artichokes, avocados, leafy greens, wheat germ, whole grains
B12	2.4 mcg	meat, poultry, fish, dairy products, eggs, fortified soy and rice milk
Biotin	30 mcg	widespread in foods
Pantothenic acid	5 mg	widespread in foods

Vitamin B supplements

To ensure you're getting your daily B vitamins, take a good-quality multi-vitamin and mineral supplement each day to supplement your healthy diet.

Magnesium

More than 300 enzymes rely on a steady supply of magnesium for optimal activity. Magnesium is part of adenosine triphosphate (ATP), the active energy compound that's used by every cell in your body. It's believed that a deficiency in magnesium can lead to the decreased energy and weakness seen in CFS. Some investigations have found low levels of magnesium in the red blood cells of patients with CFS.[12,13] When these patients were regularly given magnesium by injection, they reported more energy, less pain and more balanced emotions.

Researchers have also learned that many CFS patients who are deficient in magnesium have a decreased antioxidant status in their body. Supplementing the diet with magnesium has been shown to improve the body's magnesium stores and antioxidant levels.[14]

Many Canadian women don't meet their daily magnesium requirements. Women aged 19 to 29 need 310 milligrams of magnesium each day; women aged 30 and older require 320 milligrams. The best sources of magnesium include legumes, nuts and seeds, prunes, figs, whole grains, leafy green vegetables and brewer's yeast. Green vegetables are particularly good sources of magnesium because the centre of the chlorophyll molecule—the compound that gives green vegetables their colour—contains magnesium. See the Magnesium in Foods chart in Chapter 1, page 24, for specific foods and portion sizes that will help you meet these daily targets.

Magnesium supplements

There's no definite dose of magnesium for the treatment of CFS. Doses of 200 to 300 milligrams have been used to reduce the muscle pain and joint tenderness associated with fibromyalgia. If you want to take a supplement, buy magnesium citrate. Compared to other forms of the mineral (e.g., magnesium oxide), magnesium citrate is more easily absorbed by your body. You can also get supplemental magnesium from your calcium pills if you buy one that has magnesium added.

The daily upper limit for magnesium has been set at 350 milligrams from a supplement. That's because doses higher than this can cause diarrhea and stomach upset, common side effects of magnesium supplementation.

HERBAL REMEDIES

The following herbs have been shown to boost the body's production of infection-fighting immune compounds. Of the three I discuss, echinacea and Panax ginseng have been shown to enhance the activity of immune cells in people with CFS.[15] Echinacea can be beneficial in treating bothersome colds, while ginseng and aged garlic extract can be used longer term for immune stimulation.

Echinacea

If you suffer from frequent colds, studies have found that this herb can reduce the duration of your symptoms by as much as 50 percent. Echinacea's active ingredients enhance the body's immune system by increasing production of certain white blood cells that fight off viruses and bacteria.

Three species of echinacea are found in products—*Echinacea pupurea, Echinacea angustifolia* and *Echinacea pallida*—and all have medicinal benefits. To ensure you're getting a quality product, buy one that's standardized. Take echinacea at the first sign of cold or flu symptoms. Take 900 milligrams of standardized echinacea three to four times daily. Limit daily use to eight consecutive weeks due to concern that long-term use of echinacea might depress the immune system. Do not use echinacea if you're allergic to plants in the Asteracease/Compositae family (ragweed, daisy, marigold and chrysanthemum).

Panax ginseng

This ginseng goes by many names, including Asian, Korean and Chinese. Studies have shown the herb to have strong immune-enhancing properties. A large Italian study found that individuals taking 100 milligrams of a standardized ginseng product (G115 extract) had significantly higher levels of antibodies in response to a flu shot compared to those who did not take the herb.[16] Killer white blood cells were nearly twice as high in the ginseng group after eight weeks of supplementation. These and other white blood cells are an important part of the body's defence against viruses and foreign molecules.

The benefits of Panax ginseng on the immune system can be attributed to active compounds in the root called ginsenosides. Many ginsenosides have been identified, but ginsenosides Rg1 and Rb1 have received the most attention. Scientific research has focused on ginseng extracts standardized to contain 4 percent to 7 percent ginsenosides.

The typical dosage of a standardized extract is 100 or 200 milligrams once daily. Take ginseng for three weeks to three months, and then follow with a one- to two-week rest period before you resume taking the herb.

In some people, ginseng may cause mild stomach upset, irritability and insomnia. To avoid overstimulation, start with 100 milligrams a day and avoid taking the herb with caffeine. Ginseng should not be used during pregnancy, breastfeeding or by individuals with poorly controlled high blood pressure.

Siberian ginseng *(Eleutherococcus senticosus)*

In a study of 96 patients, those assigned to take Siberian ginseng versus placebo reported less fatigue after two months of supplementation. Treatment was most effective for patients with less severe fatigue.[17]

Unlike Panax ginseng, this herb has a much milder effect and fewer reported side effects. It's also been used in clinical studies of CFS. Pregnant and nursing women can safely take Siberian ginseng, and it's much less likely to cause overstimulation in sensitive individuals. To ensure quality, choose a product standardized for eleutherosides B and E. The usual dosage is 300 to 400 milligrams once daily for six to eight weeks, followed by a one- to two-week break.

Garlic *(Allium sativum)*

You may want to add fresh garlic to your meals more often. A daily intake of garlic and its accompanying sulphur compounds has been used to enhance the body's immune system and kill many types of bacteria and fungi (including the *Candida* organism that causes yeast infections). One-half to one clove a day is recommended.

When it comes to garlic pills, buy *aged* garlic extract. The aging process used to make this supplement increases the concentration of the special sulphur compounds that stimulate the immune system. In fact, animal studies have found that the amount of garlic equivalent to three aged garlic extract capsules dramatically increases activity of white blood cells (killer cells, macrophages and leukocytes). Generally, two to six capsules a day (one or two with meals) are recommended. You can also take aged garlic in a liquid form (Kyolic brand) that you add to foods.

OTHER NATURAL HEALTH PRODUCTS

Fish oil supplements

Based on the finding that CFS patients have depressed essential fatty acids in their blood cells, Scottish researchers had 63 adults with CFS take either fish oil (eight 500 milligram capsules per day) or placebo capsules for three months.[18] When the study was over, 85 percent of patients taking the fish oil reported a significant improvement in their symptoms. As would be expected, there was also an increase in cellular levels of essential fatty acids. Researchers from the United Kingdom tried to replicate these results among 50 patients with CFS and found no difference in symptoms between those taking fish oil and those taking a placebo.[19] Other studies have reported beneficial effects of fish oil supplementation.

Buy a product that contains both EPA and DHA omega-3 fatty acids. The brand used in clinical studies was Efamol Marine. You might also consider using a liquid fish oil supplement rather than a capsule. Per teaspoon, most brands of liquid fish oil supply twice the amount of omega-3 fatty acids as one capsule. Avoid fish *liver* oil capsules. Most supplements made from fish liver are a concentrated source of vitamin A; too much of this nutrient can be toxic when taken in large amounts for long periods.

Fish oil has a blood-thinning effect. If you take anti-clotting medication, consult your physician before taking fish oil. And follow your health care practitioner's advice for dosage.

Acetyl-L-carnitine (ALC)

This compound isn't considered an essential nutrient because the body makes it in sufficient quantities. The body obtains some carnitine from the diet, primarily from red meat and dairy products. The body can also synthesize carnitine from amino acids. In the body, ALC is converted to L-carnitine, a compound that helps all cells in the body generate energy, especially muscle cells. ALC is also used to synthesize acetylcholine, a brain chemical that aids in memory. It's possible that a deficiency of this compound can cause the fatigue associated with CFS. Studies have shown that CFS patients tend to have lower levels of carnitine in their blood, and higher levels are linked with less-severe symptoms.[20,21]

Two studies suggest supplementing with ALC can reduce CFS symptoms. In one study of 96 elderly patients with fatigue, ALC treatment significantly outperformed the placebo treatment for improving muscle pain, prolonged fatigue after exercise, sleep disorders, physical fatigue and mental fatigue.[22] Another study conducted in 90 patients with CFS found ALC to reduce mental fatigue—50 percent of the patients on the supplement showed considerable improvement in attention and concentration. In this study, the researchers also tested the effectiveness of another form of carnitine called propionyl-L-carnitine. Among patients who received this treatment, 63 percent reported significant improvement of general fatigue. Patients in the study who were given a combined supplement of ALC and propionyl-L-carnitine reported less improvement.[23]

Based on the clinical research, a dose of 2 grams of ALC or propionyl-L-carnitine has been used. If symptoms of mental fatigue trouble you most, supplement with ALC. If feelings of general fatigue are most bothersome, take propionyl-L-carnitine. Supplement for six months to evaluate its effectiveness in improving energy.

Propionyl-L-carnitine may cause the urine and breath to have a fishy odour.

Avoid products that contain D-carnitine or DL-carnitine. These forms compete with L-carnitine in the body and could lead to a deficiency. The supplement is considered safe. Occasional side effects of gastrointestinal upset have been reported.

Melatonin

Melatonin, a hormone produced in the tiny pineal gland located in the brain, regulates the body's wake-sleep cycles. Its release from the brain is stimulated by darkness: the darker the room, the more melatonin your body produces. The hormone induces sleep by interacting with melatonin receptors in the brain. Based on the observation that many patients with CFS have wake-sleep cycle disturbances, researchers have investigated the effectiveness of melatonin supplements in treating CFS.

One study conducted in 29 patients with CFS found that taking 5 milligrams of melatonin in the evening for twelve weeks improved measures of fatigue, concentration, motivation and activity.[24] However, another study reported no benefit of melatonin supplementation. These studies used different methods for assessing symptoms, which might explain the different findings.

To improve sleep disturbances associated with CFS, take a daily dose of 5 milligrams of melatonin at bedtime. The most commonly reported side effects of melatonin include daytime drowsiness, headache and dizziness. Long-term use of melatonin supplements should be avoided; studies have been brief in duration and long-term safety hasn't been evaluated. Because melatonin is a hormone, its effects, if any, may take years to develop. People taking immunosuppressive drugs and women who are pregnant or breastfeeding should not use melatonin. People with depression should avoid this supplement, as it can worsen symptoms. Since melatonin is metabolized in the liver, people with liver disease should avoid using it.

Keep in mind that not all melatonin products are safe. Most commercial melatonin is synthesized in the laboratory. However, in some cases it can be derived from the pineal glands of animals. Melatonin from animal sources should be avoided due to the possibility of contamination of bovine spongiform encephalopathy (BSE, or mad cow disease). Some preparations of synthetic melatonin contain contaminants that are associated with eosinophilia-myalgia syndrome, a sometimes-fatal flu-like disease that causes severe pain, inflammation of the tendons, fluid build-up in the muscles and skin rash.

THE BOTTOM LINE...
Leslie's recommendations for managing CFS

1. First and foremost, implement the healthiest, nutritious diet possible.
2. If your intestinal tract or skin reacts to certain foods, make an appointment with a specialist to have food-allergy tests performed. Often food sensitivities are the result of a weakened immune system.

3. To increase your intake of omega-3 fatty acids, eat oily fish such as salmon, trout, sardines and herring twice per week.

4. Ensure your daily diet includes plenty of antioxidant-rich foods to meet your requirements for vitamins C and E, beta carotene and selenium. Refer to the foods listed on page 32.

5. To ensure you're meeting your daily targets for essential nutrients, especially the B vitamins, take a multivitamin and mineral supplement each day. If you're sensitive to many foods, buy a "professional brand" that contains no binding ingredients.

6. Some evidence suggests that taking certain natural health products might ease the symptoms of CFS. In addition to eating wholesome, nutrient-dense foods, consider adding the following to your daily regime:
   - B complex vitamin formula
   - magnesium citrate, 200 to 300 milligrams
   - fish oil, 2 grams
   - aceytl-L-carnitine, 2 grams
   - melatonin, 5 milligrams

7. To stimulate your body's immune system, consider adding the following herbal remedies to your daily plan:
   - Panax ginseng (G115 extract), 100 to 200 milligrams, OR Siberian Ginseng, 300 to 400 milligrams
   - Aged garlic extract, 2 to 6 capsules

8. If you suffer from frequent bouts of the common cold, take a standardized extract of echinacea at first sign of infection. Take 900 milligrams of echinacea three to four times daily until your cold disappears. Avoid using this herb if you're allergic to plants in the Asteracease/Compositae family (ragweed, daisy, marigold and chrysanthemum).

5
Hypoglycemia

Most of us have experienced that difficult time of day when energy dips, concentration wanes and our stomach grumbles for food. But for some people, the effects of too little sugar (glucose) in the bloodstream are more debilitating—headache, shakiness, weakness, rapid heartbeat, anxiety, confusion, blurred vision—and they often occur without warning. Hypoglycemia is the medical term for low blood sugar or blood glucose, a condition that can cause many body organs to malfunction. The brain is the most susceptible because glucose is its main energy source.

Your body relies on glucose as its main source of fuel for daily activities. During the process of digestion, the carbohydrates (sugars and starches) that you eat are broken down in the intestine into glucose. Glucose is absorbed by your bloodstream and then carried to every cell in your body. Unused glucose is stored in your muscles and liver as glycogen. Your body draws on these sugar stores for energy when your blood sugar drops.

Normally, blood-glucose levels range from 4.0 to 6.0 millimoles per litre (mmol/L) of blood before eating and rise to 5.0 to 8.0 mmol/L in the two hours following a meal. Whenever you eat food, the breakdown of carbohydrates into glucose causes your blood-sugar level to rise. This triggers your pancreas, an organ located in your upper abdomen, to release a hormone called insulin. Insulin helps glucose enter body cells, where it supplies the energy to fuel most bodily functions. As glucose is absorbed into the cells, your blood-sugar level gradually drops back to a normal range.

A few hours later, when most of the available glucose supply is consumed, your blood-sugar levels start to fall below normal, indicating that your body needs more fuel. Your pancreas responds to the falling glucose levels by releasing a different hormone, called glucagon. Glucagon stimulates your liver to release its stored supply of glucose into the bloodstream, where it's circulated to the cells. Once again, your blood-sugar levels rise back to normal. Adrenaline and cortisol, hormones released by your adrenal glands, also help keep blood-glucose levels up. By relying on insulin, glucagon and several other hormones, your body keeps your blood-glucose levels under constant control and regulates your daily energy supply.

What causes hypoglycemia?

Hypoglycemia occurs when your blood-glucose levels drop too low and you no longer have enough energy to fuel your daily activities. It can be a concern for people with diabetes who are taking certain blood sugar–lowering medications, but it can also affect people who don't have diabetes. Two types of hypoglycemia can occur in people without diabetes: fasting and reactive. *Fasting hypoglycemia* happens when a person hasn't had anything to eat or drink for eight or more hours. It's usually related to an underlying illness, a hereditary hormone or enzyme deficiencies; to taking certain medications; or to binge drinking (alcohol interferes with your liver's attempts to raise blood glucose levels).

More common is *reactive hypoglycemia*, which happens when blood glucose drops abnormally low within one to four hours after eating a meal. This type of low blood-sugar reaction occurs when the pancreas releases too much insulin at once, causing your blood-sugar level to plummet below normal. If you're prone to reactive hypoglycemia, eating too many refined starchy or sugary foods can aggravate the condition. That's because large portions of processed carbohydrate-rich foods cause your blood sugar to rise very rapidly, triggering excessive insulin production and a dramatic drop in your glucose level, leaving you feeling sweaty, anxious, hungry and shaky.

Other possible causes of hypoglycemia include

- stress and anxiety
- an unbalanced diet that's high in refined grains and/or sugars
- drinking alcohol
- early pregnancy
- prolonged fasting
- long periods of strenuous exercise
- exercising while you're on beta-blocker medication (e.g., propranolol)

- liver disease
- gastric surgery that disrupts the balance between digestion and insulin release
- hereditary intolerance of foods that contain the natural sugars fructose and galactose (rare childhood conditions)

Although there are many conditions that may cause hypoglycemia, only 1 percent of hypoglycemia cases occur in people who do not have diabetes. Studies indicate that it's actually quite a rare disorder.

Symptoms

When your blood-sugar level falls, your body responds by releasing a hormone called epinephrine (adrenaline) from your adrenal glands. This hormone stimulates your liver to release its stored glucose into your bloodstream. But this adrenaline rush also produces the unpleasant symptoms that are characteristic of hypoglycemia, which include sweating, nervousness, rapid heartbeat, anxiety, hunger, faintness and trembling.

If your blood-sugar level continues to fall, the reduced glucose supply will begin to affect your brain. When hypoglycemia interferes with brain activities, you may experience headache, dizziness, rapid heartbeat, sweating, confusion, blurred vision, difficulty concentrating, anxiety, agitation, weakness or fainting and abnormal behaviour that could be mistaken for drunkenness. If your condition continues to worsen, convulsions, loss of consciousness and coma may result. Keep in mind that such life-threatening symptoms are usually caused by too much medication in people with diabetes.

Symptoms of hypoglycemia vary in severity among individuals and may progress from mild to severe in a short period of time.

Who's at risk?

Hypoglycemia is most common among people who have diabetes and take blood-sugar-lowering medication. Other factors that can predispose you to hypoglycemia include fasting, following a low-calorie diet, being pregnant, having certain medical disorders and taking certain medications.

For some people, hypoglycemia develops when they drink alcohol after a long period without eating food. As their blood-glucose levels fall, they develop a hypoglycemia-induced stupor, which makes them appear drunk and confused. This type of stupor can develop even when blood-alcohol levels are well below the legal driving limit.

Diagnosis

If you have symptoms of hypoglycemia and you don't have diabetes, your doctor may conduct some simple blood tests to measure your blood-sugar and insulin levels. Ideally, this test will be done while you are experiencing an episode of hypoglycemic symptoms. The diagnosis of hypoglycemia will be confirmed if the blood test indicates that your blood-sugar levels are below normal and your symptoms improve when you consume sugar. If your blood glucose is less than 4.0 mmol/L and your symptoms disappear when food is eaten, hypoglycemia is likely the cause.

Your doctor will also take your medical history and conduct a physical examination, and may test you for diabetes. Depending on the cause of your hypoglycemia, additional laboratory tests may be required.

For years doctors used the oral glucose tolerance test to diagnose hypoglycemia. (The test measures blood-glucose levels after an overnight fast, and then two hours after consumption of a sugary solution.) However, its use has fallen out of favour because it can produce misleading results. It's now recognized that the signs and symptoms of hypoglycemia can occur in individuals who have blood-glucose levels within the normal range. And 10 percent of people who don't have any symptoms of hypoglycemia show low blood-sugar levels when they take the oral glucose tolerance test. So relying on blood-sugar levels alone is often not enough to diagnose hypoglycemia.

One of the most useful ways to determine if you suffer from hypoglycemia is to assess your symptoms. In general, when symptoms appear three to four hours after eating and disappear after you've consumed food, hypoglycemia is a likely cause. The following question-naire is a useful tool to help you determine if you're suffering from hypoglycemia.

Hypoglycemia Questionnaire

Symptom	No	Mild	Moderate	Severe
Crave sweets	o	1	2	3
Irritable if meal is missed	o	1	2	3
Feel tired or weak if meal is missed	o	1	2	3
Dizziness if you stand suddenly	o	1	2	3
Frequent headaches	o	1	2	3
Poor memory or concentration	o	1	2	3
Feel tired an hour or so after eating	o	1	2	3
Heart palpitations	o	1	2	3
Feel shaky at times	o	1	2	3
Afternoon fatigue	o	1	2	3
Vision blurs on occasion	o	1	2	3
Depression or mood swings	o	1	2	3
Overweight	o	1	2	3
Often anxious or nervous	o	1	2	3
Total score				

Scoring
≤5   hypoglycemia is not a likely factor
6–15   hypoglycemia is a likely factor
>15   hypoglycemia is extremely likely

Source: Murray, M, and JE Pizano. *Hypoglycemia: Textbook of natural medicine*, vol. 2 (Edinburgh: Churchill Livingstone, 1999).

Conventional treatment

In most cases, the symptoms of hypoglycemia will quickly improve when you consume sugar in any form. Eating candy, sugar cubes, glucose or dextrose tablets, or drinking a glass of fruit juice, milk or sugar water will immediately raise your blood-sugar levels, making you feel much better. If you do experience a low blood-sugar reaction, treat it immediately by consuming 10 to 15 grams of carbohydrates such as five Life Savers, half a banana or 1/2 to 3/4 cup (125 to 175 ml) of fruit juice.

If you have diabetes or are prone to recurring episodes of hypoglycemia, you should always carry some candy or other type of sugar with you. Dextrose tablets are widely available in drugstores in the diet section. They are handy to have in the event of a low blood-sugar reaction when you're away from home and don't have access to food; three tablets give you 9 grams of carbohydrates. In severe cases of hypoglycemia, an injection of glucagon or intravenous glucose may be necessary to restore blood-sugar levels.

Hypoglycemia that develops after gastrointestinal surgery can often be managed by eating small, frequent meals and following a high-protein, low-carbohydrate diet. A hereditary intolerance of fructose (fruit sugar) or galactose (milk sugar) is treated by eliminating the foods that cause hypoglycemic symptoms.

Managing hypoglycemia

This section focuses on nutritional strategies that will help you maintain a consistent blood-sugar level, and so be less vulnerable to experiencing hypoglycemia. While some of my recommendations are helpful for women with diabetes, for the most part they are intended for women who have hypoglycemia that's not related to medication that lowers blood sugar.

Over the years, I've had many clients seek my help for managing their hypoglycemia. They've learned that following the proper diet is key to preventing hypoglycemia. Instead of relying on fast-acting carbohydrates to treat a low blood-sugar reaction, use the strategies below to prevent a sugar low from occurring in the first place.

DIETARY STRATEGIES
Meal timing
One of the first and most important ways to prevent a low blood-sugar reaction is to eat regularly throughout the day. After eating a meal, your blood sugar will peak in 45 to 90 minutes. After this point, your sugar level starts its decline. If you suffer from hypoglycemia, you should *eat every three hours*. That means eating *three meals and three snacks*. Here's what a meal and snack schedule might look like if you work during the day from

nine o'clock to five o'clock (note that time spans are to show the approximate time of the meal or snack, not duration):

Breakfast:	7:00–8:00 A.M.
Snack:	10:00–10:30 A.M.
Lunch:	12:00–1:00 P.M.
Snack:	3:00–4:00 P.M.
Dinner:	6:00–7:00 P.M.
Snack:	8:00–9:00 P.M. (optional)

Eating at regular intervals sounds simple, yet many people don't make this a priority—they're too busy running from meeting to meeting, working through their lunch hour or racing out the door to pick up their children. I can't tell you how often I hear people complain that they don't even have time to eat breakfast before they rush off to work.

Once you get into a consistent pattern of eating, you'll feel much better. And if you choose the right foods at your meals and snacks, chances are you'll forget you're vulnerable to hypoglycemic reactions. So now that you have your eating schedule down pat, the next step is choosing foods with longer-lasting energy.

Carbohydrates: Low glycemic index (GI)

You're already familiar with the fact that carbohydrate-containing foods (e.g., starches, fruit, milk, sugars) eventually wind up as glucose in your bloodstream. So it makes sense that you can prevent hypoglycemia by eating carbohydrates. But not all carbohydrates behave the same way when it comes to raising your blood sugar. Some carbohydrate-rich foods are digested and absorbed into your bloodstream quickly while others are broken down and converted to blood glucose slowly.

Why does this make a difference if you have hypoglycemia? Let's say you eat two slices of white toast for breakfast. White bread (and whole-wheat bread) is digested relatively quickly, causing your blood sugar to rise quickly. This rapid rise in blood glucose triggers your pancreas to release an excessive amount of insulin, causing your blood-glucose level to drop to a very low level. (Insulin is the hormone that clears sugar from your bloodstream, sending it to your cells, where it's needed for energy.) On the other hand, a bowl of high-fibre breakfast cereal with low-fat milk is digested and absorbed more slowly, causing a gradual rise in blood sugar.

Because this meal doesn't result in a quick and sizeable spike in blood sugar, you don't get a surge of insulin. As a result, your blood-sugar level won't plummet quickly after eating. Instead, you'll experience a smooth, steady blood-sugar level leading to more consistent energy levels.

The rate at which a food causes your blood sugar to rise can be measured and assigned a value. This measurement is referred to as the food's glycemic-index value. The glycemic index (GI) is a ranking from 0 to 100. The number tells you whether a food raises your blood glucose rapidly, moderately or slowly. Foods that are digested quickly and cause your blood sugar to rise rapidly have high glycemic-index values. Foods that are digested slowly, leading to a gradual rise in blood sugar, are assigned low glycemic-index values. All foods are compared to pure glucose, which is given a value of 100 (fast acting).

Now let's use the glycemic index to manage your hypoglycemia. The key is to choose carbohydrate foods that do *not* cause large increases in blood sugar.

Keep in mind the following:

- Unprocessed fresh foods such as whole grains, legumes, fruit and vegetables have a low GI value. High-GI foods are usually highly processed and may have a concentrated amount of sugar.
- Include at least one low-GI food per meal, or base two of your meals on low-GI choices. Use the list of foods below to help you choose low-GI foods.
- Pay attention to breads and breakfast cereals, since these foods contribute the most to the high-glycemic load of our North American diet.
- Avoid eating high-GI snacks like pretzels, corn chips and rice cakes, as these can trigger hunger and overeating. Opt for fresh fruit, low-fat dairy products, nuts or plain popcorn.
- Choose fruit that is more acidic (e.g., oranges, grapefruit, cherries) as these have a low GI and will lower the glycemic load of a meal.
- Use salad dressings made from vinegar or lemon juice—the acidity will further reduce the GI of your meal.

Below is a list of foods ranked by their GI value, from lowest to highest. Use this table to plan your meals and snacks. Here's what the numbers mean:

Less than 55	Low GI
55–70	Medium GI
Greater than 70	High GI

Selected Foods Ranked by Their GI Value

Bread & Crackers

Pumpernickel bread, whole grain	46
Sourdough rye bread	53
Cracked wheat	53
Linseed Rye bread, Rudolph's	55
Pita bread, white	57
Whole-meal rye bread	58
Rye crispbreads	64
Rye bread	65
Stoned Wheat Thins crackers	67
Breton crackers (original wheat)	67
Light rye, Silverstein's Bakery	68
Whole-wheat bread	69
Melba toast	70
White bread	70
Water crackers	71
Bagel, white	72
Kaiser roll	73
Wonder (enriched white bread)	73
Soda crackers	74
Rice cakes	82
Baguette, French	95

Breakfast Cereals

All-Bran Original, Kellogg's	42
All-Bran Buds cereal with Psyllium, Kellogg's	47

Red River Hot Cereal	49
Oat bran	50
Porridge made from steel-cut oats	52
Special K, Kellogg's	54
Porridge made from rolled oats, large flake	62
Cream of Wheat	66
Oatmeal, instant	66
Grape-Nuts, Post	71
Raisin Bran, Kellogg's	73
Bran flakes	74
Cheerios, General Mills	74
Cream of Wheat Instant	74
Corn Bran, Quaker	75
Shredded Wheat, Nestlé	75
Weetabix	75
Corn Flakes, Kellogg's	81
Crispix, Kellogg's	87

Cakes, Cookies & Muffins

Sponge cake	46
Banana bread	47
Oatmeal cookies	55
Blueberry muffin	59
Digestive biscuits	59
Oat bran muffin	60
Arrowroot cookies	65
Angel food cake	67
Oatmeal muffins, made from mix	69
Graham crackers	74

Grains, Pasta & Potatoes

Barley	25

Fettuccine, egg	32
Spaghetti, whole-wheat	37
Spaghetti, white	41
Rice, white, converted, Uncle Ben's	45
Bulgur	46
Corn, sweet	53
Sweet potato, mashed	54
Rice, brown	55
Rice, long-grain, white	56
Rice, basmati	58
Potato, new, unpeeled, boiled	62
Couscous	65
Millet	71
Rice, short-grain	72
Potato, french fries	75
Potato, white-skinned, baked	85
Potato, instant, mashed	86
Rice, instant	87
Potato, red-skinned, boiled	88
Potato, red-skinned, mashed	91
Legumes & Nuts	
Peanuts	14
Soybeans	18
Kidney beans	27
Lentils	30
Black beans	31
Lentil soup, canned	34
Chickpeas, canned	42
Baked beans	48
Black bean soup	64
Split pea soup	66

Fruit & Unsweetened juices

Cherries	22
Grapefruit	25
Peach	28
Apricot, dried	31
Apple	34
Pear	38
Tomato juice	38
Apple juice	40
Orange	42
Grapes	43
Orange juice	46
Mango	51
Banana	52
Kiwi fruit	53
Banana	55
Pineapple	59
Raisins	64
Cantaloupe	65
Watermelon	72
Dates, dried	103

Milk products & Milk alternatives

Yogurt, low-fat, aspartame	14
Milk, whole	27
Milk, skim	32
Yogurt, low-fat, sugar	33
Soy beverage, full-fat	33
Milk, chocolate	34
Ice cream, premium	39
Soy beverage, low-fat	44
Ice cream, regular	61

Tofu-based frozen dessert	115
Snack foods & Sugary drinks	
Potato chips	54
Popcorn	55
Cola	58
PowerBar, chocolate	58
Corn chips	72
Gatorade	78
Pretzels	83
Sugars	
Fructose (fruit sugar)	23
Lactose (milk sugar)	46
Honey	58
Sucrose (table sugar)	65
Glucose	100

Source: Foster-Powell, K, et al. International tables of glycemic index and glycemic load values: 2002. *American Journal of Clinical Nutrition* 2002; 76(1):5–56.

Soluble fibre

Many of the foods with a low glycemic-index value tend to be higher in a special kind of fibre, called soluble fibre. Dried peas, beans and lentils, oats, barley, psyllium husks, apples and citrus fruit are all good sources of soluble fibre and, as you can see from the GI table, these foods also have a low GI. When you eat these foods, the soluble fibre forms a gel in your stomach and slows the rate of digestion and absorption. That means your blood sugar will rise at a slower rate and your pancreas won't produce excessive amounts of insulin.

If you don't feel like using the GI table to choose foods, you might just plan your meals around foods rich in soluble fibre:

- Cereals: Kellogg's All-Bran Buds with Psyllium, Nature's Path SmartBran, oatmeal, oat bran
- Grains: barley
- Legumes: all (baked beans, bean soups, black beans, chickpeas, kidney beans, lentils, soybeans, etc.)

- Fruit: apples, cantaloupe, grapefruit, oranges, pears, strawberries
- Vegetables: carrots, green peas, sweet potato

Protein foods

Choosing foods based on their soluble-fibre content is a great way to lower the glycemic-index value of your meal. But there are a couple of other tricks that slow down digestion and influence the rate at which your blood sugar rises. Adding protein to your meals slows the rate at which your stomach empties its contents into the small intestine. As a result, the carbohydrate in your meal will enter your bloodstream at a slower rate.

Choose lean protein foods such as lean beef, chicken breast, turkey, pork tenderloin, centre-cut pork chops, fish, seafood and eggs. If you're a vegetarian, be sure to include vegetarian protein foods at your meals—tofu, beans, veggie ground round, tempeh, etc.

You don't need to add a lot of protein-rich foods to your meals. The daily protein requirements are as follows for women:

Recommended Dietary Allowance (RDA) of Protein

No regular exercise; sedentary	0.8 grams per kg body weight
Regular exercise; cardio 4 to 7 days/week	1.2 grams per kg body weight
Heavy exercise; cardio and weights most days	1.2–1.7 grams per kg body weight

To calculate your actual protein requirements for the day, multiply your weight (in kilograms) by your RDA for protein. For example, a 135 pound (61 kg) woman who doesn't exercise needs 49 grams of protein each day (61 kg × 0.8). If that same woman was exercising three or four times a week, she would need to eat 73 grams of protein (61 kg × 1.2).

Protein Content of Selected Foods

Food	Protein (grams)
Meat, 3 oz (90 g)	21–25 g
Poultry, 3 oz (90 g)	21 g
Salmon, 3 oz (90 g)	25 g
Sole, 3 oz (90 g)	17 g
Tuna, canned and drained, 1/2 cup (125 ml)	30 g

Food	Protein (grams)
Egg, 1 whole	6 g
Legumes, 1/2 cup (125 ml)	8 g
Milk, 1 cup (250 ml)	8 g
Yogurt, 3/4 cup (175 ml)	8 g
Cheese, cheddar, 1 oz (30 g)	10 g
Vegetables, 1/2 cup (125 ml)	2 g
Bread, 1 slice	2 g
Rice, pasta, cooked, 1/2 cup (125 ml)	2 g

Source: Data adapted from the *Canadian Nutrient File*, Health Canada (2006). Available at: http://webprod.hc-sc.gc.ca/cnf-fce/index-eng.jsp.

To help manage your blood sugar, distribute your protein throughout your day. If you need to eat 60 grams of protein each day, aim for 20 grams at each meal. As for snacks, make sure you choose low-GI foods. And don't forget that milk and yogurt have protein as well—so they're good low-GI snack choices!

One more interesting tidbit: If you enjoy a green salad with your meal, continue doing so. Just make sure you toss it with a vinaigrette dressing. Studies have found that vinegars, especially red wine vinegar, also slow the rate at which food leaves your stomach.

Caffeine and alcohol

Caffeine is known to cause a low blood-sugar reaction, especially if it has been a few hours since you ate. Researchers from the Yale School of Medicine found that consuming 400 milligrams of caffeine triggered hypoglycemia when blood-sugar levels were in the low–normal range, as might occur two to three hours after a meal.[1] If you're hypoglycemic, chances are you already know if you're sensitive to caffeine. If you are, make the switch to low-caffeine or caffeine-free beverages. One 6 ounce cup of coffee provides 110 to 175 milligrams of caffeine. Compare that to the same amount of black or green tea at 25 to 35 milligrams. It makes a difference!

Replace coffee with decaf coffee, cereal-based beverages (e.g., Ovaltine), herbal tea, weakly brewed black tea or green teas. If you don't want to part with your daily cup of coffee, make sure to drink it with a meal. That way the caffeine will be less likely to trigger a low blood-sugar reaction. Between meals, stick to vegetable juice, water, milk, herbal tea or decaf lattes.

Drinking alcoholic beverages can also impair blood-sugar control and trigger a hypoglycemic reaction in susceptible individuals. It can induce reactive hypoglycemia by interfering with glucose uptake and promoting the release of insulin from your pancreas. The drop in blood sugar that follows leads to a craving for foods, especially sweets. If you reach for sugary foods in response to this low blood sugar, you'll only aggravate your symptoms.

If you have hypoglycemia, avoid drinking alcohol on an empty stomach. Instead, enjoy your drink with a meal. The presence of food in your stomach will delay the absorption of alcohol. If you do drink alcohol, limit yourself to seven drinks per week for health protection.

VITAMINS AND MINERALS
Chromium
Supplements of this trace mineral have been promoted to manage hypoglycemia; unfortunately, research studies are few and far between. One small study was conducted in the late 1980s with 8 women who had hypoglycemia.[2] Those who took 200 micrograms of chromium for three months experienced a significantly reduced rate of low blood-sugar symptoms and had higher blood-glucose levels two to four hours after eating. Another small study conducted among 20 patients with hypoglycemia found similar results using 125 micrograms of the mineral.[3]

But this is all we have to go on. A greater number of studies have investigated the use of chromium in individuals with type 2 diabetes—and you'll read about this mineral's potential role in insulin resistance and high blood sugar in Chapter 20, Polycystic Ovary Syndrome (PCOS). Despite the lack of scientific support for the use of chromium in hypoglycemia, it's important to make sure you get enough of this mineral in your daily diet.

It appears that chromium does play an important role when it comes to regulating blood glucose. Your body needs chromium to make glucose-tolerance factor (GTF), a compound that interacts with insulin and helps maintain normal blood-sugar levels. With adequate amounts of chromium present, your body uses less insulin to do its job.

The recommended intake for chromium is 25 and 35 micrograms per day for women and men, respectively. Chromium-rich foods include apples with the skin, green peas, chicken breast, refried beans, mushrooms, oysters, wheat germ and brewer's yeast. Processed foods and refined (white) starchy foods like white bread, instant rice, white pasta, sugar and sweets contain very little chromium.

If you're concerned that you're not getting enough of this mineral through your diet, check your multivitamin and mineral supplement to see how much it contains. If it's less than 50 micrograms, consider taking a separate 100 or 200 microgram supplement each day. Studies show that chromium picolinate and chromium nicotinate are absorbed more easily than other forms (such as chromium chloride). The safe upper limit is 400 micrograms per day.

Keep in mind, though, the most important thing you can do to prevent hypoglycemia is to eat at regular intervals and choose carbohydrate foods high in soluble fibre. If you're not doing this, don't expect chromium to help manage your condition.

LIFESTYLE FACTORS
Regular exercise
When it comes to preventing hypoglycemia, I can't neglect to mention the importance of a program of regular, moderate exercise. Exercise improves many aspects of blood-sugar control. Working out enhances the body's sensitivity to insulin, improves glucose uptake by your cells and increases the concentration of chromium in your tissues. (If you have type 1 diabetes, however, it's critical to know how to manage insulin dosage and food intake to prevent an exercise-induced low blood-sugar reaction.)

You don't need to exercise vigorously to reap benefits. In fact, working out too intensely may bring on hypoglycemia. If you exercise with someone, you should be able to carry on a conversation (though you should be a little breathless). If you work out at a gym, consult with a certified personal trainer to help you find your target heart-rate zone. Staying within this range while you exercise will prevent you from overdoing it. Good activities include brisk walking, jogging, stair climbing, swimming, rowing and cycling. Aim to exercise four times per week, with each session at least 30 minutes long. If you're not exercising this much, gradually work up to it.

Plan your snacks around your exercise session. If you eat lunch at noon and exercise at 3 P.M., you'll want a snack about 30 minutes before you begin. At 2:30 P.M., eat an apple, some yogurt or a sports energy bar. Depending on what time you eat dinner, you'll likely need to eat another small snack around 4:30 P.M., after your workout session.

THE BOTTOM LINE...
Leslie's recommendations for managing hypoglycemia

1. Eat every three hours to prevent your blood-sugar level from plummeting. If you tend to get so involved in what you're doing that you forget to eat, set a timer on your computer or watch.
2. At meals and snacks, choose carbohydrate foods with a low glycemic-index value.
3. Include a source of protein foods at your meals, since this nutrient helps to slow down digestion.
4. Enjoy a tossed salad with a vinaigrette dressing at lunch and dinner. Studies have shown that vinegar slows the rate at which food leaves your stomach.
5. As much as possible, avoid caffeinated beverages and alcohol, especially on an empty stomach.
6. Boost your intake of chromium-rich foods such as unpeeled apples, green peas, chicken breast, refried beans, mushrooms, oysters, wheat germ and brewer's yeast. Intakes of 125 to 200 micrograms per day might help reduce symptoms of hypoglycemia. If your multivitamin and mineral supplement contains less than 50 micrograms of chromium, consider adding a 200 microgram supplement to your daily nutrition regime.
7. Exercise at a moderate pace four times a week for at least 30 minutes in duration.

6

Insomnia

Do you wake up after a full night's sleep feeling tired and listless? Do you have difficulty falling asleep despite how tired you feel? Or perhaps you can't seem to stay asleep, tossing and turning throughout the night. If any of these symptoms ring true for you, you may very well be suffering from insomnia.

Sleep is a basic human need. When we sleep, our minds and bodies rest and restore vital energy. Adults need between seven and eight hours of restful sleep each night to maintain good health and to feel mentally alert during the day, and children and teenagers need nine to ten hours each night. A lack of sleep can result in decreased productivity, increased motor vehicle and job-related accidents and higher rates of mental and physical illness.

Insomnia affects up to one-third of all Canadians and is one of the most common sleep complaints among Canadians. Women tend to experience insomnia more frequently than men because of our biological factors such as menstruation, pregnancy and menopause.

There are a variety of ways to treat insomnia, but the best results come from lifestyle management techniques that improve your ability to relax and manage stress.

What causes insomnia?

Insomnia, the inability to sleep, is a term that refers to a number of different sleep disruptions and disturbances, including:

- difficulty falling asleep
- waking up early in the morning and being unable to return to sleep
- waking up frequently during the night or having difficulty staying asleep
- waking up after a full night's sleep and not feeling rested

Every once in a while, we all toss and turn through a sleepless night. This is known as short-term or *transient insomnia*, and is rarely a cause for concern. Only when your sleep habits are disturbed regularly for more than three weeks are you considered to be suffering from *chronic insomnia*. Insomnia usually results from a combination of factors and is often a symptom of some other physical or mental condition that's affecting you.

Insomnia is often associated with psychiatric disturbances and is especially common in people with depression and anxiety disorders. Alzheimer's disease and other forms of dementia can also disturb sleep and cause repeated nighttime awakening. People suffering from arthritis, kidney or thyroid disease, asthma, restless leg syndrome, sleep apnea and gastrointestinal disorders will frequently experience pain and discomfort severe enough to interfere with normal sleep patterns. As well, medications used to treat these and other health conditions may trigger insomnia as an unwanted side effect.

Our sleep patterns change as we age. Research indicates that sleep efficiency decreases from a high of 95 percent in adolescence to less than 80 percent in old age. Consequently, older people have more difficulty falling asleep or staying asleep, and often find that sleep is not as refreshing as it used to be. But there are also many lifestyle and environmental factors that can lead to chronic insomnia, such as:

- drinking excessive amounts of alcohol or taking recreational drugs
- drinking coffee or caffeinated beverages before bedtime
- smoking cigarettes before bedtime
- taking long naps in the daytime or evening
- engaging in shift work that disrupts your day/night (or wake/sleep) cycle or in ongoing work travel that results in jet lag
- experiencing chronic tension or stress, or worrying excessively
- sleeping in a noisy environment
- sleeping in a room that's too warm or too cold

These factors are often responsible for the development of sleep problems and they may also prolong the symptoms of existing insomnia. Simple adjustments in sleep habits and lifestyle can go a long way towards helping you get a good night's sleep.

Insomnia is much more common in women than it is in men. In general, women tend to sleep fewer hours and to experience a poorer quality of sleep, especially as they get older. Fluctuating hormone levels are the primary culprits. As the levels of estrogen and progesterone hormones change in response to menstrual cycles, pregnancy and menopause, women are more likely to suffer ongoing sleep disturbances that rob them of energy, health and mental agility.

1. **Menstruation.** Poor-quality sleep is often associated with the beginning of the menstrual cycle, when bleeding starts. Some women feel particularly sleepy and fatigued right after ovulation, when progesterone levels rise. As the menstrual cycle continues, progesterone levels begin to fall rapidly, signalling the start of menstruation. This is a time when many women are quite wakeful and find it difficult to fall asleep at night.

2. **Premenstrual syndrome (PMS).** During the latter part of the menstrual cycle, some women struggle with the debilitating symptoms of PMS. In addition to bloating, moodiness, abdominal cramps and irritability, women with PMS may find it hard to get to sleep or to stay asleep, or they may sleep excessively. Insomnia and the associated daytime tiredness are common symptoms of PMS.

3. **Pregnancy.** The physical and emotional demands of pregnancy often lead women to report more disturbed sleep. Rising levels of progesterone in the first trimester are known to increase sleepiness. In the early stages of pregnancy, sleep patterns may also be disrupted by the need to urinate frequently. In the second trimester, sleep quality tends to improve but is still worse than before pregnancy. Most pregnancy-related sleep problems develop during the third trimester, when the fetus puts pressure on the bladder, increasing the need to go to the bathroom during the night. Heartburn, sinus congestion and leg cramps are also common in the later stages of pregnancy and can cause enough physical discomfort to disturb sleep. Once the baby is born, a mother's sleep is interrupted often, and the resulting sleep deprivation may trigger emotional problems such as a mild depression known as *postpartum blues*.

4. **Menopause.** As a woman ages, her levels of estrogen and progesterone begin to drop, and eventually she stops menstruating. This transition to actual menopause (cessation of menstruation) is the time when

women report the highest levels of sleep disruptions. In many cases, insomnia is brought on by night sweats, which are hot flashes that occur during sleep. Women in menopause often experience daytime tiredness and chronic fatigue.

Who's at risk?

It's estimated that 3.3 million—1 in 10—Canadians suffer from insomnia.[1] Although anyone can experience insomnia, it seems that women experience it more frequently than men and are more willing to seek treatment. Insomnia is also common among the elderly. Studies have indicated that people coping with stressful situations, such as divorce or unemployment, or who have medical or emotional conditions are much more prone to insomnia. Those who have sleep disturbances that persist for more than twelve months are also more likely to develop depression, anxiety disorders and alcohol dependency.

Diagnosis

Insomnia can be difficult to diagnose. The need for sleep varies from individual to individual. Some people require much less sleep than others to function effectively. This makes it challenging to develop sleep standards and norms for effective diagnosis. Generally, you'll be diagnosed with insomnia if your sleep disturbances are severe enough to noticeably affect your daytime mood and activities. Determining the frequency, intensity and duration of your sleep disruptions is also helpful in making an accurate diagnosis.

Because insomnia is so often a symptom of another disorder, the Canadian Medical Association recommends that the real emotional, physical or environmental causes of insomnia be diagnosed and treated before any other steps are taken to treat insomnia complaints. To do this, your doctor will evaluate your sleep patterns, your drug use (including alcohol, nicotine and caffeine), your psychological and physical condition and your level of physical activity. In some cases, you may be sent to a sleep clinic for further testing.

Conventional treatment

Naturally, the treatment of insomnia depends on the underlying cause of the condition. Making simple lifestyle changes is often the best way to treat insomnia. Some recommendations for improving your sleep habits include the following:

- **Exercise.** Regular, moderate-intensity exercise is known to improve sleep quality. Take a brisk walk, do some gardening or join an exercise class. You'll find it much easier to fall asleep naturally if you add some activity to your day. Just avoid exercise in the late evening before bedtime because it may overstimulate your body.
- **Change your diet.** Avoid big meals late at night and limit your use of alcohol and tobacco. Foods that are high in sugar or high in caffeine, such as coffee, tea and caffeinated beverages, should also be restricted. Some people find that their sleep improves if they avoid eating spicy or high-fat foods in the evening. Limiting fluid intake may also reduce your need to go to the bathroom during the night, allowing you a more restful sleep. You'll read much more about these and other nutritional approaches below.
- **Control your weight.** If obstructive sleep apnea is the cause of your sleep disturbances, losing excess weight can help you get a good night's sleep. Obstructive sleep apnea—the most common form of sleep apnea—occurs when the upper airway gets completely or partially blocked during sleep and breathing momentarily stops. These breathing pauses, or apneas, can last up to 30 seconds and can happen many times throughout the night. The brain senses this breathing difficulty and briefly rouses you from sleep to reopen your airway. Symptoms of sleep apnea include excessive daytime sleepiness, loud snoring, memory loss and difficulty staying asleep.

  Fat deposits around the upper airway can obstruct breathing during sleep. Losing 10 percent of your body weight can greatly reduce the number of sleep apnea episodes each night.
- **Control your sleep environment.** Keep your bedroom dark and quiet, and make sure it isn't too warm or cold. Use your bedroom mainly as a place to sleep; don't use it for watching television, eating, exercising, working or doing other activities associated with wakefulness.

- **Establish a regular bedtime routine.** Go to bed at the same time each night. Even more important, you should try to get up at the same time in the morning, both during the week and on the weekends. Following a regular routine of brushing your teeth, washing your face and setting your alarm—even when you're away from home—will help you to set the mood for sleep in the evening. Avoid daytime naps that might interfere with your nighttime sleep schedule.
- **Relax.** Stress and worry play an important role in triggering symptoms of insomnia. Relax at bedtime by taking a warm bath, enjoying a cup of herbal tea or reading until you feel sleepy. And try to avoid worrying about daytime problems. Some people find that alternative therapies, such as biofeedback, muscle relaxation, behavioural therapy or psychotherapy help them to achieve a more restful sleep.

If your insomnia can't be managed using these basic techniques, your doctor may recommend medications to help you sleep. These drugs are called hypnotics, but you may hear them referred to as sedatives, barbiturates or tranquilizers. All hypnotics present a risk of overdose, addiction, tolerance and withdrawal symptoms. For this reason, your doctor will prescribe the lowest dose possible. You should use hypnotic drugs only a few times a week and only for a short time (two to four weeks) to avoid future problems.

If you're using hypnotic drugs and suddenly stop taking them, you may experience a condition known as *rebound insomnia*. This insomnia is temporary but it can create a vicious cycle of drug use and insomnia symptoms if not properly managed. Hypnotic drugs should be discontinued gradually to avoid this problem.

Managing insomnia

DIETARY STRATEGIES

Caffeine

This may sound simple, but eat and drink less caffeine-containing foods and you'll sleep better. Caffeine stimulates the central nervous system and increases the metabolic rate. Researchers have found that older adults suffering from insomnia report higher caffeine intakes. Studies have reported increased sleep problems in people consuming 240 to

400 milligrams of caffeine versus abstainers.[2-7] Although one or two cups of coffee in the morning can boost your mental alertness, drinking more can overstimulate your body and cause insomnia. Studies have shown that less caffeine (one or two small cups of coffee) consumed in the morning can affect the quality of sleep that same night.[8,9] Caffeine blocks the action of adenosine, a natural sleep-inducing brain chemical.

Health Canada's safe daily upper limit for caffeine is 450 milligrams, but this recommendation is based on studies that have investigated the effect of caffeine on blood pressure and other health conditions, not your ability to sleep soundly. If you have insomnia, aim for no more than 200 milligrams of caffeine a day, and preferably none. (One 8 ounce/250 ml cup of coffee has 80 to 175 milligrams of caffeine; the same serving size of tea has 45 milligrams.) See Chapter 1, page 11, for a detailed list of caffeine-containing beverages and foods. Avoid caffeine in the afternoon. Replace caffeinated beverages with caffeine-free or decaffeinated beverages such as herbal tea, mineral water, fruit and vegetable juice or decaf coffee.

Alcohol

The effects of alcohol are detrimental to sleep. Alcohol worsens insomnia and can rob you of a good night's sleep even if you don't have a sleep disorder. Once absorbed into the bloodstream, alcohol is metabolized at a set rate by your liver. If you drink more alcohol than your liver can keep up with (i.e., more than one drink an hour), alcohol arrives in your brain, where it interferes with brain chemicals called neurotransmitters. Alcohol has been shown to impair REM (rapid eye movement) sleep, the portion of sleep associated with dreaming and thought to be important for memory.

Alcohol also dehydrates you, which can make you feel fatigued the next day. It does so by depressing the brain's ability to produce a hormone called antidiuretic hormone. This causes your body to lose water through your kidneys. Water enables your body to generate energy; to digest, absorb and transport nutrients; and to regulate your body temperature. So when you're dehydrated after an evening of drinking alcohol (or even after a few drinks), your cells and tissues receive nutrients less efficiently and your body can't properly regulate its temperature. Both lead to fatigue.

A review of sixty studies suggests that up to two to three standard drinks consumed before bedtime initially promotes sleep, but that these effects diminish in as few as three continuous days of such alcohol consumption. The vast majority of studies support a relationship between sleep disturbances and alcohol use.[10]

When it comes to reducing your risk for cancer, women should consume no more than seven drinks per week. But if you're suffering from insomnia, I recommend that you eliminate alcohol from your diet altogether. Instead of having a glass of wine, pour yourself a glass of sparkling mineral water with a slice of lime. Or try some of the non-alcoholic wines or beers available in the supermarket. If you're looking for a cocktail, order a virgin Caesar, a tomato juice or a glass of cranberry and soda.

To lessen alcohol's effect on your ability to sleep, drink alcohol with a meal or snack. If you drink alcohol on an empty stomach, about 20 percent is absorbed directly across the walls of your stomach and reaches the brain within a minute. But when the stomach is full of food, alcohol has a lesser chance of touching the walls and passing through, so the effect on your brain is delayed.

If you're out socially or you're entertaining at home, don't drink more than one alcoholic beverage per hour. Since the liver can't metabolize alcohol any faster than this, drinking slowly will ensure your blood-alcohol concentration doesn't rise. To slow your pace, alternate one alcoholic drink with a non-alcoholic drink or a glass of water. One drink is equivalent to 5 ounces (145 ml) of wine, 12 ounces (340 ml) of beer or 1-1/2 ounces (45 ml) of liquor.

Carbohydrate before bed

If you've ever heard that a glass of warm milk can help you sleep, you might give it a try—there's some science to back this claim. A carbohydrate-rich snack like milk, a small bowl of cereal or a slice of toast provides the brain with an amino acid called tryptophan. The brain uses tryptophan as a building block to manufacture a neurotransmitter called *serotonin*. Serotonin has been shown to facilitate sleep, improve mood, diminish pain and even reduce appetite.

To see if eating a little bit of carbohydrate helps you fall asleep, eat something *small* or drink a glass of low-fat milk or soy beverage. Try it for a week. If your insomnia hasn't improved, look at other factors that may be disrupting sleep.

VITAMINS AND MINERALS
Vitamin B12

Many studies have found that vitamin B12 promotes sleep in people who suffer from sleep disorders. In a randomized double-blind study, Japanese researchers determined that a daily dose of 1.5 to 3 milligrams of the vitamin restored normal sleep patterns in such patients.[11] German researchers have also found that sleep quality, concentration and "feeling refreshed" were significantly correlated with the blood level of vitamin B12 in healthy men and women.[12]

Researchers believe that B12 helps you sleep by working with melatonin, a natural hormone in the body. Melatonin is involved in maintaining the body's internal clock, which regulates the secretion of various hormones. In so doing, melatonin helps control sleep and wakefulness. Secretion of this hormone is stimulated by darkness and suppressed by light. Vitamin B12 appears to directly influence the action of melatonin and the vitamin may prevent disturbances in melatonin release.

Women need 2.4 micrograms of B12 each day. Vitamin B12 is found exclusively in animal foods: Meat, poultry, eggs, fish and dairy products are all good sources. Fortified soy and rice beverages also contain vitamin B12. You'll find a list of foods and their B12 content in Chapter 1, page 33.

If you fall into one of the following categories, I recommend you supplement your diet with vitamin B12:

- If you're 50 years of age or older. Up to one-third of older adults don't produce enough stomach acid to properly absorb vitamin B12 from their diet. Therefore, it's recommended that you take a daily multivitamin supplement or consume foods fortified with the vitamin.
- If you're taking antacid medication for reflux or a stomach ulcer. Any medicine that blocks your body's ability to produce stomach acid will impair your ability to absorb B12 from food (this doesn't include foods fortified with B12).
- If you're a strict vegetarian who eats no animal foods and you don't drink at least 2 servings of a fortified soy or rice beverage each day or take a multivitamin supplement.

You can get additional B12 from a multivitamin and mineral, a B complex formula or single supplements of the vitamin (these come in 500 or 1000 microgram doses). For sleep disorders due to a deficiency of vitamin B12 (have your doctor measure your B12 stores), a dose of 500 to 1000 micrograms three times daily can be used.

Vitamin B12 is considered safe and non-toxic, even in large amounts. However, there have been rare reports of B12 supplements causing diarrhea, itching, swelling, hives and, rarely, anaphylactic reactions. If you're taking high doses of vitamin B12, or any supplement, be sure to inform your health care practitioner.

HERBAL REMEDIES
Valerian *(Valeriana officinalis)*
This native North American plant acts like a mild sedative on the central nervous system. Studies show that valerian root makes getting to sleep easier and increases deep sleep. Unlike conventional sleeping pills, the herb doesn't lead to dependence or addiction. Valerian promotes sleep by interacting with certain brain receptors called GABA receptors and benzo-diazepine receptors. Compared to drugs like Valium and Xanax, valerian binds very weakly to these receptors.

In one double-blind study from Germany, 44 percent of those taking valerian root reported perfect sleep and 89 percent reported improved sleep compared to those taking the placebo pill.[13] Another small study found that individuals with mild insomnia who took 450 milligrams of valerian experienced a significant decrease in sleep problems.[14] The same researchers studied 128 individuals and found that compared to the placebo, 400 milligrams of valerian produced a significant improvement in sleep quality in people who considered themselves poor sleepers.[15]

Scientists attribute the herb's effectiveness to essential oils in the root. To make sure you're getting a sufficient amount of the active ingredient, buy a product that's been standardized to contain at least 0.5 percent essential oils or 0.8 percent *valerenic acid.* Take 400 to 900 milligrams in capsule or tablet form, two hours before bedtime. If you wake up feeling groggy, reduce the dose. Don't expect results overnight. The herb works better when it's used over a period of time; it may take four weeks to notice an improvement in sleep.

Valerian is not recommended for use during pregnancy or breast-feeding, since it hasn't been studied in these conditions. Long-term use may result in sleeping-pill-like withdrawal symptoms when the herb is discontinued.

THE BOTTOM LINE...
Leslie's recommendations for managing insomnia

1. Cut back your caffeine intake to a maximum of 200 milligrams per day. If you've done this and you're still having trouble sleeping, eliminate caffeine completely for two weeks, and see if your sleep and/or your energy level during the day improve.
2. If you drink alcohol and you don't want to give it up (which I do recommend if you're experiencing sleep problems), aim for no more than seven drinks a week or one drink a day. To lessen alcohol's effect on your brain, have your drink with a meal or snack.
3. Try a light carbohydrate-rich snack 30 minutes before bed to increase the level of sleep-promoting serotonin in your brain.
4. Make sure you get enough vitamin B12 in your diet. If you can't get enough B12 through food, or if you don't produce enough stomach acid for its absorption, take a daily B12 supplement of 500 micrograms.
5. Consider taking 400 to 900 milligrams of valerian root extract. Buy a product that is standardized to contain at least 0.5 percent essential oils or 0.8 percent valerenic acid. Take the herb 1 to 2 hours before going to bed.
6. Consider other possible causes of sleep disturbances: a lack of exercise, too much stress or a possible medical problem. If you've tried everything you can and you still have fitful sleep, consult your family physician.

7
Migraine headaches

Migraine is one of the most common and misunderstood of all diseases. It has disabling effects on millions of people, yet it's very often misdiagnosed and has no definitive cure. Women are two to three times more likely to suffer from migraines than men—a factor that may be related to the hormonal changes that occur during the menstrual cycle.

A migraine is a type of headache that results from inflammation of the blood vessels and nerves surrounding the brain. The exact causes of migraine headaches are not known, but they seem to be set off by changes in brain activity. Very often, specific substances, actions or stimuli in your body or environment may trigger migraines.

Although the symptoms, frequency and intensity of migraines vary widely, they are often acutely painful and incapacitating. Over 80 percent of migraine sufferers cope with some degree of headache-related disability. Treatment of migraines usually involves a two-pronged approach: Therapies focus on providing relief of symptoms and preventing or reducing future headache attacks.

What causes a migraine?

Migraine headaches are caused by a combination of vasodilation (enlargement of the blood vessels) and the release of chemicals from nerves that wrap around the blood vessels. During a migraine, the temporal artery, which lies outside the skull just under the skin of the temple, enlarges. This triggers the surrounding nerves to release chemicals that cause inflammation, pain and further enlargement of the artery, which intensifies the pain. Migraine headaches also stimulate your sympathetic nervous system, and that can induce nausea, vomiting, diarrhea and delayed stomach emptying.

Symptoms

The pain of migraine headaches is usually felt on one side of the head, but it can change sides from one attack to the next. About one-third of migraines are bilateral, with pain felt on both sides of the head. The pain is typically aggravated by daily activities such as walking up stairs. It's common for migraine headaches to be accompanied by nausea, vomiting, diarrhea, facial pallor, cold hands, cold feet and sensitivity to light and sound.

Warning symptoms, which can last hours or days, precede up to 60 percent of migraine attacks. Such symptoms may include fatigue, irritability, depression or food cravings. About 20 percent of migraines are associated with an aura, which is a set of neurological symptoms that occurs approximately 10 to 30 minutes before the headache starts. During the aura phase, you may experience visual disturbances, such as flashing lights or geometric patterns in front of your eyes, or you may even suffer a brief vision loss. It's not uncommon to feel dizzy and confused or to have some facial tingling and muscle weakness as the aura progresses.

Most migraines don't conform to a typical pattern. Some people suffer a migraine only once in a while; others are incapacitated by attacks as often as three times a week. The intensity of pain can vary from reasonably mild to completely debilitating. Migraines also vary in length, from a brief 15-minute episode to an attack that can last a week. On average, the duration of a migraine ranges between four and seventy-two hours. For up to twenty-four hours after an attack, migraine sufferers may feel drained of energy and may continue to be sensitive to light and sound.

Who's at risk?

Migraine is a universal condition that affects approximately 6 percent of men and 15 percent to 18 percent of women.[1] As many as 50 percent to 70 percent of all migraine sufferers have a family history of the disease, indicating that these headaches may be hereditary. However, a specific migraine gene has not yet been found.

Diagnosis

Because of the wide variation in symptoms, migraines are quite difficult to diagnose. Migraine generally begins in childhood to early adulthood. Although migraines can start after age 50, advancing age makes other types of headaches more likely. For this reason, migraine headaches in older adults can often be confused with tension, sinus or other kinds of headaches. It's reasonable to assume you suffer from migraines if your headaches have some of the following characteristics:

- a sequence of at least five attacks that last between two and seventy-two hours
- pain that is located on one side of your head, sometimes spreading to both sides
- pain that is pulsating or throbbing
- pain that prohibits or limits daily activity
- pain that is aggravated by physical activity
- nausea or vomiting during headache attacks
- sensitivity to light, noise or smell during headache attacks

If you have very severe headaches, or if there's a significant change in the nature of the headache or the presence of other symptoms such as vision or hearing loss, your doctor may order additional medical tests such as blood testing or brain scanning (CT or MRI).

Migraine triggers

In some cases, certain stimuli or triggers that you experience as part of your normal life can provoke migraines. By avoiding these triggers, you may be able to reduce the frequency or severity of your attacks. Although triggers don't actually cause a migraine, they do seem to influence the activities in your brain that stimulate the disease. Often, you'll be sensitive to the combined effect of more than one trigger.

There are many common migraine triggers and you must determine which ones affect you. Keeping a migraine headache diary is a good way to identify the circumstances that set off your migraines. Keep in mind, however, that triggers don't always lead to a headache and avoidance of triggers doesn't always prevent a headache from occurring.

- **Diet.** Certain foods and food additives are well-known migraine triggers. Alcoholic beverages (especially red wine), foods treated with MSG (monosodium glutamate), foods that contain tyramine (e.g., aged cheeses, soy sauce) or aspartame (NutraSweet) and foods preserved with nitrates and nitrites all may provoke migraines. Chocolate, caffeine, citrus fruit and dairy products are other known culprits.
- **Lifestyle.** Changes in your behaviour or your surroundings can encourage migraines. If you alter your eating or sleeping habits, experience high levels of stress or smoke cigarettes, you may find yourself struggling with more frequent migraines.
- **Environment.** Some people find that bright lights or loud noises bring on a migraine. Weather or temperature changes and physical exertion are common triggers, and even changing time zones may affect your headache frequency. Strong odours, perfume, high altitudes and computer screens are other recognized triggers.
- **Female hormones.** Women may be more susceptible to migraines because of the estrogen cycles associated with menstruation. Migraines become more prevalent in females after puberty, reaching a peak at age 40, and then declining in frequency as women age. But almost two-thirds of women who suffer from migraines will experience a worsening of their headaches during their period. Up to 15 percent of women get migraines only during their period—what is called *true menstrual migraine*. Menstrual migraines are typically without aura and last longer than other migraines. They are also more difficult to treat. To prevent these debilitating headaches, it's extremely important for women to avoid migraine triggers during the premenstrual week (you'll find a list of dietary triggers later in the chapter).
- **Oral contraceptives and estrogen therapy.** These seem to make migraines worse. If you take these medications and suffer from migraines, you may want to speak to your doctor about being on a low-dose estrogen regimen.
- **Pregnancy.** Migraines are more common in early pregnancy but usually improve by the second trimester. In a small group of women, *pregnancy migraines* will worsen throughout the trimesters. During pregnancy, women should pay special attention to avoiding dietary and environmental triggers, sticking to regular sleeping and eating schedules, getting regular exercise and managing stress (as should all women with migraines).

Conventional treatment

When a migraine strikes, the light, noise and pain may be overwhelming when you are around other people. Most migraine sufferers retreat to a quiet, dark room and try to sleep through it. The disabling effects of migraines often result in work loss and may seriously curtail social and family activities.

When migraines begin to have a negative impact on your life, your doctor may prescribe drug therapy. People respond to a variety of different medications and you may have to experiment to find the one that works best for you.

MIGRAINE RELIEF MEDICATIONS

These medications target the pain of an attack and should be taken as soon as you sense that a headache is beginning. General analgesics (painkillers) and NSAIDs (non-steroidal anti-inflammatory drugs) are frequently used to relieve the discomfort of mild and moderate migraine attacks. One of the most effective drugs is sumatriptan (Imitrex), a drug that specifically targets the receptors for serotonin. It acts quickly to reduce pain and is effective for over 70 percent of migraine sufferers. Some combination medications may also be useful in cases where other drug therapies are not effective. Because migraines are usually accompanied by extreme nausea, your treatment plan may include an anti-nausea drug to relieve these symptoms.

Among other side effects, both analgesics and NSAIDs are known to cause stomach problems that may eventually lead to internal bleeding and ulcers. Overuse of these drugs may also cause you to experience rebound headaches. Rebound headaches are not migraines but are medication induced and may quickly become chronic.

Severe migraine attacks that result in incapacitating pain may be treated with opiates, which are very powerful painkillers. However, they are also highly addictive and are usually prescribed only in extreme cases.

MIGRAINE PREVENTION THERAPIES

As with migraine relief medications, these drugs work with varying success. A "good" response is defined as a 50 percent reduction in the severity and frequency of migraine attacks. The main types of prevention medications are:

- **Beta blockers.** These have a 60 percent success rate. They stabilize serotonin levels and reduce the dilation of blood vessels.
- **Ergot drugs.** Usually as effective as beta blockers, these also affect serotonin levels and blood vessel dilation.
- **Calcium channel blockers.** These are thought to modulate neurotransmitters. The effects are gradual and the success rate is lower than with beta blockers.
- **Antidepressants.** The positive effect on serotonin levels makes these effective, but they may have serious interactions with other medications.

All of the migraine prevention medications produce side effects that may have negative consequences for your overall health. Most of these drugs are contraindicated during pregnancy. When you're experimenting with preventive therapies, you should try only one drug at a time, so that you and your physician can carefully monitor the positive and negative effects. Dosage should begin at a low level and move upwards only as needed.

ALTERNATIVE TREATMENTS
There's a growing body of evidence to indicate that alternative therapies have a positive effect on the symptoms and frequency of migraine attacks. Resting in a quiet, dark room and applying ice or pressure often helps to relieve pain. Avoiding triggers through diet and lifestyle changes is also very beneficial in preventing the onset of migraines. Other therapies that have shown some success in alleviating migraines are:

- relaxation therapy
- biofeedback
- acupuncture
- stress-management training
- psychotherapy
- hypnosis
- physiotherapy, osteopathy and chiropractic

Managing migraines

DIETARY STRATEGIES

Food triggers

A number of foods and beverages have been reported to trigger a migraine attack.[2-7] One study found that when people who suffer migraines eliminate these foods from their diet, about one-third experience fewer headaches and up to 10 percent become headache-free.[8] The following are the most common foods to trigger a migraine, or make one worse:

- cheese, especially aged cheese
- chocolate
- coffee, tea
- eggs
- fish
- garlic
- hot dogs
- milk
- wine, especially red

The following foods and food additives have also been reported to bring on a headache:

- alcoholic beverages
- artificial sweeteners
- citrus fruit
- corn
- foods with MSG
- foods with nitrites/nitrates (processed meats, smoked fish, some imported cheeses, beets, celery, collards, eggplant, lettuce, radishes, spinach, turnip greens)
- lima beans
- nuts
- overripe bananas
- peanuts, peanut butter
- soybeans
- shellfish
- tomato

Some migraine sufferers have actual food allergies. It's thought that certain immune compounds formed in response to an offending food can trigger a migraine headache. If you find that certain foods are triggering migraines, it might be worthwhile to have your doctor refer you to an allergy specialist for food testing.

Whether a food allergy or some other food response is responsible for your migraines, consult a registered dietitian who specializes in food sensitivities (www.dietitians.ca). He or she can plan an elimination and challenge diet for you, a very useful tool to identify food triggers. You can also do this on your own. Begin by keeping a food and headache diary. List all foods, beverages, medications and dietary supplements taken. Note the date of your menstrual period, since hormones may precipitate a migraine too. You should keep this diary for at least two weeks, or long enough to cover at least three migraine attacks. Once you've completed this exercise, look for patterns. Did you eat the same food before each migraine? Did your migraines hit you after a night of drinking wine?

Once you've identified possible culprits, eliminate them from your diet for a period of four weeks, or longer if you experience migraines less frequently. If you're migraine free during this period, it's very likely that you've found your triggers. The next step is to confirm if all, or only some, of the foods are the actual culprits. One by one test each food by adding it to your diet. Wait three days before testing the next food on your list. Keep in mind that this process may not give you clear-cut results. A combination of events may be required to bring on a migraine. For instance, you may get a migraine only when you eat the food at a specific time in your menstrual cycle. Or the combination of stress or weather and a food trigger may be required to cause a migraine.

VITAMINS AND MINERALS
Vitamin B2 (riboflavin)

To prevent a migraine headache from coming on, you might want to reach for more riboflavin. Riboflavin facilitates the release of energy from all body cells. Studies reveal that migraine sufferers have less efficient energy metabolism in their brain cells, so it's thought that by increasing your riboflavin intake and, therefore, the potential of your brain cells to generate energy, you might keep migraines at bay. Looks like this strategy might work. Well-controlled studies have found that a daily 400 milligram supplement of riboflavin was effective at reducing the frequency of headache attacks. One study demonstrated 400 milligrams of riboflavin to be as effective as certain drugs used to treat migraines.[9,10] Although most clinical studies have given patients a 400 milligram dose, one trial found that 25 milligrams of riboflavin taken daily for three months significantly reduced the number of migraines and migraine days and the level of migraine pain.[11]

You don't need much riboflavin to prevent a deficiency. The recommended daily intake for women is 1.1 milligrams per day. During pregnancy and breastfeeding you need 1.4 and 1.6 milligrams, respectively. Riboflavin is found in many foods, including milk, meat, eggs, nuts, enriched flour and green vegetables. If you take a multivitamin or B complex supplement, you're getting even more riboflavin, as much as 100 milligrams.

If you're striving to get 400 milligrams each day in the hopes of preventing a migraine, you'll need to buy a separate supplement of this B vitamin. B2 supplements are available in 25, 50, 100, 500 and 1200 milligram doses. Chances are, you won't find this supplement at a drugstore. You'll have to visit your local health food or supplement store. It may take up to three months to notice an improvement in your headache frequency. Riboflavin supplements are non-toxic and very well tolerated.

Magnesium

Researchers have established an important link between magnesium levels in the body and migraine attacks. Evidence shows that during a migraine headache up to 50 percent of sufferers have low magnesium levels in their brain and red blood cells. It's thought that a deficiency of magnesium in the brain can cause nerve cells to be overly excited, triggering a migraine attack. (A few medications, including estrogen, estrogen-containing birth control pills and certain diuretics, can deplete magnesium stores.)

If you increase the amount of magnesium in your tissues and red blood cells, can you prevent a migraine? According to some studies, the answer is yes. In one study, German researchers gave 81 migraine sufferers either 600 milligrams of magnesium or a placebo pill once daily for three months. In the second month of the study, the frequency of migraine attacks was reduced to 42 percent in the magnesium group, compared to only 16 percent in the placebo group. What's more, the duration of a migraine and drug use significantly decreased among those people who took magnesium supplements.[12] Another study conducted in children and teenagers found that taking a daily magnesium supplement didn't prevent migraine, but led to a significant reduction in headache days.[13]

Magnesium is the second most abundant mineral in the body (after calcium). It plays a crucial role in over three hundred cellular reactions. Among its many roles, magnesium helps cells generate energy, moves important compounds in and out of cells and transmits impulses from nerve to nerve. To help prevent a low magnesium level and resulting migraine, first make sure you're getting enough from your daily diet. Women aged 19 to 29 need 310 milligrams of magnesium daily; older women require 320 milligrams.

The best sources of magnesium are whole foods including unrefined grains, nuts, seeds, legumes, dried fruit and green vegetables. See Chapter 1, page 24, for a list of selected foods and their magnesium content.

Magnesium supplements

If you're going to try to ward off your migraines by boosting your intake of magnesium, you'll need to take a supplement. The randomized controlled trial I discuss above used 600 milligrams per day. Buy a magnesium citrate supplement: Compared to other forms of the mineral (e.g., magnesium oxide), magnesium citrate is more readily absorbed by the body. Split your dose over the course of the day. Depending on what dose you can find in your health food or supplement store, take a 300 milligram supplement twice daily or 200 milligrams three times a day. You may be able to get your extra magnesium from calcium supplements if you buy a 1:1 formula—that means each tablet gives you an equal amount of calcium and magnesium.

The daily upper limit for magnesium from a supplement has been set at 350 milligrams because doses higher than this can cause diarrhea and stomach upset, common side effects of magnesium supplementation. Taking 600 milligrams in divided doses may help ease intestinal upset.

HERBAL REMEDIES

Feverfew *(Tanacetum parthenium)*

Scientific evidence tells us that, when used properly, the leaves of this herb can significantly reduce the frequency and severity of migraine headaches. The link between feverfew and migraine become popular in England back in the 1970s, when a doctor's wife noticed that her migraines were much improved once she started chewing fresh feverfew leaves. As the story goes, after one year of faithfully taking the leaves, she almost forgot she ever suffered from migraines.

Since then, this herbal remedy has been the focus of a number of studies in people with migraines. Of these trials, one hailing from Nottingham, England, was a randomized controlled trial (the gold standard among researchers). In this study, 76 people who experienced migraines were given either whole feverfew leaf or a placebo for four months, and then the treatments were reversed for another four-month period. The results were impressive. Without knowing what treatment they received, 59 percent of the people taking feverfew identified the treatment during the feverfew period as more effective, compared to 24 percent who chose the placebo period. The herbal remedy reduced the number of classic migraines (with aura) by 32 percent and common migraines (without aura) by 21 percent.[14]

The herbal remedy has also been shown to reduce symptoms of migraine, including pain, nausea, vomiting and sensitivity to light and noise. It's thought to be more effective in people who suffer more frequent migraine attacks. Researchers believe that feverfew reduces the frequency and intensity of migraines by preventing the release of substances called prostaglandins, which dilate blood vessels and cause inflammation. It was once thought that an active ingredient in the herb called parthenolide was responsible for feverfew's beneficial effect. But when researchers made a special alcohol extract that contained the same amount of parthenolide as an effective dose of feverfew leaf, there was no effect on migraine headaches. It seems that other compounds in the leaf of the plant are responsible for feverfew's effect on migraines.

To prevent a migraine, the recommended dose of feverfew is 50 to 100 milligrams daily of powdered feverfew leaf. We know that whole feverfew leaf is effective, so don't buy an alcohol extract made up of parthenolide. Instead, buy capsules of powdered feverfew leaf. You can also try taking the herb at the onset of a migraine to ease the symptoms.

Feverfew is deemed to be very safe, as it rarely causes side effects other than mild gastrointestinal upset. The herb may cause an allergic reaction in people sensitive to plants in the Asteracease/Compositae family (ragweed, daisy, marigold and chrysanthemum). Like many other herbs, the safety of feverfew has not been studied in pregnant or nursing women, or in those with liver or kidney disease.

THE BOTTOM LINE...
Leslie's recommendations for managing migraines

1. Identify possible food triggers. If you're not sure which component of your diet might be a culprit, try an elimination and challenge diet. You might also consider getting tested for food allergies.
2. To prevent a migraine, boost your intake of riboflavin (vitamin B2). Take a 400 milligram supplement each day.
3. Consider supplementing with magnesium to avoid a migraine attack. Research indicates that 600 milligrams of the mineral in supplement form may prevent headaches. Buy magnesium citrate supplements and take 600 milligrams per day in divided doses.
4. If you're looking for an herbal remedy to prevent and lessen the severity of your migraines, reach for feverfew. Take 50 to 100 milligrams of dry powdered leaf once daily. Feverfew may cause allergic reactions in people sensitive to ragweed, daisies, marigolds and/or chrysanthemums.

8

Lupus

Lupus is the name of a group of chronic autoimmune diseases that targets mainly women during their childbearing years, causing inflammation in many different body systems. An autoimmune disease develops when the body begins to harm its own healthy cells and tissues.

The most common and serious type of lupus is *systemic lupus erythematosus (SLE)*. It has been identified as a systemic disease because it can target any tissue in the body, including the skin, muscles, blood, joints, lungs, heart, kidneys or brain. SLE affects each woman differently and symptoms vary depending on which tissues and body organs become inflamed. The disease is chronic and is characterized by recurring periods of illness, called flares, which alternate with periods of wellness or remission.

Other types of lupus include:

- **Discoid lupus erythematosus (DLE)**, which primarily affects the skin, causing a red, scaly rash on your face, scalp, ears, arms and/or chest. Extreme sun sensitivity is a common symptom of this disease.
- **Subacute cutaneous lupus erythematosus (SCLE)**, which causes rashes and sun sensitivity. However, the rashes develop only on the arms and upper body, and the disease rarely affects other organs.
- **Drug-induced lupus erythematosus**, which is very similar to SLE. The symptoms usually disappear when the medication is discontinued.
- **Neonatal lupus**, which affects infants born to women with immune disorders such as SLE.

What causes lupus?

Normally, your immune system protects your body from germs, viruses and bacteria by producing antibodies to fight these dangerous invaders. With lupus, the immune system malfunctions and begins to produce antibodies that attack its own body parts. This causes inflammation and tissue damage that result in a wide variety of disabling symptoms that affect the joints, skin, kidneys, heart, lungs, blood vessels and brain. Some scientists believe that with lupus the immune system is more easily stimulated by external factors like viruses or ultraviolet light. Sometimes, symptoms of lupus can be precipitated or aggravated by only a brief period of sun exposure.

Current research indicates that lupus doesn't have a single cause but, rather, is triggered by a combination of genetic, environmental and hormonal factors. High levels of estrogen may accelerate the progress of the disease. Lupus also seems to run in families, which may indicate a hereditary basis for the illness.

Recent evidence from studies conducted in mice suggests that the inability of a key enzyme, called DNase1, to dispose of dying cells may contribute to the development of SLE. DNase1 normally eliminates "garbage DNA" by chopping it into tiny fragments for elimination from the body. It's thought that a genetic mutation in a gene that could disrupt the body's cellular waste disposal may be involved in the onset of lupus.

Symptoms

Lupus affects each woman in a different way, with symptoms ranging from fairly mild to severe, disabling or even fatal. Generally, lupus develops slowly, with symptoms appearing over a period of weeks, months or years. Initially, the disease is quite active and symptoms steadily increase in severity, often requiring medical attention and treatment. This phase is known as a flare. After a flare, lupus will frequently move into a chronic phase, in which symptoms are less severe, though they don't disappear entirely. Women with lupus may also experience periods of remission, when the disease is inactive and symptoms subside.

The following symptoms may be early warning signs of SLE:

* fatigue—often extreme and overwhelming
* weight changes—an unexpected weight loss of more than 5 pounds (2.3 kg) may signal SLE activity; a sudden weight gain may be caused by swelling associated with SLE damage to heart and kidney tissue
* fever
* swollen glands—a sudden, unexplained swelling of the lymph glands might be an immune system response triggered by SLE
* joint pain, stiffness and swelling

There are also a number of specific symptoms that indicate the presence of lupus. Although the list of lupus symptoms below is extensive, it's rare for anyone to experience more than a few of these complications.

* **Photosensitivity.** At least 50 percent of people with lupus develop an abnormal skin reaction to sunlight, causing a rash on exposed skin.
* **Butterfly rash (malar rash).** A red rash appears on the cheeks and over the nose of nearly 50 percent of all people with SLE.
* **Mucosal ulcers.** Small sores often appear on the mucous lining of the mouth or nose.
* **Arthritis.** Almost all women with SLE eventually develop arthritis. The arthritis associated with lupus doesn't usually cause crippling or deformities in the joints.
* **Pleuritis or pericarditis.** Inflammation of the lining around the lungs (pleuritis) or inflammation of the lining around the heart (pericarditis) affects nearly half of all people with SLE, causing chest pain and painful breathing.
* **Kidney damage.** Lupus can cause serious kidney damage; in fact, one of the leading causes of death among people with lupus is kidney failure.
* **Seizures.** SLE-caused damage to the central nervous system can produce problems such as epileptic seizures, delusions, hallucinations and behavioural changes.
* **Blood cell disorders.** The immune system may produce antibodies that will attack the red blood cells, causing a type of anemia. It can also reduce the number of white blood cells and may interfere with blood clotting.

- **Discoid rash**. This is a raised, red, scaly rash that appears on the chest, arms, face, scalp or ears of approximately one-quarter of people with lupus. The rash will worsen if exposed to sunlight.

Who's at risk?

Lupus mainly strikes women between the ages of 15 and 45. Systemic lupus erythematosus (SLE) is eight to ten times more common in women than men.[1] Women who have a relative with some type of autoimmune disease are also at greater risk of developing lupus. Lupus is more common in blacks and Asians than in Caucasians. Long-term use of certain prescription drugs may also trigger a form of lupus called drug-induced lupus erythematosus in a small percentage of people.

Diagnosis

Because women with SLE can have a wide variety of symptoms and different combinations of organ involvement, there's no single test used to diagnose lupus. A person with four or more of the following eleven criteria is likely to have SLE:

- "butterfly" rash over the cheeks of the face
- discoid skin rash (patchy redness that can cause scarring)
- photosensitivity (skin rash in reaction to sunlight exposure)
- spontaneous ulcers of the lining of the mouth, nose or throat
- two or more swollen, tender joints of the extremities
- pleuritis or pericarditis (inflammation of the lining tissue surrounding the lungs or heart, usually associated with chest pain when breathing or changing body position)
- abnormal amounts of urine protein or clumps of cellular elements called casts
- brain irritation manifested by seizures and/or psychosis
- low counts of white or red blood cells, or platelets, on routine blood testing
- abnormal immune blood tests
- anti-nuclear antibodies in the blood (positive ANA antibody test)

Sometimes, SLE may be diagnosed in women who exhibit only a few of these criteria. Among those women, some may later develop other signs and symptoms, but many never do.

Doctors may use other tests to determine the severity of organ involvement in SLE. These include blood tests to detect inflammation, analysis of body fluids and tissue biopsies.

Conventional treatment

The treatment for lupus varies from person to person, depending on the severity of the disease and the type of symptoms involved. Because there's no cure, the goal of treatment is to bring the disease under control so that patients can lead a relatively normal life. Women with a mild case of lupus may not require any medical treatment. If the disease is more advanced, a variety of treatment options is available.

The most important factor in managing lupus is avoiding circumstances that trigger flares, such as excessive fatigue and high levels of stress. Following a healthy diet, quitting smoking and engaging in regular exercise can help keep the disease under control. As well, it's important that you learn to recognize the warning signs of a flare, such as increased fatigue, pain, rash, stomach upset, headache and dizziness.

In some cases, medications are used to manage the symptoms of lupus; one of the primary drugs is a corticosteroid called prednisone. Because corticosteroids act rapidly to suppress inflammation in your tissues, they're usually prescribed when symptoms are severe or life threatening. Corticosteroids are potent drugs with serious side effects such as high blood pressure, osteoporosis, weight gain, acne and stomach ulcers.

Non-steroidal anti-inflammatory drugs (NSAIDs) are helpful in decreasing the inflammation that causes joint pain, fever and swelling. The arthritis pain often associated with SLE can usually be controlled with a mild pain-relief medication such as acetaminophen. Some people also find that their lupus symptoms respond well to antimalarial drugs, which suppress some of the immune responses that cause joint pain, fatigue, skin rashes and lung inflammation. If the nervous system or kidneys are affected, immunosuppressive drugs may be prescribed to restrain an overactive immune system.

Managing lupus

Once medication brings lupus under control, a number of lifestyle changes can minimize the possibility of future flares. Whereas a poor diet, excessive use of alcohol and smoking can contribute to lupus flares, regular exercise can help prevent them, as well as reduce pain and help you manage stress.

DIETARY STRATEGIES

It's important to eat a healthy, low-saturated-fat diet that provides plenty of fibre and fresh fruit and vegetables. These foods contain protective vitamins, minerals and antioxidants that can keep you healthy. The following dietary guidelines should be followed:

- **Emphasize plant foods** in your daily diet. Fill your plate with grains, fruit and vegetables. If you eat animal-protein foods like meat or poultry, choose lean sources and make sure they take up no more than one-quarter of your plate. Eat vegetarian sources of protein, like beans and soy, more often.
- **Eat fish twice per week.** Oily fish such as salmon, trout, Arctic char, sardines and herring are rich in omega-3 fatty acids, which may help reduce the inflammation of lupus. (See Fish Oil Supplements below.)
- **Choose foods and oils rich in essential fatty acids.** Nuts, seeds, flaxseed and flaxseed oil, canola oil, omega-3 eggs, wheat germ and leafy green vegetables are good choices.
- **Choose foods rich in vitamins, minerals and protective plant compounds.** Choose whole grains as often as possible. Eat 7 to 10 servings of fruit and vegetables every day. Select a variety of different-coloured fruit and vegetables in your daily diet to increase your intake of phytochemicals, many of which have anti-inflammatory properties.
- **Eliminate sources of refined sugar** as often as possible: that means cookies, cakes, pastries, frozen desserts, soft drinks, sweetened fruit juices, fruit drinks and candy.
- **Buy organic produce or wash fruit and vegetables** to remove pesticide residues.
- **Limit foods that contain chemical additives.**

- **Limit or avoid caffeine** (caffeine can worsen fatigue by interrupting sleep patterns).
- **Drink at least 9 cups (2.2 L) of water every day.**
- **Avoid alcohol.** If you drink, consume no more than one drink per day, or seven per week.

Alfalfa

Alfalfa seeds contain an amino acid called L-canavanine that has been shown to provoke lupus in animals.[2-5] There have also been reports that alfalfa can worsen symptoms or cause a flare in women with lupus. Avoid eating alfalfa sprouts and don't use any herbal supplements that contain alfalfa.

Flaxseed

The seed of the flax grain contains plant estrogens called lignans and the essential fatty acid alpha-linolenic acid. Research indicates that flaxseed may inhibit the action of platelet-activating factor, a substance involved in SLE kidney disease. Two small studies found that women with lupus who consumed 30 grams of ground flaxseed each day experienced improved kidney function, less inflammation and reduced blood-cholesterol levels.[6,7] Add 1 to 2 tablespoons (15 to 30 ml) of ground flaxseed to yogurt, breakfast smoothies, applesauce, hot cereal and baked goods.

VITAMINS AND MINERALS
Vitamin C

There's some evidence that higher intake of vitamin C from the diet may reduce the risk of a lupus flare. In a study of 279 women with SLE, those who consumed the most vitamin C from foods were significantly less likely to have active lupus.[8]

The recommended daily intake of vitamin C is 75 milligrams for women and 90 milligrams for men. If you smoke, you need an additional 35 milligrams each day. The best food sources of vitamin C include citrus fruit, kiwi, mango, strawberries, cantaloupe, Brussels sprouts, cabbage, cauliflower, bell peppers and tomato juice. Include at least two vitamin C–rich foods in your daily diet.

Vitamin D

Numerous studies have reported insufficient blood levels of vitamin D in women with lupus. Research has also revealed that the severity of SLE appears to be linked with low levels of vitamin D.[9-11] These findings suggest that vitamin D deficiency may be a risk factor for SLE and the nutrient could play a role in the prevention and/or treatment of the disease. Among its many roles, vitamin D helps regulate the immune system and, in doing so, may help suppress autoimmune conditions such as lupus. An adequate intake of vitamin D may also help reduce the risk of osteoporosis, for which people with lupus have an increased risk.

It's recommended that Canadian adults take 1000 international units (IU) of vitamin D each day in the fall and winter, and year-round if you're over 50, if you have dark-coloured skin, if you don't expose your skin to sunlight in the summer months or go outdoors often, or if you wear clothing that covers most of your skin. (Exposure to sunlight—without the use of sunscreen—triggers the synthesis of vitamin D in the skin.) People with lupus should take 1000 IU of vitamin D throughout the year, regardless of age, since too much sun exposure can trigger flares. If a blood test has determined you have insufficient vitamin D in your blood, you may be advised to take a higher dose. See Chapter 1, page 13, for more information on vitamin D supplementation.

Vitamin E

Some experts believe that free radical damage may play a role in the development of lupus. Studies have shown that lupus is associated with an increased level of oxidized blood fats and lower levels of circulating vitamin E.[12,13] Treatment with corticosteroid medication can further increase free radical injury. Preliminary animal research has found that supplemental vitamin E can slow the progress of lupus.[14] A small preliminary study conducted in women with SLE found that 150 to 300 IU of vitamin E taken together with prednisone suppressed the formation of lupus autoantibodies.[15] (Autoantibodies are immune compounds that mistakenly target and damage specific tissues or organs of the body.)

The recommended dietary allowance for vitamin E is 22 IU. The best food sources include wheat germ, nuts, seeds, vegetable oils, whole grains and kale. To supplement, take 200 to 400 IU of natural source vitamin E. The daily upper limit is 1500 IU. If you have heart disease or diabetes, don't take high-dose vitamin E supplements.

Calcium

Women with SLE have a higher risk of low bone mass and osteoporosis, which are thought to be related to the duration of lupus.[16,17] Corticosteroid drugs used to treat lupus also cause bone loss and are associated with the development of low bone density. To protect your bones, make sure you meet your daily requirements for this essential nutrient.

The recommended dietary allowance is 1000 to 1500 milligrams. Best food sources are milk, yogurt, cheese, fortified soy beverages, fortified orange juice, tofu, salmon (with bones), kale, bok choy, broccoli and Swiss chard. If you take calcium supplements, be sure to take them in divided doses during the day; don't take more than 500 or 600 milligrams of calcium at one time. See Chapter 1, page 16, for more information about calcium supplements.

OTHER NATURAL HEALTH PRODUCTS

DHEA (dehydroepiandrosterone)

The hormone DHEA is produced by the two triangular-shaped adrenal glands, which sit above the kidneys. The secreted DHEA is a building block in the making of estrogen and testosterone. DHEA supplementation seems to change circulating levels of estrogen and progesterone. In women, DHEA increases blood levels of male sex hormones called androgens without increasing blood levels of estrogens. The effects of DHEA on circulating hormone levels may be responsible for its health benefits.

A number of studies have found DHEA supplements, in conjunction with conventional medication, reduce SLE disease activity, the frequency of flares and the dose of corticosteroid medication needed to manage the disease. DHEA may also help SLE symptoms such as muscle ache and oral ulcers. The supplement has also been shown to increase bone mineral density in women being treated with high-dose corticosteroids.[18-25]

DHEA supplements consist of a hormone manufactured from compounds found in soybeans. It's sold as a dietary supplement in the United States but isn't allowed for sale in Canada.

The recommended dose for lupus is 200 milligrams per day as an adjunct to conventional medication. DHEA is considered safe when taken for the short term. However, at doses of 200 milligrams per day, DHEA frequently causes adverse effects such as acne and hirsutism (excessive hair growth on the face or body) in women.

Fish oil supplements

Researchers have found that fish oils have anti-inflammatory effects in women with lupus. Studies have found that women with lupus who take fish oil supplements experience symptom improvement, longer periods of remission and a lowering of blood-triglyceride levels.[26-31] Some researchers even suggest that fish oil may reduce free radical damage and help regulate the body's production of antioxidant enzymes.[32]

Fish oil capsules are a concentrated source of two omega-3 fatty acids, DHA (docosahexanaenoic acid) and EPA (eicosapentanoic acid). These fats inhibit the body's production of inflammatory compounds called leukotrienes.

The typical dosage used in lupus studies is 3 grams of fish oil per day. Buy a fish oil supplement that provides both EPA and DHA. Do not buy fish *liver* oil supplements, which are usually concentrated sources of vitamin A. (A prolonged intake of excess supplemental vitamin A can harm your bones.) Fish oil supplements can cause belching and a fishy taste; taking an enteric-coated product can help prevent these side effects. Because fish oil has a blood-thinning effect, use caution if you're taking blood-thinning medication such as aspirin, warfarin (Coumadin) or heparin.

THE BOTTOM LINE...
Leslie's recommendations for managing lupus

1. Adopt a diet that's low in saturated fat and contains plenty of nutrient- and antioxidant-rich fruit and vegetables. Include oily fish in your diet twice per week to get anti-inflammatory omega-3 fatty acids. Avoid alfalfa sprouts, as they may trigger lupus symptoms.
2. Add 1 to 2 tablespoons (15 to 30 ml) of ground flaxseed to your daily diet.
3. Include at least two vitamin C–rich foods in your daily diet, such as cantaloupe, citrus fruit, kiwi, mango, strawberries, bell peppers, Brussels sprouts, cabbage, cauliflower and tomato juice.
4. To help regulate your immune system, supplement with 1000 international units (IU) of vitamin D each day, year-round.
5. To help combat the harmful effects of free radicals, increase your intake of vitamin E–rich foods such as wheat germ, nuts, seeds,

vegetable oils, whole grains and kale. To supplement, take 200 to 400 IU of natural source vitamin E.

6. Ensure you're meeting your daily calcium requirements of 1000 or 1500 milligrams, depending on your age. Add calcium-rich foods like dairy, soy beverages and leafy greens to your diet. If your diet falls short of the mineral, take a calcium supplement once or twice daily.

7. To help reduce inflammation, consider supplementing your diet with 3 grams of fish oil per day.

PART 3

BREAST, BONE AND HEART HEALTH

9
Breast cancer

Breast cancer is the most common type of cancer among Canadian women, affecting 22,400 women in 2009. One in nine women will develop breast cancer in her lifetime. This lifetime risk represents the average risk for the population of Canadian women.[1] If you have certain risk factors for breast cancer, like a family history or a poor diet, this number underestimates your risk. If you have no risk factors at all for the disease, this lifetime risk overestimates your chances of getting breast cancer.

Sadly, 102 Canadian women die from breast cancer every week.[2] But the good news is that the death rate from breast cancer has decreased since the mid-1990s. This is largely because more and more women are having mammograms, allowing for earlier detection and treatment.

What causes breast cancer?

Simply put, cancer is a disease in which abnormal cells grow out of control. When enough of these cells accumulate, a tumour forms. Finally, if the cancer cells are able to break away from the tumour, they can circulate through the body and take up residence in another organ, a process called metastasis.

Every cell has a genetic blueprint, called DNA (deoxyribonucleic acid). The DNA of cells contains genes that program cell reproduction, growth and repair, affecting all body processes. Sometimes genes can become damaged and this damage can result in cancer. There are three ways in which your genes can become faulty:

1. A mutation can occur during normal cell division, such that the newly formed cell contains an abnormal gene. This can happen randomly or if the cell is exposed to some other agent.

2. Cells can be exposed to an environmental agent, a carcinogen that harms the DNA. For instance, cigarette smoke is a carcinogen that causes lung cancer.

3. Flawed genes can be inherited from your parents, though the incidence of this is rare.

Cancer is not explained by genetics alone. Experts agree that cancer is the result of an interaction between genes and environmental factors. For instance, you might have a mutated gene that predisposes you to breast cancer, but because you eat a low-fat diet with plenty of fruit and vegetables, the cancer may never express itself.

The breast is composed of fatty tissue and milk glands called lobes and lobules. Lobes and lobules empty into ducts, small passageways that carry milk to the nipple. Breast cancer begins with a single cell, usually in the lobule or duct, that runs amok. These are two areas where cells are rapidly dividing during the normal menstrual cycle. Estrogen and progesterone stimulate the breast cells to begin dividing each month, preparing the body for pregnancy. If conception doesn't occur, breast cell receptors receive a message to stop cell division. The process begins again the following month, and each month until menopause. With cell division regularly occurring for such a span of years, there's a greater chance for a genetic mutation to occur. Although most breast cancers aren't detected until after menopause, it's believed that they actually begin to develop in the premenopausal years.

Very few cancers—and only 5 percent to 10 percent of breast cancers—are the result of inherited genes. Families that have genetic defects in one of two genes—breast cancer gene 1 (BRCA1) or breast cancer gene 2 (BRCA2) have a much greater risk of developing both breast and ovarian cancer.

Who's at risk?

The clearest risk factors for breast cancer are associated with hormonal and reproductive factors. It's thought that estrogen promotes the growth and development of mutated breast cells. It seems that the longer your breast tissue is exposed to your body's circulating estrogen, the greater the risk for breast cancer. Some risk factors, such as age and family history, you can't change; others, including weight and diet, are within your control. The following risk factors make a woman more susceptible to breast cancer. Keep in mind, however, that just because you have one or more risk factors doesn't mean you'll get the disease.

- **Age.** Breast cancer is more common in women over 50 years of age. More than 75 percent of breast cancers occur in post-menopausal women. Increasing age also makes it more likely that other risk factors discussed below will occur. When two or more risk factors are combined, your risk is greater than with the one risk factor alone.
- **Previous breast cancer.** A history of breast cancer increases the odds that a woman will get breast cancer again, in the same or in the opposite breast.
- **Family history of breast cancer.** If you have a first-degree relative (a mother, sister or daughter) with breast or ovarian cancer, you have a greater chance of also developing breast cancer. In general, the more relatives you have who were diagnosed with breast cancer before menopause, the higher your own risk. If you have one first-degree relative who developed breast cancer before the age of 50, your own risk is doubled.
- **Age of first pregnancy.** Women who have children before 30 years of age have a lower risk of breast cancer. Women who have their first child after 30 have a higher risk, and women who never have children are at an even greater risk. Many experts believe that the important factor here is the amount of time between menarche (the age when you began menstruating) and first pregnancy. The theory is that the developing breast tissue is most sensitive to carcinogens during this time. Pregnancy hormones mature the breast cells and make them more resistant to carcinogens. It may be that these same pregnancy hormones stimulate mutated breast cells in a woman who has her first baby after 30 years of age.
- **Genetic predisposition.** Defects in one of several genes, especially BRCA1 or BRCA2 genes, increase your risk of developing breast (and ovarian) cancer. Normally, these genes inhibit cancer development by making proteins that keep cells from growing out of control. Mutated genes are less effective at protecting from cancer.
- **Age of first period (menarche).** Onset of your period before 12 years of age is associated with a slightly higher risk of breast cancer. It's believed that the longer breast tissue is exposed to endogenous

estrogen (estrogen that's made in your body), the greater the chance for cells to become cancerous.

- **Late menopause.** Women who menstruate for longer than forty years have a slightly higher risk of breast cancer. Like early menarche, late menopause influences the amount of time breast cells are exposed to estrogen.
- **Exposure to radiation.** Ionizing radiation from X-rays taken at a younger age may increase the risk for breast cancer later in life. However, experts feel exposure to radiation is probably a minor contributor to your overall risk.
- **Use of hormones.** Short-term use of hormone replacement therapy (HRT) for menopausal symptoms is considered safe. But taking the hormone combination of estrogen and progesterone for more than four years increases the risk of breast cancer. HRT also makes breast tumours harder to detect on a mammogram, leading to a cancer that's more advanced and harder to treat. Estrogen-alone hormone therapy hasn't been shown to increase the risk of breast cancer in post-menopausal women.
- **Diet.** A growing body of research is finding a link between certain diet factors and the risk of breast cancer. Diet affects breast cancer development either by initiating cancer growth and causing a genetic mutation, or by promoting the growth of cancerous cells.
- **Alcoholic beverages.** Women who drink more than one alcoholic beverage per day have a greater risk of breast cancer than women who don't drink. Even consuming one drink per day is thought to slightly increase risk.
- **Excess weight.** Carrying extra body weight increases the risk of breast cancer, especially if that weight was gained during adolescence. The risk is even greater if weight gain occurs after menopause. Carrying excess weight around the abdominal area (i.e., apple shape) also increases the risk.

Diagnosis

Beginning at age 20, all Canadian women should be performing monthly breast self-exams to detect physical changes in their breasts. Use the pads of your fingers to examine the tissue in your breasts and in your armpits.

Be sure to also look carefully at your breast for any noticeable physical changes, such as a lump in the breast or underarm area, unusual breast swelling, change in colour or texture of skin on the breast, blood leakage from the nipple or inversion of the nipple. Any of these changes should prompt a visit to your family doctor.

Women aged 40 to 49 should have a clinical breast examination by a trained health care professional every two years. If you have a higher-than-average risk for breast cancer, you will likely be screened more often and earlier (before age 40).

It's recommended that all Canadian women between the ages of 50 and 69 years have a mammogram every two years in addition to a clinical breast exam. A mammogram is a special X-ray of the breast that can catch breast cancer early and lead to a significant improvement in the chance of survival. Mammograms show detailed images and views of the breast taken from different angles.

Your doctor may advise a diagnostic procedure such as an ultrasound or biopsy to further characterize an abnormality found on a screening mammogram. An ultrasound uses sound waves to create an image of the breast. A biopsy is a small sample of tissue removed from the breast for analysis in a laboratory.

Preventing breast cancer

When it comes to breast cancer, dietary factors such as fat, alcohol, fibre, fruit and vegetables have all been well studied. Below, I list nutrition recommendations based on our current body of scientific evidence. Some of these strategies have strong research to support their adoption; others have evidence to suggest that they *may* be helpful. Although scientists are still learning the role of nutrition in the risk of breast cancer, making these dietary changes will improve your overall well-being, not to mention possibly lower your chances of developing breast cancer.

DIETARY STRATEGIES
Dietary Fat
It's long been thought that dietary fat may increase breast cancer risk by affecting estrogen metabolism. Studies have found that women who follow a low-fat, high-fibre diet have lower levels of circulating estrogen and less

breast cancer.[3,4] A high-fat diet may lead to breast cancer by promoting weight gain and body fat accumulation, which increase the risk of breast cancer.

Although the hypothesis that a low-fat diet guards against breast cancer has existed for decades, only recently was it tested in a randomized controlled trial. The Women's Health Initiative Dietary Modification Trial, the largest long-term trial ever conducted, followed 48,835 post-menopausal women aged 50 to 79 from across the United States for eight years. Researchers assigned 40 percent of the women to a low-fat diet (20 percent of calories from fat) and an increased amount of fruit and vegetables (at least 5 servings per day) and grains (6 or more servings per day). The remaining women were assigned to the comparison group and were asked to not make any changes to their diets. After eight years of follow up, there was no overall difference in risk of breast cancer between women in the low-fat diet group and the comparison group. There were, however, signs that a woman's risk of disease could be modified by dietary change. Women in the low-fat group were 9 percent less likely to develop breast cancer than their peers in the comparison group, although this finding was not deemed statistically significant (it could have been due to chance). That difference in risk means that out of 10,000 women, 42 following the low-fat diet and 45 following their normal diets developed breast cancer each year.

The researchers did find, however, that the low-fat diet was associated with a 15 percent reduction in circulating levels of the hormone estradiol, the form of estrogen that increases the risk of breast cancer. Significant results were seen among women in the low-fat diet group who were consuming the most fat when the study began. Women in this category were 15 percent to 22 percent less likely to be diagnosed with breast cancer compared to women following their normal diets. Adopting a low-fat diet may help guard against breast cancer, especially among women who have a relatively high fat intake to begin with.[5]

A low-fat diet has also been shown to improve survival in women diagnosed with breast cancer. The Women's Intervention Nutrition Study, conducted among 2437 women aged 48 to 79 with early-stage breast cancer, demonstrated that a low-fat diet consisting of 15 percent fat calories, or 33 grams of fat per day, can influence body weight and decrease breast cancer recurrence in women with estrogen receptor (ER)–negative breast cancer.[6] Cells with estrogen receptors grow and multiply when estrogen attaches to the receptors. After a breast cancer tissue is removed, the cancer cells are tested to see if they have hormone receptors. If either estrogen or progesterone receptors are present, a response to hormonal therapy is very possible. About 75 percent of breast cancers are ER-positive and 25 percent are ER-negative.

Although the evidence isn't concrete that reducing your fat intake will reduce breast cancer risk, it's prudent to limit your fat intake to 20 percent of daily calories if you're a post-menopausal woman. Women who have been diagnosed with ER-negative breast cancer should consume no more than 15 percent of daily calories from fat.

Saturated fat

Some studies show that higher meat intakes are linked with a greater risk of breast cancer. The harmful effect may be due to meat's saturated fat content, or to the way it's prepared. Cooking meat at high temperatures forms compounds called heterocyclic amines, which have been shown to cause breast tumours in animals. This may hold true for women too. A University of Minnesota study found that women who ate hamburger, steak and bacon cooked well done were more than four times as likely to have breast cancer than women who enjoyed their meat cooked rare or medium-done.[7] Until we know more about the effect of cooked meat, breast cancer experts advise that we consume no more than 3 ounces (90 g) of meat per day.

Omega-3 fatty acids

Research suggests that consuming plenty of fish for many years is associated with a lower risk of breast cancer. Studies conducted in the laboratory and in animals have demonstrated the ability of omega-3 fatty acids from fish to slow the growth of breast cancer and increase the effectiveness of certain chemotherapy drugs.[8] Three studies have reported lower risks of breast cancer among women who consume the most fish.[9] Aim to eat fatty fish like salmon and trout two times a week. If you don't like fish, consider taking a fish oil capsule that supplies 500 milligrams of DHA and EPA, the two omega-3 fatty acids found in fish.

Carbohydrates: Low glycemic index

Some evidence suggests that eating a low-glycemic diet guards against breast cancer. (The glycemic index is a measure of the rate at which a carbohydrate-containing food—starchy foods, fruit, milk and yogurt—are converted to glucose in the bloodstream. Low-glycemic foods release their sugar slowly and are linked with better health. See Chapter 5, page 93, for more information on the glycemic index.) A Canadian study of 49,613 women who were followed for nearly seventeen years revealed that post-menopausal women who followed a high-glycemic diet were 87 percent more likely to develop breast cancer than women whose diet included mainly low-glycemic foods.[10] Glycemic index didn't alter the risk of breast cancer among premenopausal women. It's thought that diets rich in high-glycemic carbohydrates lead to higher blood-glucose and insulin levels, which, in turn, increases breast cancer risk. Insulin may impact breast cells directly or increase the growth of cancerous cells.

Reduce your intake of foods with a high glycemic index such as white bread, white rice, white potatoes, refined breakfast cereals, cookies, cakes and candy. Instead choose low-glycemic options such as stone-ground whole-wheat bread, steel-cut oats, brown rice, pasta, legumes, citrus fruit, apples, pears and yogurt.

Soy foods

Epidemiological studies reveal that Asians, who typically eat a high-soy diet, have lower rates of breast cancer. Researchers attribute soy's possible protective effect to naturally occurring compounds called isoflavones. Once in the body, isoflavones behave like weak estrogen compounds and are able to attach to estrogen receptors in the breast. In so doing, they can block the ability of a woman's own estrogen from taking that spot. This means that breast cells have less contact with estrogen. A handful of studies have shown that a regular intake of soy isoflavones may lower circulating levels of estrogen, and this might reduce a woman's future risk of breast cancer. Other studies show that consuming a soy-rich diet can lengthen a woman's menstrual cycle, thereby influencing how much estrogen her breast cells are exposed to.

Whether increasing your intake of soy foods will reduce the risk of breast cancer in Canadian women remains to be seen. Keep in mind that Asians generally have a low-fat diet and eat more fish and vegetables than

North Americans do. It's also thought that Asian women might be more responsive to the effects of soy. But what might be most important is when you start consuming soy. Research conducted among women living in China and the United States suggests that consuming soy during childhood and adolescence is associated with a lower risk of breast cancer in adulthood. Soy isoflavones may confer their protective effects during puberty when breast cells are maturing and are more vulnerable to cancer-causing substances.[11,12]

Yet many women worry that because isoflavones have estrogen-like effects in the body, consuming soy may increase breast cancer risk. The concern is that soy isoflavones could increase a woman's total estrogen levels and encourage the growth of estrogen-dependent breast cancer, especially in women who already have the disease. Some studies conducted in animals and test tubes indicate that isoflavones inhibit the development of breast cancer, while others suggest they may increase breast cancer growth. It depends on the particular isoflavone studied (soybeans are rich in two different isoflavones) and the amount used. There's no compelling evidence that soy foods increase breast cancer, but research is ongoing.

Because we lack sufficient reliable information about the effect of soy foods in women with breast cancer, a history of breast cancer or a family history of breast cancer, soy should be used cautiously. Until more is known, avoid consuming large amounts of soy each day, and avoid using soy protein powders and isoflavone supplements. Consuming soy foods three times a week as part of a plant-based diet is considered safe. If you want to start eating soy foods because they might help reduce your risk of breast cancer, and because they have other potential health benefits (such as protecting from heart disease), try the following tips to enjoy more soy:

- **Try a calcium-fortified soy beverage.** Pour it on cereal, add it to soups, use it in baking or enjoy it on its own. Find a product that you like—depending on how they're made, brands can taste very different.
- **Snack on roasted soy nuts.** These are crunchy and full of phytoestrogens and have less fat and more fibre than other nuts. Enjoy them as a snack or sprinkle them over your salad. They also come in flavoured varieties.
- **Cook with canned soybeans.** Check out the canned bean aisle of your grocery store for these no-fuss beans. If you can't find them there, look

in the ethnic food section. If you have the time, buy them dried, soak them overnight, and then simmer them for an hour or so. Add canned or home-cooked soybeans to chilies, pasta sauces, soups and salads.

- **Use soy deli meats** in place of pepperoni or salami on pizzas and in sandwiches.
- **Try soy ground round** in your next pasta or burrito recipe.
- **Bake with soy flour.** You'll find defatted soy flour at your local health food store. Replace one-quarter to one-half of the all-purpose flour in recipes with soy flour.
- **Try cooking with tofu or tempeh.** For recipes, information and free brochures on soy foods, visit www.soybean.ca.

Flaxseed

These tiny whole-grain brown and golden seeds contain natural plant estrogens called lignans. Once in the body, phytoestrogens from flaxseed have a weak estrogen action, and they're able to bind to estrogen receptors (just like soy isoflavones). In so doing, they appear to block the action of our body's own estrogen on breast cells. Animal studies conducted at the University of Toronto found that flaxseed has anti-cancer properties.[13,14] Researchers have demonstrated that giving women 1 or 2 tablespoons (15 to 30 ml) of ground flaxseed each day significantly lowered circulating estrogen levels.[15] In a study of post-menopausal women with newly diagnosed breast cancer, consuming 25 grams of flaxseed per day in the form of a muffin, versus a placebo muffin, significantly slowed the growth of breast tumours.[16] Lignans in whole grains may also inhibit the action of enzymes that are involved in the body's production of estrogen. To date, research on flaxseed has focused on ER-negative breast cancers. The effect of flaxseed on ER-positive breast cancer is unknown.

Aim to get 1 to 2 tablespoons (15 to 30 ml) of ground flaxseed each day. Grind your flaxseed in a clean coffee grinder or use a mortar and pestle. You can also buy pre-ground flaxseed at supermarkets and natural food stores. Once you grind flaxseed, store it in an airtight container in the fridge or freezer, since the natural fats in flaxseed go rancid quickly if exposed to air and heat. Ground flaxseed can be stored in an airtight container for several months.

Ground flaxseed can be added to many foods and recipes. Here are a few ways to add crunch and a nutty flavour to your meals:

- Add ground flaxseed to hot cereals, muffin batters and cookie mixes.
- Blend ground flaxseed into a smoothie and enjoy at breakfast or as a snack.
- Mix ground flaxseed into a single serving of yogurt or applesauce.
- Sprinkle flaxseed on salads and soups.
- Add ground flaxseed to casseroles.
- Try a loaf of flaxseed bread from your local bakery or supermarket.
- Try Red River Hot Cereal, another good source of flaxseed.

Vegetables

Hundreds of studies from around the world have shown that a diet high in vegetables lowers the risk of many cancers, including breast cancer. Researchers from Harvard University studied more than 89,000 women and found that those who ate more than 2.2 servings of vegetables a day had a 20 percent lower risk of breast cancer compared with those who ate less than 1 serving a day.[17] Another study in premenopausal women found that high total vegetable intake lowered the risk of breast cancer by 54 percent.[18]

Several studies hint that cruciferous vegetables such as broccoli, cauliflower and cabbage might be especially protective. Researchers have reported that women diagnosed with breast cancer have significantly lower intakes of cruciferous vegetables than their cancer-free peers. Triggered by the observation that breast cancer risk of Polish women rose threefold after they immigrated to the United States, scientists from Michigan State University recently decided to evaluate the diets of Polish immigrant women living in Chicago and Detroit. They found that women who ate at least 3 servings of raw or lightly cooked cabbage and sauerkraut had a significantly lower risk of breast cancer compared with those who ate only 1 serving per week. Interestingly, cabbage cooked for a long time had no bearing on breast cancer risk.[19]

Cruciferous vegetables contain phytochemicals called glucosinolates, potent protectors against cancer development. When you eat cruciferous vegetables, glucosinolates are broken down by bacteria in the digestive tract and transformed into compounds called isothiocyanates and indole-3-carbinol. Isothiocyanates help eliminate cancer-causing substances by regulating the body's detoxification enzymes. Researchers suspect that the various compounds in cruciferous vegetables work together to promote a greater cancer-fighting effect.

Make sure you get at least 7 to 10 servings of fruit and vegetables each day. One serving is 1/2 cup (125 ml) of cooked or raw vegetable, 1 cup (250 ml) of raw greens or one medium-sized whole fruit. Aim for a minimum of 5 vegetable servings. Include 1 serving of cruciferous vegetable in your diet five times per week. Cruciferous vegetables include bok choy, broccoli, broccoli sprouts, broccoflower, broccolini, Brussels sprouts, cabbage, cauliflower, rutabaga and turnip.

Fibre and wheat bran

Evidence suggests that a high-fibre diet may offer protection from breast cancer. Toronto researchers found that 20 grams of fibre per day (the amount found in about 1 cup/250 ml of 100% bran cereal) was associated with lower risk.[20] Fibre may help lower the risk of breast cancer by binding to estrogen in the intestine and causing it to be excreted in the stool. Every day, your intestine reabsorbs estrogen from bile, the compound that's released into your intestine from your gallbladder to help digest fat. If dietary fibre can attach to this estrogen and facilitate its removal from the body, your body has to take estrogen out of your bloodstream to make more bile. The net result is a lower level of circulating estrogen. It's possible that following a high-fibre diet for many years could lower your risk for breast cancer.

High-fibre diets also tend to be higher in antioxidant nutrients and lower in fat, both of which might help protect from breast cancer. People who eat plenty of fibre also tend to maintain a healthy weight. The studies suggest that dietary fibre works best if you follow a low-fat diet. So adding foods rich in wheat bran to a diet that's high in fat and low in fruit and vegetables probably won't do you much good.

Foods contain two types of fibre, soluble and insoluble. Both types are present in varying proportions in different plant foods, but some foods may be rich in one or the other. And each type of fibre functions differently in your body to promote health. Foods like wheat bran, whole grains and some vegetables contain mainly insoluble fibres and may help reduce circulating levels of estrogen.

Soluble fibre, plentiful in oats, oat bran, barley, psyllium and legumes, is also thought to reduce breast cancer risk by controlling blood sugar, insulin and insulin-like growth factors, all of which have been linked to a greater risk of breast cancer. Insulin may impact breast cells directly or increase the growth of cancerous cells.

To boost your intake of total dietary fibre, try the following:

- Strive for at least 7 servings of fruit and vegetables every day. Citrus fruit and apples are good sources of soluble fibre.
- Leave the peel on fruit and vegetables whenever possible.
- Eat at least 5 servings of 100% whole-grain foods each day.
- Buy a high-fibre breakfast cereal. Gradually add 1/2 to 1 cup (125 to 250 ml) of 100% bran cereal to your morning meal; a 1/2 cup (125 ml) portion contains 12 grams of fibre. To increase soluble fibre, look for a psyllium-enriched breakfast cereal like Kellogg's All-Bran Buds or Nature's Path SmartBran. Cooked oatmeal and oat bran are also excellent sources of soluble fibre.
- Add legumes such as lentils, chickpeas, black beans and kidney beans to salads, soups, pasta sauces and casseroles.
- Add 2 tablespoons (30 ml) of natural wheat bran or oat bran to cereals, yogurt, casseroles and soup.
- Add nuts and seeds to salads.
- Reach for high-fibre snacks like popcorn, nuts, dried apricots or dates.

To avoid intestinal distress, build up your fibre intake gradually. Be sure to drink 8 ounces (250 ml) of fluid with every high-fibre meal and snack.

Green tea

A growing body of evidence suggests that drinking green tea protects from certain cancers, including breast cancer. Recently, scientists combined the results from four studies examining the link between green tea and breast cancer—three from Japan and one from Los Angeles—and concluded that green tea is indeed protective. Compared to women who consumed less than 1 cup (250 ml) of green tea per day, those who drank at least 5 cups (1.2 L) daily were 22 percent less likely to develop breast cancer.[21]

Drinking green tea might also improve a woman's prognosis once diagnosed with breast cancer. Japanese researchers discovered that among women with stage I and stage II breast cancer, drinking five or more daily cups lowered the risk of the cancer coming back by 46 percent. The researchers suspect that phytochemicals in green tea somehow modify breast cancer, making it easier to successfully treat.[22]

Like fruit and vegetables, green tea is a plant food, and as such it contains natural chemicals that act as powerful antioxidants. The antioxidants in green tea leaves belong to a special class of compounds called catechins. By mopping up harmful free radical molecules in the body, catechins in tea may prevent damage to the genetic material of breast cells.

There are three main types of tea: green tea, black tea and oolong. All three come from the same tea plant, but they're processed differently. Herbal teas aren't made from tea leaves and, therefore, they don't have the antioxidant properties of green tea. Aim to drink 1 to 3 cups (250 to 750 ml) of green tea each day. Here are a few tips to help you increase your intake of green tea:

- If you drink coffee or a diet soft drink in the afternoon, replace it with green tea, hot or iced.
- The next time you're at the grocery store, pick up a box of green tea bags.
- If you're preparing an Asian meal at home, serve it with a pot of green tea. Use bags or buy loose tea.
- The next time you're at your local coffee shop, try a green tea latte made with non-fat milk or soy milk.

Alcoholic beverages

The evidence is convincing that drinking alcoholic beverages increases the risk of breast cancer before and after menopause. A pooled analysis of 98 studies concluded that one drink per day increased a woman's risk by 10 percent.[23] Studies have also determined that the more drinks consumed, the greater the risk of breast cancer. The Million Women Study published in 2009 found that for every additional drink regularly consumed per day, the risk of breast cancer increased by 12 percent. All types of alcoholic beverages—wine, beer and spirits—increased the risk equally.[24]

Alcohol may increase breast cancer risk in a number of ways. One of its metabolic byproducts, acetaldehyde, may be carcinogenic. Alcohol may also make breast cells more vulnerable to the effects of carcinogens or it may enhance the liver's processing of these substances. Alcohol may inhibit the ability of cells to repair faulty genes and may also increase estrogen levels in the body.

Nutrition and cancer experts recommend that women not drink alcohol. If consumed at all, alcoholic drinks should be limited to one a day or seven per week. If you do drink, ensure you're meeting your daily requirements of folate, a B vitamin that may help protect breast cells from alcohol's harmful effects. See Chapter 1, page 18, for more information on folate requirements and best food sources.

Weight control

Gaining weight after menopause is clearly linked with a higher risk of breast cancer. Among post-menopausal women, those who are obese have a risk of breast cancer about 50 percent higher than that of lean women. Women who are overweight and sedentary have an even greater risk. In a study of 38,660 women aged 55 to 74, those with the highest calorie intake, the highest body mass index (BMI) and the least physical activity had double the risk of breast cancer compared with women who reported eating the fewest calories, having the lowest body mass index and engaging in the most physical activity.[25-31] The relationship between excess weight and breast cancer risk is most clearly seen after the age of 60. Obesity is thought to influence breast cancer risk by increasing circulating estradiol, the most potent form of estrogen in the body. Estradiol is positively associated with the risk of breast cancer in post-menopausal women.

World cancer experts advise maintaining your weight within a healthy BMI throughout adulthood. Steps should be taken to avoid adult weight gain and increases in waist circumference. If you are overweight or have gained excess weight since menopause, I strongly advise that you take action to lose weight. Start by determining your BMI (see Chapter 2, page 37).

VITAMINS AND MINERALS

Carotenoids

A number of studies show that women who get the most beta carotene in their diet have a lower risk of breast cancer. The Harvard Nurses' Health Study found that premenopausal women who ate 5 or more daily servings of high-carotenoid fruit and vegetables had a lower risk of breast cancer than women who ate less than 2 servings a day.[32]

More recently, the Women's Health Initiative Observational Study from Los Angeles, California, revealed that among nearly 85,000 women, those with the highest intakes of beta carotene and lycopene were less likely to develop ER-positive breast cancer compared to those who consumed the least. Other research has shown that women with higher blood levels of beta carotene and lycopene—a reflection of dietary intake—had about half the risk of breast cancer compared with women who had the lowest blood levels.[33,34] A diet rich in beta carotene fruit and vegetables may also improve breast cancer survival.

More than six hundred types of carotenoid compounds exist in plants, with beta carotene in carrots, sweet potato and winter squash being the most plentiful. Other important carotenoids include alpha carotene, lycopene and lutein. Beta carotene and lycopene have an antioxidant effect in the body, which can help protect our genes from oxidative damage caused by free radicals. Some beta carotene is also converted to vitamin A inside the body. This vitamin is essential for proper cell growth and development and the normal functioning of the body's immune system. Research also suggests that these two carotenoids may trigger cancer cell death and inhibit the growth of breast cancer cells.

Dietary carotenoids aren't that well absorbed—but you'll absorb more of them if you eat these foods with a little fat. Try a yogurt dip with carrot sticks, a little olive oil in lycopene-rich pasta sauce or a splash of salad dressing on your roasted red pepper.

Use the list below to increase your daily intake of carotenoid-rich fruit and vegetables. Every day, aim for 5 servings of 1/2 cup (125 ml) each.

Carotenoid-Rich Fruit and Vegetables

Beta carotene	Lycopene	Lutein
Carrots	Tomato juice	Beet greens
Red pepper	Tomato sauce	Collards
Squash	Tomatoes	Corn
Sweet potato	Grapefruit, red and pink	Kale
Cantaloupe	Giava	Okra
Mango	Watermelon	Red pepper
Nectarine		Romaine lettuce
Papaya		Spinach
Peach		

Vitamin C

Although the research findings on vitamin C are less consistent than for beta carotene, there's evidence to suggest you should be getting more in your diet. The vitamin may keep women stay healthy by acting as an antioxidant or it may work by enhancing the body's immune system. Vitamin C also plays an important role in the synthesis of collagen, an important tissue in the breast.

For women, the recommended daily intake for vitamin C is 75 milligrams (if you smoke you need 110 milligrams). This amount is easy to get from your diet. The best food sources of vitamin C are citrus fruit, strawberries, kiwi, cantaloupe, broccoli, bell peppers, Brussels sprouts, cabbage, tomatoes and potatoes.

Vitamin C supplements

At this time, there's no evidence to warrant vitamin C supplements for breast cancer prevention; however, it won't do harm if you're already taking one. But before you take a supplement every day, make sure you add one or two vitamin C–rich foods to your daily diet. Fruit and vegetables have plenty of other protective compounds that may work in tandem with vitamin C to keep you healthy. If you find your diet lacks these foods, or you want to increase your vitamin C intake further, use the following guide when taking vitamin C supplements.

- Take 500 or 600 milligrams of vitamin C once or twice daily. Taking more than 200 milligrams of vitamin C at once won't increase your blood levels further. I've recommended 500 or 600 milligrams because these are the most common doses you'll find. If you want to take more, you're better off splitting your dose over the course of the day.
- If you prefer a chewable supplement, make sure it's made from calcium ascorbate or sodium ascorbate. These forms of the vitamin are less acidic, so they're easier on the enamel of your teeth.

Vitamin D

Many studies have reported that higher levels of vitamin D in the bloodstream are linked with a lower risk of breast cancer. A study of 34,321 postmenopausal women also found that consuming more than 800 international units (IU) of vitamin D daily—versus less than 400 IU—

was associated with protection from breast cancer.[35] Once consumed from foods or synthesized in the skin from sunlight, vitamin D acts like a hormone in the body and has been shown to have anti-cancer effects. In 2007, the first randomized controlled trial demonstrated vitamin D's cancer-fighting properties in women. In the four-year study of 1179 healthy, post-menopausal women, researchers found that those taking 1110 IU of vitamin D per day, in conjunction with calcium, were 60 percent less likely to get cancers than their peers taking placebos.[36]

This finding—and the fact that Canadians don't produce enough vitamin D from sunlight from October to March—prompted the Canadian Cancer Society to recommend adults take 1000 IU of vitamin D per day in the fall and winter. Older adults, people with dark skin, those who don't go outdoors often and those who wear clothing that covers most of their skin should take the supplement year-round. To learn more about vitamin D supplements, see Chapter 1, page 13.

Folate

If you drink alcohol, be sure to meet your daily requirement for the B vitamin folate. A Harvard University study found that, among women who consumed 15 grams of alcohol per day (about a glass and a half of beer or wine), those with the highest daily intake of folate (600 micrograms) had a 45 percent lower risk for breast cancer compared with women who consumed the least folate (150 to 299 micrograms a day).[37] It's thought that alcohol interferes with the transport and metabolism of folate and may deprive body tissues of this B vitamin, which is essential to DNA synthesis.

The best food sources of folate include spinach, broccoli, lentils, orange juice, asparagus, artichokes and whole-grain breads and cereals. To supplement, take a multivitamin and mineral that supplies 400 micrograms (0.4 milligrams) of folic acid. I don't advise taking more than 400 micrograms from a supplement since some research hints that high intakes of folic acid might stimulate the growth of certain pre-cancerous lesions. For more information about folate and folic acid, see Chapter 1, page 18.

To help you meet the recommended daily intake of 400 micrograms a day, practise the following:

- Eat spinach, broccoli, asparagus and artichokes more often. These vegetables have the most folate, with spinach leading the pack.
- Drink a glass of orange juice with your morning meal.

- Use lentils and other legumes in pasta sauces, chilies and tacos.
- Most often, choose whole-grain breads and cereals.
- Take a multivitamin and mineral supplement or a B complex supplement that contains 0.4 milligram of folic acid to ensure you're meeting your needs.
- If you take separate folic acid supplements, be sure to buy one that has vitamin B12 added (folic acid, found in vitamin pills and fortified foods, is the synthetic form of folate; folate refers to the vitamin as it occurs naturally in foods).

THE BOTTOM LINE...
Leslie's recommendations for preventing breast cancer

1. Reduce your intake of saturated fat, especially from meat:
   - Eat no more than 3 ounces (90 g) of meat per day.
   - For protein, choose lean poultry, fish, beans and soy foods most often.
   - When you do eat meat, avoid cooking it well-done.
   - To help you eat an overall low-fat diet, choose 1% or skim milk, yogurt with 1% milk fat (MF) or less and cheese with 15% MF or less.
2. To get more omega-3 fatty acids, eat fish two times a week.
3. When choosing carbohydrate-rich foods, opt for low-glycemic choices such as grainy bread, brown rice, pasta, sweet potato, bran cereals and steel-cut or large-flake oatmeal.
4. Eat one soy food each day to boost your intake of soy protein and isoflavones. Encourage your daughters to incorporate these foods into their diet, since researchers believe that it's a lifetime intake that offers protection from breast cancer.
5. To get plant estrogens called lignans, add 1 or 2 tablespoons (15 to 30 ml) of ground flaxseed to your foods and recipes.
6. Eat at least 7 to 10 servings of fruit and vegetables every single day.
   - Make sure 5 servings are foods brimming with carotenoid compounds.
   - To boost your intake of vitamin C, eat one or two foods packed with this vitamin.

7. Gradually increase your daily dietary fibre intake to 21 or 25 grams. To help lower blood levels of your body's own estrogen, focus on foods rich in wheat bran, such as whole-grain breads, 100% bran cereals and whole-wheat pasta.

8. Drink more green tea to get a source of catechins, natural antioxidant compounds found in tea leaves.

9. Avoid alcoholic beverages. If you do drink, consume no more than one drink per day.

10. Manage your weight before and after menopause.

11. Supplement your diet with 1000 IU of vitamin D every day during the fall and winter, and year-round if you're 50 or older.

12. Get more B vitamins into your diet every day, especially folate. If you drink alcoholic beverages, be sure to boost your intake of folate. To ensure you're meeting your needs, take a multivitamin and mineral supplement each day.

10
Fibrocystic breast conditions

Formerly called fibrocystic breast disease, this disorder affects about one-half of all women. If you've ever felt a lump in your breast, you know how frightening the experience can be—it's only natural to worry that the lump could be a sign of breast cancer. Fortunately, most breast lumps are not cancerous. Many women live a normal, active life with breasts that are tender and lumpy.

Fibrocystic breast conditions may include breast nodules, breast swelling, tenderness and pain. Doctors often refer to this condition as nodular or glandular breast tissue. A woman may experience breast pain only, lumpiness only, or both. Although these breast conditions can be painful, and suspicious lumps can cause anxiety, most don't increase a woman's risk of breast cancer.

The main symptoms of fibrocystic breast conditions are swelling and pain in the breasts, which waxes and wanes with the menstrual cycle. However, women who are severely affected by these conditions complain of continuous discomfort. And up to 50 percent of women with breast pain report that it interferes with their sex life and physical activity. Occasionally, a woman may develop breast cysts that require medical attention.

What causes fibrocystic breast conditions?

The exact cause of this disorder is not known. Most women eventually develop some lumpiness in their breasts. Breast changes usually appear during the years a woman menstruates, and regress with the onset of menopause. In most cases, the small, round lumps appear in the breasts because of hormonal changes associated with menstruation. The hormones estrogen and progesterone that control your menstrual cycle trigger physical responses that make your breasts become lumpy, or fibrocystic, and painful. It's thought that a deficiency of progesterone and an excess of estrogen in the last fourteen days of a woman's menstrual cycle are responsible for breast changes.

These symptoms are collectively referred to as fibrocystic breast conditions. You may also hear breast pain and tenderness called cyclic mastalgia or mastitis. Because fibrocystic breast conditions are influenced by hormonal cycles, a woman will find that her breasts become increasingly tender and painful as her body prepares for menstruation. The discomfort normally subsides once her period starts. Over time, breast lumps may develop into cysts, which fill with fluid, causing swelling and pain. Up to 20 percent of women with fibrocystic breast conditions say that their symptoms spontaneously improve over time.

Fibrocystic breast conditions are often associated with the symptoms of premenstrual syndrome (PMS). Some researchers believe that hormone-like compounds called prostaglandins are responsible for causing breast changes. A handful of studies indicate that the development of lumpy breasts may also be stimulated by a diet that includes higher levels of caffeine and dietary fat. Despite these other theories, most of the clues about the cause of fibrocystic breast conditions suggest that estrogen is the key.

Symptoms

Breast lumpiness is one of the main characteristics of fibrocystic breast conditions. A woman may discover only one lump, but it's more common to have multiple lumps. The lumps are tender, come in different sizes and usually move freely within the breast tissue. A woman may also experience some breast pain and swelling, which becomes worse just before her menstrual period. Some women who are severely affected by these conditions complain of continuous discomfort. Up to 50 percent of women with breast pain report that it interferes with their sex life and physical activity. Occasionally, a woman may develop breast cysts that require medical attention.

Who's at risk?

Fibrocystic breast conditions can affect women from puberty to old age. However, these conditions affect approximately 50 percent of women between the ages of 30 to 50 years. Breast symptoms usually disappear with menopause, and it's quite rare to find the disorder in post-menopausal women unless they're taking hormone replacement therapy.

Diagnosis

Up to 85 percent of breast lumps are found by patients through breast self-examination. The Canadian Cancer Society recommends that all Canadian women, beginning at age 20, should be examining their breasts regularly every month. (Go to www.breastselfexcam.ca for a detailed guide to breast self-examination.) The self-examination should be done five to ten days after menstruation, at the same time each month. Using the pads of your fingers, you should examine all of your breast tissue and the tissue under your armpits. You should also examine your breasts visually, looking for physical changes or differences between your breasts. This practice should be continued even when you no longer menstruate. It's also recommended that once a woman turns 50, she have a mammogram (specialized breast X-ray) once every two years to determine overall breast health.

Fibrocystic breast conditions can sometimes imitate the symptoms of true breast cancer or can hide the presence of cancerous growths. Fibrocystic breast lumps and cysts normally feel soft or slightly firm, tender and painful. This distinguishes them from cancerous growths, which tend to be hard and don't usually cause tenderness and pain. However, if a woman's fibrocystic breast condition becomes more advanced, chronic inflammation may cause the soft, fluid-filled cysts to harden and thicken. When this happens, it becomes increasingly difficult to tell the difference between non-cancerous and cancerous growths.

To distinguish hardened cysts from breast cancer, your doctor may order some specific diagnostic tests. He or she will begin by taking a medical history and conducting a physical examination. Your doctor may then order radiological tests, such as a mammogram or an ultrasound (sound wave picture), which are useful in identifying breast cysts. In some cases, your doctor may feel that a biopsy is necessary. A small piece of tissue from the lump will be surgically removed and sent to a laboratory for microscopic examination. This procedure will determine if the cells in the lump are benign (non-cancerous) or malignant (cancerous).

Conventional treatment

If fibrocystic breast changes don't cause symptoms or cause only mild symptoms, no treatment is required. Women who suffer from painful breasts at certain times during the month may find that applying cold compresses on the tender areas and wearing a well-fitting, supportive bra both day and night will relieve some of the discomfort. Your doctor may recommend pain relievers to treat the aches and pains. If fibrocystic breast conditions cause severe pain, medications such as danazol, a mild, synthetic male hormone, may be used. Because these drugs can produce side effects, they should be used for a short time only. Oral contraceptives, which lower menstrual cycle hormones, may also be prescribed. Or your doctor may perform a simple procedure called a needle aspiration; fluid is removed from the lump using a small, hollow needle and then tested. Needle aspiration is also used to relieve pressure on surrounding breast tissue by draining the contents of large, fluid-filled cysts. In rare cases, surgery may be required to remove a persistent cyst that doesn't resolve after other treatment.

Managing fibrocystic breast conditions

DIETARY STRATEGIES

At this time, there's only weak evidence pointing to dietary factors as the cause of fibrocystic breast conditions. However, certain food and food components may very well aggravate symptoms. And since a high level of estrogen, or an increased sensitivity to estrogen, seems to be the dominant theory, any dietary modification that's able to reduce the circulating level of estrogen may help lessen your symptoms. The first three dietary tips—reduce fat, increase fibre and eat more soy—address this point.

Dietary fat

If you have a fibrocystic breast condition, reducing the amount of fat you eat—from the typical North American intake of 35 percent of calories to 15 or 20 percent—may be beneficial. Although studies haven't investigated the effect of a low-fat diet on fibrocystic breast conditions per se, there's indirect evidence to support this strategy. Research in women with breast dysplasia (abnormal growth of breast cells) has found a low-fat diet to have a positive effect on the density of breast tissue and the composition of breast fluid.[1]

Eating a high-fat diet is also associated with higher levels of circulating estrogen and cholesterol, a building block of hormones. Studies reveal that when women reduce their fat intake, their blood-estrogen levels also decline. The strongest theory for fibrocystic breast conditions is an imbalance between estrogen and progesterone, and excessive levels of estrogen seem to be a key factor. In two small studies, women with fibrocystic breast conditions who followed a 21 percent fat diet for three months experienced a significantly lower level of circulating estrogen and cholesterol.[2,3] The low-fat diet did not alter progesterone levels.

To understand how dietary fat influences the amount of estrogen that circulates throughout your body, let me take you on a brief course in estrogen metabolism (don't worry, it's very brief!). Your liver attaches estrogen to a molecule of glucuronic acid or a sulphate residue, compounds that make estrogen easier to eliminate from the body. Your liver then puts almost one-half of these estrogen compounds into your bile, a digestive aid that's released into your intestinal tract once you eat a meal. Once in your intestine, bacterial enzymes break the bond between estrogen and glucaronic acid or sulphate residues. Many of these free estrogens are then reabsorbed into your bloodstream.

It seems that a high-fat diet can increase the activity of these bacterial enzymes, which means that more free estrogens are reabsorbed, increasing the amount of circulating estrogen. Low-fat diets, on the other hand, may slow the action of these intestinal enzymes and reduce the amount of estrogen that re-enters your bloodstream.

Here are a few tips to help you cut back to a 20 percent–fat diet:

1. Choose lower-fat animal foods.

Instead of...	Choose...
Whole milk	Skim, 1% milk fat (MF) milk
Yogurt	Products with less than 1.5% MF
Cheese, 31% MF or more	Products with less than 20% MF
Cottage cheese, 2% or 4% MF	Products with 1% MF
Sour cream, 14% MF	Products with 7% MF or less

Instead of...	Choose...
Cream, 10% or 18% MF	Evaporated, 2% or skim milk
Red meat, higher-fat cuts	Flank steak, inside round, sirloin, eye of round, extra lean ground beef, venison
Pork, higher-fat cuts	Centre-cut pork chops, pork tenderloin, pork leg (inside round, roast), baked ham, deli ham, back bacon
Poultry, dark meat	Skinless chicken breast, turkey breast, ground turkey
Eggs, whole	Egg whites (2 whites replace 1 whole)

2. Use added fats and oils sparingly, even if it's olive oil. Invest in a few high-quality non-stick pans to reduce the need for cooking oil. I'm sure you're already well versed in low-fat eating, but there are probably a few things you can do to cut back on fat.

Instead of...	Choose...
Butter on toast	Sugar-reduced jam
High-fat spreads on sandwiches	Mustard
Mayonnaise in tuna salad	Yogurt, plain
Butter on your baked potato	Low-fat sour cream
Salad pre-tossed with dressing	Order dressing on the side
Oil to prevent sticking in a stir-fry	Chicken broth or apple juice

3. Read nutrition labels on packaged foods like crackers, frozen entrées, snack foods, cookies and cereals. A food that provides no more than 20 percent of calories from total fat will have no more than 2 grams of total fat per 100 calories.

Dietary fibre

Just like dietary fat, fibre may influence your circulating estrogen levels. Although most of the research on fibre intake and estrogen levels has focused on breast cancer risk, the findings may be relevant to fibrocystic breast conditions. There have been a few recent studies that show higher-fibre diets reduce estrogen levels in the body. Two studies conducted in premenopausal women suggest that diets high in wheat bran are effective in lowering circulating estrogen.[4,5] In one study, both a 10 and a 20 gram wheat bran supplement significantly lowered estrogen after four weeks. The total daily fibre intake of these women was between 20 and 32 grams.

Scientists think that fibre may work through its ability to bind estrogen in the intestinal tract, making the hormone less available for absorption into the bloodstream. High-fibre diets cause more estrogen to be excreted. Boosting your fibre intake may also change the acidity of your intestinal tract, slowing the activity of the bacterial enzymes that make estrogen ready for absorption.

Wheat bran belongs to a class of fibres referred to as insoluble, which means they're unable to dissolve in water. They pass through the intestinal tract intact and, in the process, are able to bind compounds, including estrogen. Soluble fibres found in oatmeal, oat bran, dried beans, lentils and psyllium-enriched breakfast cereals also have this ability, although they have not been specifically studied for their effect on estrogen levels.

It's estimated that Canadians eat on average 14 grams of fibre per day—not quite the 20 grams that may lower estrogen levels. You certainly don't need to rely on a fibre supplement to get more wheat bran into your daily diet. All it takes is a bowl of high-fibre breakfast cereal each morning.

See the table in Chapter 1, page 29, for more high-fibre foods. Use the list to gradually add higher-fibre foods to your diet. Too much fibre too soon can cause bloating, gas and diarrhea, so spread fibre-rich foods out over the course of the day. And don't forget that fibre needs fluid to work, so drink at least 8 ounces (250 ml) of fluid with each high-fibre meal and snack.

Soy foods

As is the case with fat and fibre, the research findings on soy intake and estrogen levels provide indirect evidence that soy foods may be beneficial in preventing fibrocystic breast conditions. Many studies have found that a diet rich in soy foods lowers the level of circulating estrogen in women.[6–9] Soybeans contain natural chemicals called isoflavones, a class of plant compounds that have weak estrogen activity in the body. One of the main isoflavones in soybeans, called genistein, is able to compete with a woman's own estrogen for binding to estrogen receptors. In so doing, soy isoflavones are able to reduce the amount of estrogen that contacts breast cells.

One study found that women who added soy isoflavones to their diet experienced significantly less breast tenderness than women who added a milk-protein placebo. Another study of 64 premenopausal women revealed that after one year of daily supplementation with a soy protein powder, women and their physicians reported a consistent reduction in breast tenderness and fibrocystic breast changes.[10,11]

Here are a few ideas to help you add soy foods to your menu:

- Pour a calcium-fortified soy beverage on breakfast cereal or in a smoothie, and use it in cooking and baking (soups, casseroles, muffins, pancake batters).
- Cube firm tofu and add it to canned or homemade soups.
- Grill firm tofu on the barbecue. Brush tofu and vegetable kebabs with hoisin sauce or marinate them in teriyaki sauce.
- Substitute firm tofu for ricotta cheese in recipes.
- Use soft tofu in creamy salad dressing or dip recipes.
- Throw canned soybeans, drained and rinsed, in a salad, soup or chili.
- Replace up to one-half of all-purpose flour in a recipe with soy flour.
- Buy roasted soy nuts in health food stores. They come in plain, barbecue, garlic or onion flavours. Enjoy 1/4 cup (60 ml) as a midday snack. Toss roasted soy nuts in a green salad.
- Replace ground meat with soy ground round in chili, pasta sauce and tacos.

Flaxseed

Ground flaxseed is a rich source of lignans, natural plant compounds that help to lower circulating levels of estrogen and, as a result, may help ease breast symptoms. A Canadian review of treatment strategies for fibrocystic breast conditions concluded that flaxseed should be considered a first-line treatment for cyclic mastalgia.[12] Add 2 tablespoons (30 ml) of ground flaxseed to your daily diet. Add ground flaxseed to hot cereal, smoothies, yogurt, applesauce, casseroles, muffin and pancake batters, and other baked-good recipes.

Caffeine

It's been thought for some time that caffeine plays a role in fibrocystic breast conditions. The interest in caffeine dates back to the late 1970s and early 1980s, when researchers noted higher intakes of caffeine in women with fibrocystic breast conditions. It has been hypothesized that caffeine causes an abnormally high level of energy compounds called cAMP in cells, which may lead to symptoms.

Studies over the past decade have failed to find a relationship between caffeine intake and the development of fibrocystic breast conditions. Drinking coffee may, however, make your symptoms worse. A study from Duke University in Durham, North Carolina, asked 147 women with fibrocystic breast conditions to abstain from caffeine-containing foods, beverages and medication. Among those women who successfully removed caffeine for one year, 69 percent reported a decrease or absence of breast pain.[13]

Cutting back on caffeine certainly can't hurt. In addition to easing breast symptoms, removing caffeine can also help you sleep better (read chapter 6, Insomnia). Currently, Health Canada recommends a daily maximum of 450 milligrams of caffeine for good health. Although your goal is to limit caffeine intake as much as possible, use this amount as a benchmark to see how much you're consuming now. A list of caffeine-containing foods and beverages can be found in Chapter 1, page 11. Eliminate caffeine for three months before you assess its effect on reducing your symptoms.

VITAMINS AND MINERALS
Vitamin E
This nutrient has long been promoted to help alleviate fibrocystic breast conditions; its use in treating this disorder dates back to the 1960s. Vitamin E has been claimed to alter blood levels of certain hormones, especially progesterone, but this hasn't yet been proven. A few small studies from the early 1980s did find that vitamin E was effective in reducing symptoms.[14,15] However, subsequent well-designed studies that looked at the effect of 150, 300 and 600 international units (IU) of vitamin E in larger numbers of women found no effect on breast pain or lumps. These studies lasted only two or three months, and it's possible that vitamin E might be beneficial if taken for a longer period of time.

Although the evidence doesn't support the use of vitamin E supplements for managing fibrocystic breast conditions, it's certainly worth a try. If you decide to take them, here's what you need to know:

- Take a supplement that provides 400 IU per day. Some research hints that high doses of vitamin E may do more harm than good, especially in people who have diabetes or heart disease. If you have existing cardiovascular disease or diabetes, avoid high-dose vitamin E supplements; if you do take a supplement, take no more than 100 IU per day.
- Buy a natural source vitamin E supplement (look for *d-alpha-tocopherol* on the label; synthetic forms are labelled *dl-alpha tocopherol*). Although the body absorbs both synthetic and natural forms equally well, studies suggest that your liver prefers the natural form. It incorporates more natural vitamin E into transport molecules.
- The daily upper limit for vitamin E is 1000 IU (natural) or 1500 IU (synthetic).
- If you're on blood-thinning medication like Coumadin (warfarin), don't take vitamin E since it also has slight anti-clotting properties. Talk to your doctor before adding any supplement to your regime.
- Don't forget about food. Although dietary sources of vitamin E can't give you 400 IU per day, vitamin E–rich foods like vegetable oils, nuts, seeds, wheat germ and leafy green vegetables have plenty of other protective nutrients and natural plant compounds.

HERBAL REMEDIES
Evening primrose *(Oenothera biennis)* oil
This over-the-counter nutritional supplement is derived from a native North American plant with brightly coloured yellow flowers. The oil from evening primrose is a rich source of a fatty acid called gamma linoleic acid (GLA). GLA is an omega-6 fatty acid our bodies produce from linoleic acid, an essential fat found in corn, sunflower and safflower oils.

By providing the body with GLA, evening primrose oil may ease breast pain and tenderness in two ways. GLA is a polyunsaturated fat, which means it belongs to a class of fats with a different chemical structure from saturated fats (found in meat and dairy products). As a result, they behave differently in the body. Taking evening primrose oil is thought to increase the ratio of polyunsaturated to saturated fats in the body. Some experts believe that if saturated fats dominate, your body will be overly sensitive to hormones like estrogen. That's because hormones made from saturated fat are more potent and attach more readily to receptors. What's more, a diet that's high in saturated fat is also believed to impair the conversion of dietary linoleic acid to GLA inside the body. Interestingly, research has found abnormally high levels of saturated fatty acids in women with fibrocystic breast conditions.

Supplementing with evening primrose oil may also alter your body's production of hormone-like compounds called prostaglandins. There are many prostaglandins made in the body: Some are inflammatory and may cause breast pain; others are considered friendly, as they don't lead to inflammation. GLA produces a special class of friendly prostaglandins called PGE1. These prostaglandins are also thought to reduce the activity of prolactin, a hormone that may be involved in fibrocystic breast conditions.

There's some research to support using evening primrose oil for breast pain and tenderness. An early review of studies conducted in 291 women with persistent breast pain found evening primrose oil to be beneficial in easing symptoms.[16] However, more recent trials have not found evening primrose oil to be any more effective at reducing breast tenderness and pain than the placebo treatment. Despite this, many women do find supplementing with evening primrose oil eases their symptoms, so if you experience cyclic breast pain, it's worth trying.

The recommended dose of evening primrose oil is 3 to 4 grams daily. Take two 1000 milligram capsules twice daily. The capsules are available in 500 milligram and 1000 milligram (1 gram) doses. Buy a supplement that's standardized to 9 to 10 percent GLA.

Evening primrose oil is very safe; it has been used in many studies without reports of side effects. Keep in mind that it may take three menstrual cycles before you feel the effects of evening primrose oil, and up to eight months for the supplement to reach its full effect.

Ginkgo biloba

Besides protecting your brain cells from the hands of time, ginkgo might also help reduce symptoms of fibrocystic breast conditions. French researchers studied 143 women with PMS and found that ginkgo biloba significantly reduced PMS-related breast tenderness (as well as abdominal bloating and swollen hands, legs and feet).[17] The women took ginkgo on day 16 of their cycle and continued until day 5 of the next cycle, at which time they stopped. They resumed taking the herb again on day 16.

The recommended dose of ginkgo is 80 milligrams taken twice daily. Start on day 16 (counting from the first day of your period) and continue until day 5 of the next cycle. This means you'll take ginkgo for roughly eighteen days each month. To buy a high-quality product, choose one standardized to 24 percent ginkgo flavone glycosides.

On rare occasions, ginkgo may cause gastrointestinal upset, headache or an allergic skin reaction in susceptible individuals. Ginkgo shouldn't be taken with blood-thinning drugs such as Coumadin (warfarin) or heparin without medical supervision. Ginkgo may enhance the blood-thinning effect of other natural health products (like vitamin E or garlic), so be sure to inform your physician and pharmacist if you're taking a number of these supplements.

THE BOTTOM LINE...
Leslie's recommendations for fibrocystic breast conditions

1. Adopt a low-fat diet. Start by using little or no added fats with foods and in cooking. Read labels on packages of commercial foods—look for no more than 2 grams of fat per 100 calories (this means it has 20 percent fat from calories).
2. Boost your intake of dietary fibre, especially wheat bran. Start by reaching for a bowl of high-fibre breakfast cereal.
3. To help lower the amount of estrogen that comes in contact with your breast cells, consider adding soy foods to your daily diet.
4. If you suffer from breast pain, swelling or lumpiness, eliminate all sources of caffeine from your diet for at least three months.
5. If you're not already taking this supplement, consider adding 400 international units (IU) of vitamin E to your daily nutrition regime. Buy a natural source vitamin E pill. Consider a vitamin E that provides "mixed tocopherols" or "mixed vitamin E." The daily upper limit for vitamin E is 1000 IU (natural) or 1500 IU (synthetic). Don't take single vitamin E supplements if you have heart disease or diabetes.
6. If you have cyclic or non-cyclic breast pain, take evening primrose oil. Buy a product standardized to contain 9 percent GLA. Take 1-1/2 to 2 grams in the morning and 1-1/2 to 2 grams in the evening for a total of 3 to 4 grams per day. Wait at least three menstrual cycles to see if your symptoms improve.

7. Consider trying ginkgo biloba. Buy a product standardized to 24 percent ginkgo flavone glycosides. Take 80 milligrams twice daily. Start on day 16 of your cycle (counting from the first day of your period) and continue until day 5 of the next cycle. Don't use ginkgo if you're pregnant or breastfeeding.

11

Osteoporosis

Osteoporosis can strike women at any age, but it's more prevalent after menopause. One in every four Canadian women over the age of 50 has osteoporosis, a disease of fragile, brittle bones that are more likely to break. Bone fractures are increasing at a faster rate than ever. By the age of 50, the average Caucasian woman has a 40 percent chance of suffering at least one fracture caused by brittle bones. In fact, the risk of getting a fracture is at least five times the risk of developing breast cancer. You may not realize it, but more women die each year as a result of fractures from osteoporosis than from breast and ovarian cancer combined.

What causes osteoporosis?

Osteoporosis is characterized by low bone density, or mass, and deterioration of existing bone tissue. Bones become weaker and more susceptible to fractures. The definition of osteoporosis emphasizes not only low bone density but also fracture risk. Although many bone fractures are not life threatening, the impact that fractures have on health is underappreciated. For instance, hip fractures lead to death in 20 percent of cases. And close to one-half of elderly women who fracture their hips lose their ability to live independently.

Throughout childhood, bones grow in length and density. At some point in adolescence, bones stop growing in length but continue to increase in density, though at a slower rate. Then, by around age 25, bones achieve what's called their peak mass and stop building density. Peak bone mass is determined largely by genetics, but nutrition and other lifestyle factors, such as medications, determine whether or not you'll achieve your body's genetically programmed peak bone mass.

Once achieved, peak bone mass is maintained for about ten years. After age 35, both men and women normally lose 0.3 percent to 0.5 percent of their bone density per year. For women, though, when estrogen levels drop after menopause, bone loss accelerates and they can lose up to 4 percent of their bone density each year.

Ten years after menopause, the rate of bone loss diminishes to about 0.5 percent per year, but during that decade women have the potential to very quickly lose up to 25 percent to 30 percent of their bone density. Accelerated loss of bone density after menopause is a major cause of osteoporosis.

Despite its "dead" appearance, bone is very active tissue that contains two types of cells. *Osteoclasts* are bone cells that break down bone tissue by removing its mineral content—a process called bone resorption. For example, osteoclasts go to work when your diet lacks calcium; these bone cells release calcium from the bone into the blood for important body functions. *Osteoblasts* are cells that form bone; they're responsible for building the support structure of bones, as well as adding minerals to strengthen bones. Your bones are constantly going through a bone-remodelling cycle: Osteoclast cells resorb bone and osteoblast cells build bone.

HORMONES AND BONE HEALTH

By affecting how your body uses calcium, many different hormones influence whether bones are being broken down or rebuilt. The main players in calcium and bone metabolism are parathyroid hormone, vitamin D, calcitonin and thyroid hormones, but steroid drugs and estrogen also play a role.

1. **Parathyroid hormone** (PTH) is secreted by your parathyroid gland. Its job is to keep your blood-calcium level stable. Because calcium is critical for blood clotting, muscle contraction and the transmission of nerve impulses, a constant amount of the mineral must be circulated throughout your body at all times. When blood calcium falls too low because you're not consuming enough calcium in your diet, PTH tells your kidneys to stop excreting calcium. PTH also activates vitamin D in your body, and vitamin D, in turn, causes your intestine to absorb more dietary calcium. And finally, PTH instructs your osteoclasts (bone breakdown cells) to release calcium from your bones into your bloodstream. The net result is bone loss.

2. **Calcitonin** is secreted by your thyroid gland in response to a high calcium level in the bloodstream. This hormone lowers calcium to a

normal level by stopping the action of osteoclasts and stimulating the osteoblasts to build new bone. The osteoblasts take calcium from the blood to increase bone density. Calcitonin levels decline with age and with menopause.

3. **Thyroid hormones** can also have an impact on bone loss. Too much of this hormone from an overactive thyroid gland (hyperthyroid) or too much thyroid medication causes a higher rate of bone breakdown. If you take Synthroid (levothyroxine) for an underactive thyroid gland (hypothyroid), your doctor will check your thyroid hormone levels regularly. If your level is too high, your medication will be adjusted.

4. **Steroid drugs** such as glucocorticoids (e.g., prednisone), used to treat inflammatory conditions like rheumatoid arthritis, lupus and colitis, also increase the rate of bone loss. A side effect of these drugs is their ability to enhance the action of PTH on bone. Given how PTH works, that means your bones will mobilize more calcium into your bloodstream.

5. **Estrogen**, on the other hand, acts to protect bones. This hormone seems to be able to prevent the osteoclasts from releasing calcium from the bone into the bloodstream. Estrogen also causes calcitonin and vitamin D to be released, stimulating new bone growth.

Symptoms

Osteoporosis is a silent disease because bone loss occurs without symptoms. A woman may not know she has the disease until she breaks a bone. The outward signs of osteoporosis are usually not apparent until the disease is quite advanced. Signs that you may have osteoporosis include:

- a broken wrist or rib from a slight blow
- a broken hip
- back pain in the mid to lower spine
- loss of more than 1 inch (2.5 cm) of height
- a stooped or hunched-over appearance
- a hump forming in the upper back

You may notice your clothes, which once fit properly, now fit or hang differently due to a loss of height, more rounded shoulders or a change in your posture.

Who's at risk?

The strength of your bones is determined by (1) their bone mineral density, (2) their rate of self-healing and (3) the integrity of their support structures. Anything that jeopardizes these three factors can increase the odds of getting osteoporosis. Here's a list of known risk factors:

- older age
- low bone density
- being female
- thin and small body frame
- deficiency of estrogen (early or surgical menopause)
- cigarette smoking
- low intake of calcium
- vitamin D deficiency
- excessive alcohol and caffeine consumption
- lack of exercise
- certain medications (e.g., corticosteroids, chemotherapy)
- prolonged immobilization
- family history of osteoporosis
- previous bone fracture as an adult
- certain health conditions (e.g., kidney failure, hyperthyroidism, rheumatoid arthritis, malabsorption states)

Diagnosis

The only way doctors can get a sense of what's happening to your bone is by taking repeated measures of your bone mineral density using a test called the dual-energy X-ray absorptiometry (DEXA). The DEXA test can detect as little as a 1 percent change in bone density. What this test can't do, however, is detect bone fractures. And it doesn't measure bone density in the upper spine, where a series of small fractures can result in shrinking and a dowager's hump, the characteristic hunching of the spine seen in osteoporosis. Doctors use X-rays to detect these types of fractures in your upper spine.

The DEXA test is simple, fast and absolutely painless. You don't even have to undress. To have your lower spine or hip scanned, you lie comfortably on a flat, padded table. Food doesn't interfere with the test results, so you don't have to fast the night before the test. However, you shouldn't take a calcium supplement right before since an undigested pill can be measured as part of your bone density—when you're lying down, your intestines lie on top of your spine.

Once you have the scan, you'll receive a DEXA bone density report. This is a computer-generated image of four vertebrae in your lower spine (L1, L2, L3 and L4). The computer calculates how much bone mineral is present in each single vertebrae and then calculates an average bone mineral density (BMD) for the three vertebrae L2–L4.

Your DEXA bone density test results are then compared to the bone density of a healthy 30-year-old woman. If your Young Adult Comparison for your lower spine (L2–L4) is 88 percent, this means that your bone density is 88 percent of that of the average 30-year-old woman. In other words, you've lost 12 percent of your bone density. Compared to a woman who still has the bone density of a 30 year old, your risk of bone fracture doubles for every 10 percent loss of bone density.

Bone density results are also presented as a T score. The T score is the number of levels (standard deviations) your bone density is away from that of a 30-year-old woman. If you're one level away, your T score is 1.0, and you're considered to have osteopenia, or decreased bone mass. If your test results show that your bones are more than 2.5 levels away, you have osteoporosis. If your score is higher still and you have one or more tiny fractures, then you're considered to have severe osteoporosis. If you're over 65 years old, osteopenia doubles your risk for fracture, osteoporosis quadruples it and severe osteoporosis increases the risk of bone fracture twentyfold.

You'll also notice an Aged Matched Comparison on your report. This compares your bone density to what is expected for your age. If your Aged Matched Comparison is unusually low, your doctor will endeavour to determine what's causing this bone loss.

If you've not yet had a DEXA test, speak to your doctor about having the test if you fall into one of the following categories:

• You're approaching menopause and deciding about hormone replacement therapy (HRT). A bone density test can help you decide whether or not HRT is needed to prevent osteoporosis.
• You have a strong family history of osteoporosis or multiple bone fractures.

- You have premature menopause (younger than 45 years old).
- You've been on corticosteroid drugs for a medical condition for three months or longer (e.g., 7.5 milligrams of prednisone).
- You've experienced long-standing malnutrition or malabsorption (e.g., history of anorexia nervosa, celiac disease, Crohn's disease).
- You have a low body weight.
- You have hyperthyroidism.

Your first bone density test serves as a baseline that your future test results will be compared to. If at the age of 50 your first test indicates low bone mass, that doesn't mean you have osteoporosis. It may be that you're a slow loser, and later tests will find that your bone mineral content has not changed very much. Bone density tests must be repeated every two years to detect a bone loss of 2 percent to 3 percent. If future tests show that your bone density has declined rapidly between tests, your doctor will likely recommend drug treatment to slow the rate of bone loss.

Conventional treatment

The goal of osteoporosis treatment is to prevent bone fractures by stopping bone loss and increasing bone density and strength. In addition to the medications listed below, lifestyle changes such as quitting smoking, moderating alcohol intake and exercising regularly play important roles in the treatment—and prevention—of osteoporosis. (If you have osteo-porosis, speak to your doctor about which types of exercise are safe and won't injure already weakened bones.)

HORMONE REPLACEMENT THERAPY (HRT)

Many studies have shown that hormone replacement therapy (HRT) protects the bones of women. Both estrogen pills and estrogen patches have been found to decrease bone loss, reduce fractures and prevent the loss of height. Estrogen replacement prevents bone loss at any point a woman starts to take it. However, the longer a woman waits after menopause, the greater the chance she'll lose some bone permanently. And once a woman stops taking estrogen, bone loss occurs: Estrogen's protec-tive effect lasts only as long as the estrogen is taken.

Although studies do find that estrogen delays bone loss, recent clinical trials have not found this medication to be effective in preventing bone fractures. The Heart and Estrogen/Progestin Replacement Study (HERS) followed over 2700 post-menopausal women who didn't have osteoporosis and found no significant difference in hip or spine fracture rates among women taking HRT and those not taking the drugs.[1] Experts believe that HRT may reduce bone fractures only in women who have defined osteoporosis when they start on the medication.

Although estrogen therapy might be effective in treating osteoporosis, due to adverse effects such as increased risks of heart attack, stroke, blood clots and breast cancer, HRT is no longer recommended for long-term use in osteoporosis. Rather, it's used in the short term for relief of menopausal hot flashes.

BISPHOSPHONATES

This class of non-hormonal drugs offers an alternative to HRT for both men and women with low bone density or osteoporosis. Bisphosphonate drugs prevent bone breakdown by binding to the bone surface and inhibiting the activity of osteoclasts, the cells that strip down old bone. Studies have demonstrated their ability to reduce the risk of fracture to the hip, wrist and spine in post-menopausal women with osteoporosis. Types of bisphosphonates include Didrocal (etidronate and calcium carbonate), Fosamax (alendronate) and Actonel (risedronate).

SELECTIVE ESTROGEN RECEPTOR MODULATORS (SERMs)

Often called "designer estrogen," these medications offer all the beneficial effects of estrogen (bone protection, cholesterol lowering) without any of its negative effects (increased breast cancer risk, endometrial bleeding). SERMs such as Evista (raloxifene) have the favourable effects of estrogen on bone and act as an anti-estrogen in the breast and the lining of the uterus. Because of the anti-estrogen effects, hot flashes are a common side effect.

Managing and preventing osteoporosis

Ideally, every woman's goal should be to eat well and exercise regularly in order to (1) build bone density in her teens and twenties to achieve her peak bone mass, and (2) slow down, as much as possible, age-related bone loss during her thirties, forties and fifties so that bone-sparing medication is not necessary after menopause. Unfortunately, this isn't always the case.

Some women with low bone density and/or fractures do require drugs to halt bone loss and reduce the risk of bone fracture. Even if you're taking medication for osteoporosis, diet and nutrition can still influence your bone density. Here are some key nutrition strategies to help you delay bone loss. Remember, it's never too late to start paying attention.

DIETARY STRATEGIES
Soy foods

Soybeans contain naturally occurring compounds called isoflavones, a type of plant estrogen. Genistein and daidzein are the most active isoflavones in soy, and have been the focus of much research. Isoflavones have a chemical structure similar to estrogen and so they're able to bind to estrogen receptors in the body. It's the action of isoflavones on estrogen receptors in the bone that scientists believe may be responsible for soy's potential bone-preserving effect.

The interest in soybeans and osteoporosis began when researchers observed that populations that consume soy foods on a regular basis report much lower rates of hip fracture. Since then, soy foods and their naturally occurring phytoestrogens have been the focus of many studies. Although some studies find soy has no effect on bone loss, others show a significant bone-sparing effect.

A three-month study conducted at Iowa State University found that 40 grams of phytoestrogen-rich soy protein powder prevented bone loss in post-menopausal women.[2] Women in this study who instead were given whey protein powder (a protein made from milk) showed significant bone loss in the lower spine. Another study from the Department of Obstetrics and Gynecology, Internal Medicine and Pediatrics at the University of Cincinnati College of Medicine found that 60 to 70 milligrams of soy isoflavones, consumed as So Good soy beverage and soy nuts, significantly decreased bone turnover in post-menopausal women.[3] The researchers found that osteoblast (bone building) activity increased by 10.2 percent and osteoclast (bone breakdown) activity decreased by 13.9 percent. Reduced bone turnover was seen after four weeks of eating soy foods.

More recent research has also revealed favourable effects of soy on bone health. A 2008 review of nine studies with a total of 432 participants found that soy isoflavones significantly inhibited bone breakdown and stimulated bone formation.[4] Another combined analysis of ten studies conducted in 608 subjects concluded that soy isoflavones were effective in slowing bone loss of the spine in menopausal women. This effect became more pronounced when more than 90 milligrams of soy isoflavones were consumed each day.[5] However, one recent clinical trial conducted in 237 healthy early post-menopausal women found that consuming 110 milligrams of soy isoflavones each day didn't prevent post-menopausal bone loss.[6]

To reap the potential bone-preserving benefits of soy, aim for a daily intake of 90 milligrams of isoflavones. To keep your blood levels of isoflavones up through the day, consume soy foods twice daily. Depending on the food you eat, your blood-isoflavone levels will peak four to eight hours later. Twenty-four hours after eating a soy food, your body will have excreted these isoflavones. (If you're at high risk for breast cancer, don't add soy to your daily diet. See Chapter 9, Breast Cancer, for a discussion on soy and breast cancer risk.)

Soy foods vary with respect to the amount of isoflavones they contain. Even the same type of food made by different manufacturers can differ in isoflavone content. Here's a general guide to soy foods and their isoflavone content.

Isoflavone Content of Selected Soy Foods

Soy food	Serving size	Isoflavone content (milligrams)
Roasted soy nuts	1/4 cup (60 ml)	40–60 mg
Soybeans, cooked or canned	1/2 cup (125 ml)	14 mg
Soy flour	1/4 cup (60 ml)	28 mg
Soy beverage, most brands	1 cup (250 ml)	20–25 mg
Soy beverage, So Nice	1 cup (250 ml)	60 mg
Soy hot dog	1	15 mg
Soy protein isolate powder	1 oz (30 g)	30 mg
Tempeh, cooked	3 oz (90 g)	48 mg
Texturized vegetable protein, dry	1/2 cup (125 ml)	30–120 mg
Tofu, firm	3 oz (90 g)	22 mg
Tofu, soft	3 oz (90 g)	28 mg

Source: USDA Database for the Isoflavone Content of Selected Foods, Release 2.0, September 2008. Available at: www.ars.usda.gov/SP2UserFiles/Place/12354500/Data/isoflav/Isoflav_R2.pdf.

Protein-rich foods

Eating too much protein may be part of the reason why North American women have high rates of osteoporosis, despite our moderate-to-high calcium intakes. Studies have shown that high levels of dietary protein cause calcium to be excreted by the kidneys. The effect of eating large quantities of protein is rapid, and it appears that the body doesn't correct for this by absorbing more calcium from food. The protein effect may be very important for people who consume very little calcium or for those who, because of intestinal problems, absorb very little calcium.

While eating very large amounts of protein may not be good for your bones, eating too little isn't healthy either. Protein is an important structural component of bone, and studies have shown that missing out on this important nutrient might actually increase the risk of hip fracture. The Iowa Women's Health Study found that dietary protein protected post-menopausal women from hip fracture. Women who ate the most protein had a 69 percent reduced risk of hip fracture compared to women who ate the least.[7] Another study found that consuming 72 grams of protein each day was associated with high bone densities among women who consumed more than 400 milligrams of calcium daily.[8] Women who ate the most protein had a 69 percent reduced risk of hip fracture compared with women who ate the least. Studies have also found that when protein supplements are given to patients with hip fracture, bone density is increased and the rate of complications and death are reduced immediately after surgery and for six months afterward.[9,10]

Based on these studies, it seems clear that it's important to be meeting your daily requirement for protein. Women at risk for protein deficiency include:

- those who seldom eat meat, chicken or fish
- those who frequently grab quick meals during the day—bagels, pasta, low-fat frozen dinners
- vegetarians who don't eat animal foods and don't regularly incorporate high-quality vegetable protein sources, such as legumes and soy, into their diet
- those who engage in heavy exercise and fall into any of the above categories

To find out how much protein you need every day, see Chapter 5, page 98.

Alcoholic beverages

Many studies have determined that chronic alcohol abuse depletes bone density. Alcohol acts directly on your bones and suppresses bone formation. Consuming alcohol also increases the risk of falls in post-menopausal women and is associated with an increased incidence of hip fractures. If you drink alcohol, limit your intake to no more than seven drinks per week.

Caffeine

Drinking coffee, tea or colas increases the amount of calcium your kidneys excrete in your urine. This increased calcium excretion continues up to three hours after consuming caffeine. For every 6 ounce (180 ml) cup of coffee you drink, approximately 48 milligrams of calcium is leached from your bones.

The effects of caffeine are likely most detrimental for women who aren't meeting their requirements for calcium. One study found that 400 milligrams of caffeine caused calcium loss in women whose daily diet had less than 600 milligrams of calcium.[11] Another study, from Tufts University in Boston, found that women who consumed less than 800 milligrams of calcium and 450 milligrams of caffeine (about three small cups of coffee) had significantly lower bone densities than women who consumed the same amount of caffeine but more than 800 milligrams of calcium.[12] Interestingly, researchers found that habitual caffeine intake was not linked to lower bone densities in young women aged 14 to 40.[13]

If you consume caffeinated beverages, the following strategies will help maintain bone density:

- If you drink coffee, make sure you're meeting your calcium requirements of 1000 or 1500 milligrams a day, depending on your age.
- Add 3 tablespoons (45 ml) of milk or calcium-fortified soy beverage (58 mg calcium) to every cup of regular coffee you drink.
- Don't consume more than 450 milligrams of caffeine a day. If you have osteoporosis, aim for no more than 200 milligrams (see Chapter 1, page 11, to find out how foods and beverages rate with respect to caffeine content).

- If you drink caffeine-containing beverages throughout the day, cut them out after noon. Instead, try water, herbal tea, vegetable juice, milk or a glass of soy beverage.
- Replace coffee with tea, which has substantially less caffeine.
- Instead of black coffee, try a calcium-rich latte made with milk or fortified soy beverage.

VITAMINS AND MINERALS
Calcium
The fact that calcium is the most abundant mineral in the body and that 99 percent of it is housed within the bones and teeth underlines the importance of dietary calcium to bone health. During the bone-building process, the osteoblast cells secrete bone mineral, consisting of calcium and phosphorus, which strengthens the bone. By providing structural integrity to bones, dietary calcium plays a critical role in preventing osteoporosis.

The remaining 1 percent of the body's calcium circulates in the bloodstream and is vital to the functioning of the heart, nervous system and muscles. The body keeps this circulating pool of calcium at a constant level. If your diet lacks calcium and your blood-calcium level drops, your body releases parathyroid hormone (PTH), which returns calcium to your blood by taking it from the bones. When you shortchange your diet of calcium, you shortchange your bones too.

Research supports using calcium supplements to lower the risk of osteoporosis. Researchers at the University of Texas Southwestern Medical Center in Dallas found that a 400 milligram calcium citrate supplement taken twice daily increased bone density in healthy post-menopausal women.[14] In contrast, women in the placebo group experienced a 2.38 percent bone density reduction in the lower spine.

Scientists at the University of Massachusetts studied 98 pre-menopausal women (average age 39) and found that those who received 500 milligrams of calcium carbonate daily increased their bone density by 0.3 percent per year.[15] The women in the placebo group lost bone at a rate of 0.4 percent per year in the hip and 0.7 percent in the neck. A number of studies have also shown that older women who take calcium and vitamin D supplements have a lower incidence of non-vertebral fractures.

The recommended dietary allowance (RDA) for calcium is 1000 milligrams (women aged 19 to 50) or 1500 milligrams (women aged 50 and older) per day. However, if you are under 50 and have low bone density, be sure to get 1500 milligrams of calcium daily. The best food sources include milk, yogurt, cheese, fortified soy beverages, fortified orange juice, tofu, salmon (with bones), kale, bok choy, broccoli and Swiss chard. (See Chapter 1, page 15, to learn the calcium content of various foods.)

Your body doesn't absorb calcium from all foods equally well. Although many plant foods contribute calcium to the diet, some natural compounds in vegetables prevent some of this calcium from being absorbed. Studies show that dairy products contain the most absorbable form of calcium. The following strategies will help you enhance your body's absorption of calcium:

• Cook green vegetables in order to boost their calcium content by releasing calcium that's bound to oxalic acid.
• Don't take iron supplements with calcium-rich foods, as iron competes with calcium for absorption.
• Drink tea between rather than during meals. Tannins, natural compounds in tea, inhibit calcium absorption.
• Make sure you're meeting dietary requirements for vitamin D each day (as you read earlier in this chapter, vitamin D stimulates the intestine to absorb dietary calcium).

Calcium supplements

Studies support using calcium supplements to lower your risk of osteoporosis. Also, supplementation may reduce the risk of bone fracture among people with osteoporosis. A recent review of 29 studies concluded that taking calcium alone, or in combination with vitamin D, reduced the rate of bone loss and fractures of all types in people aged 50 and older.[16]

Most women I see in my private practice aren't meeting their daily calcium needs and should be taking a calcium supplement. Women may find it difficult to meet their calcium goals if they are lactose intolerant, don't like dairy products, are following a vegan diet or have poor eating habits. In these cases, supplements are often the only way that I can ensure a client is meeting her calcium needs. Which calcium product you choose will depend on convenience, absorbability and tolerance. In Chapter 1, page 17, you'll find a description of common calcium supplements and guidelines for supplementing safely.

Vitamin D

In addition to getting too little calcium, experts cite a silent epidemic of vitamin D deficiency as a contributing factor to osteoporosis. Vitamin D makes calcium and phosphorus available in the blood that bathes the bones, so that they can be deposited as bones harden or mineralize. Vitamin D raises blood levels of calcium in three ways: It stimulates your intestine to absorb more dietary calcium; it tells your kidneys to retain calcium; and it withdraws calcium from your bones if your diet is lacking this mineral. A vitamin D deficiency speeds up bone loss and increases the risk of fracture at a younger age.

Vitamin D is different from any other nutrient because the body can synthesize it from sunlight. When ultraviolet light hits the skin, a pre–vitamin D is formed. This compound eventually makes its way to the kidneys, where it's transformed into active vitamin D. However, the long winter months in Canada result in very little vitamin D being synthesized by the skin. Researchers from Tufts University in Boston have demonstrated that blood levels of vitamin D are at their lowest between February and March and peak in June and July.[17] (Although this is an American study, the findings hold true for Canadians.) But even in the summer, your body might not be making enough vitamin D, since sun protection factor (SPF) in sunscreen blocks production of the vitamin. To help you meet your vitamin D requirements, expose your hands, face and arms to sunlight without sunscreen for 10 to 15 minutes, two or three times a week.

The recommended daily intake is 1000 international units (IU) for adults and 400 IU for children. Best food sources are fluid milk, fortified soy and rice beverages, oily fish, egg yolks, butter and margarine. However, it's not possible for adults to consume 1000 IU each day from foods alone. For this reason, it's necessary to take a vitamin D supplement in the fall and winter, and year-round if you are over the age of 50, have dark-coloured skin, don't expose your skin to sunshine in the summer months or go outdoors often, or wear clothing that covers most of your skin.

To determine the extra dose of vitamin D you need to take, add up how much you're already getting from your multivitamin and calcium supplements; the difference between that and the daily recommended 1000 IU is the extra dosage of vitamin D you need. Choose a vitamin D supplement that contains vitamin D3 instead of vitamin D2, which is less potent. Vitamin D is typically sold in 400 IU and 1000 IU doses; there's no need to be concerned if your intake exceeds 1000 IU slightly. The current safe upper limit—which vitamin D experts feel is far too low—is set at 2000 IU per day.

Other nutrients

Calcium and vitamin D are critical to healthy bones, but other nutrients are also important components of the nutrient team that orchestrates the continual process of bone building and bone breakdown.

Vitamin A

This vitamin supports bone growth and development. Degradative enzymes in osteoclast cells use vitamin A to break down old bone in order to build new bone. Bone growth relies on this vitamin, as evidenced by children with a vitamin A deficiency who fail to grow properly.

However, although we need some vitamin A for good health, too much may actually decrease bone density and increase the risk of hip fracture.[18,19] Researchers from Harvard University found that among 73,000 post-menopausal women, those who consumed more than 1.5 milligrams (5000 IU) of vitamin A each day, from food and supplements combined, had a significantly higher risk of hip fracture than women who consumed less than 0.5 milligrams (1665 IU) each day.[20] A study from Sweden found similar results with respect to the harmful effects of too much vitamin A. The researchers found that women who consumed more than 1.5 milligrams versus less than 0.5 milligrams of vitamin A each day had lower bone densities of the neck and spine and were twice as likely to suffer a hip fracture.[21]

High blood levels of vitamin A stimulate bone breakdown and, based on a growing body of evidence, increase the risk of bone fracture. Vitamin A is found preformed in animal foods such as fortified milk, cheese, butter, eggs and liver. It's absorbed as retinol, the most active form of vitamin A. Unless you eat liver frequently or drink in excess of five glasses of milk each day, your diet is unlikely to cause high levels of vitamin A in your body. Taking vitamin A supplements, however, can result in excessive vitamin A accumulating in the body. Don't take single vitamin A supplements; choose a multivitamin that contains no more than 2500 IU of vitamin A (as retinol or retinyl palmitate).

Beta carotene–rich fruit and vegetables also contribute to our daily vitamin A requirements, since some beta carotene is converted to vitamin A in the body. The best sources of beta carotene include carrots, winter squash, sweet potato, spinach, broccoli, rapini, romaine lettuce, apricots, peaches, mango, papaya and cantaloupe. There's no evidence that beta carotene is harmful to bones.

Vitamin C

A number of studies of post-menopausal women have linked higher intakes of vitamin C with having a higher bone density. One study revealed that women aged 55 to 64 who had taken vitamin C supplements for at least ten years had significantly higher bone mass compared to women who had not supplemented their diet.[22] Vitamin C is important for the formation of collagen, a tissue that lends support to bones. This vitamin may also protect bones by acting as an antioxidant and modifying the negative effect of cigarette smoking on bones—many studies have shown that cigarette smoking reduces bone density and increases the risk of fracture.

To get more vitamin C in your diet, reach for citrus fruit, cantaloupe, mango, strawberries, broccoli, Brussels sprouts, cauliflower, red pepper and tomato juice. The RDA is 75 milligrams for non-smoking women and 110 milligrams for smokers. To put that in perspective, one medium orange gives you 70 milligrams of vitamin C, and 1/2 cup (125 ml) of red pepper packs 95 milligrams. If you don't think you consume enough vitamin C in your diet, take a multivitamin and mineral pill each day.

Vitamin K

You've probably heard very little about this fat-soluble vitamin. One of the reasons for its low profile is that vitamin K deficiency is hardly ever seen—the millions of bacteria in our intestinal tract synthesize the vitamin. Once we absorb this manufactured vitamin K, it's stored in the liver. The vitamin is not a part of the bone mineral complex. Instead, it helps make a bone protein called osteocalcin. Doctors can measure the amount of osteocalcin in your blood. A high level indicates that your osteoblasts are busy making new bone. Without enough vitamin K, the bones produce an abnormal protein that cannot bind to the minerals that form the bones. The best food sources of vitamin K are leafy green vegetables, cabbage, milk and liver.

When it comes to bone health, the importance of vitamin K shouldn't be underestimated. The large, ongoing Nurses' Health Study from Harvard University found that women with the highest intake of vitamin K had a significantly lower rate of hip fracture compared with women who consumed the least. Eating lettuce was also linked with fewer hip fractures: Lettuce accounted for most of the vitamin K in their diet. Those women who ate 1 or more servings of the leafy green each day (versus 1 or fewer servings a week) had a 45 percent lower risk of hip fractures.[23] A study of elderly men and women also reported low vitamin K intakes were associated with a greater risk of hip fracture.[24]

The best sources of vitamin K are leafy green vegetables, including arugula, beet greens, kale, rapini, Swiss chard and spinach. Most of us don't get enough vitamin K in our diet. The recommended daily intake of vitamin K is 90 and 120 micrograms for women and men, respectively. This amount is designed to help our blood clot, not protect our bones. Scientists speculate it takes about 200 micrograms per day to protect bones from thinning—that can be accomplished by eating 1 serving (1/2 cup or 125 ml) of cooked leafy greens each day.

Boron

Although there's no recommended daily intake for boron, studies suggest that a higher intake of this trace mineral may slow down loss of calcium, magnesium and phosphorus through the urine. And that's not all. Boosting your boron intake may also increase your blood-estrogen level. Scientists aren't exactly sure how boron keeps calcium in balance, but they think that boron is needed for activation of vitamin D.

A daily intake of 1.5 to 3 milligrams of boron is more than adequate to meet your requirements for bone growth and development. The main food sources are fruit and vegetables, but boron content depends on how much of the mineral is in the soil in which the produce grew. If you want to take a supplement, 3 to 9 milligrams per day is a very safe amount. Intakes greater than 500 milligrams a day can cause nausea, vomiting and diarrhea. However, boron supplements aren't available in Canada (but are in the United States).

Magnesium

One-half of the body's magnesium stores are in the bone. But before I continue, I'd like to clear up one piece of misinformation: Magnesium does *not* help your body absorb calcium. I can't begin to count the number of times I've heard that it does; on occasion, I've even seen it written in books. Without magnesium, you absorb calcium just fine, but you don't form healthy bones. This mineral helps make parathyroid hormone, an important regulator of bone building. Animal studies show that a lack of dietary magnesium causes increased bone breakdown and decreased bone synthesis.

It's difficult to say to what extent magnesium plays a role in osteoporosis, since very few studies have actually looked at the effect of dietary magnesium and bone loss. Most of the studies that support the use of magnesium supplements have found that osteoporosis is more common in people who have other health problems that cause a magnesium deficiency, like alcoholism and hyperthyroidism. Interestingly, scientists have found that magnesium levels in bone are actually higher, not lower, in people with osteoporosis. However, there's preliminary evidence that taking magnesium supplements can prevent bone loss in post-menopausal women. One study also found that among 2038 men and women aged 70 and older, higher magnesium intakes were associated with greater bone densities.[25]

A woman's recommended dietary allowance (RDA) for magnesium is 310 or 320 milligrams per day depending on your age (see the RDA chart in Chapter 1, page 34). The best food sources are wheat bran, whole-grain breads, cereals and pasta, legumes, nuts, seeds and leafy green vegetables.

There's no question in my mind that most people need to step up their magnesium intake. Switching from refined starches like white bread and white pasta to whole-grain products is a good place to start. If you use calcium supplements, buy one with magnesium added—in a 2:1 ratio (two parts calcium for one part magnesium) to avoid gastrointestinal upset. The daily upper limit for magnesium from a supplement is 350 milligrams.

Phosphorus

This mineral is an important component of the bone mineral complex. In fact, about 85 percent of phosphorus in the body is found in the bone. It appears that both too little and too much dietary phosphorus can result in bone loss. A high level in the blood causes the release of parathyroid hormone (PTH). If you recall, PTH turns off vitamin D production and, as a result, your intestine absorbs less calcium. Scientists believe that a long-standing imbalance of phosphorus and calcium, caused by too much dietary phosphorus and too little dietary calcium, may contribute to bone breakdown.

On the other hand, if your diet lacks phosphorus and your blood levels become low, your body will release the mineral from your bones in an effort to keep your blood level constant, the same way that blood-calcium levels remain stable at the expense of your bone. One of the symptoms of a phosphorus deficiency is bone pain. A low blood-phosphorus level can result from poor eating habits, excessive use of phosphorus-binding antacids and intestinal malabsorption.

The recommended daily intake of phosphorus is 700 milligrams. Most of the phosphorus in our diet comes from additives in cheese, bakery products, processed meats and soft drinks. Other food sources include wheat bran, milk, fish, eggs, poultry, beef and pork. As you can probably guess, most people don't have a problem getting enough phosphorus. Just make sure you meet your calcium requirements so that you keep these two minerals in balance.

Manganese, zinc and copper

These are important helpers (cofactors) for enzymes that are essential to making bone tissue. The impact of these nutrients on bone loss has been studied in post-menopausal women. The women who received a daily supplement of calcium, manganese, copper and zinc did not experience any bone loss of the spine at the end of the two-year study.[26] The placebo group, on the other hand, lost 3.5 percent of their bone mass. Manganese is widely available in foods, and deficiencies haven't been seen in humans. Meat and drinking water are your best bets for copper. When it comes to zinc, reach for wheat bran, wheat germ, oysters, seafood, lean red meat and milk.

Sodium

Like caffeine, sodium causes the kidneys to excrete calcium. This means that you need to limit the amount of sodium you consume each day—and meet daily calcium requirements. A study in post-menopausal women determined that a maximum intake of 2000 milligrams of sodium (the amount found in about 3/4 teaspoon/3.75 ml of salt) and 1000 milligrams of caffeine minimized bone loss.[27]

To reduce sodium intake, keep your daily intake less than 2300 milligrams. Read nutrition labels to choose packaged foods that are lower in sodium. Eat more meals prepared at home rather than in restaurants. Avoid the saltshaker at the table and minimize your use of salt in cooking. You'll find additional strategies to help reduce sodium intake in Chapter 1, page 9.

OTHER NATURAL HEALTH PRODUCTS
Fish oil supplements
Although preliminary, there's evidence that omega-3 fatty acids in fish oil guard against osteoporosis.[28] Data from animal studies suggest that fish oil may reduce post-menopausal bone loss. Higher intakes of omega-3 fats have been linked with higher bone density. Studies in humans have found that a higher intake of omega-3 fats—and a lower intake of omega-6 fats found in corn and soybean oils—is associated with increased bone densities.[29] Findings from a study conducted in men suggest that high levels of omega-3 fatty acids in the blood—a reflection of one's dietary intake—favourably impact bone health.[30] Supplementation with fish oil reduces the production of inflammatory immune compounds and helps increase calcium absorption and bone mineral density.

In addition to eating oily fish such as salmon or trout twice per week, take a daily fish oil supplement that supplies 300 to 600 milligrams of DHA + EPA combined, the two omega-3 fatty acids contained in fish oil. You'll find this information on the ingredient list.

LIFESTYLE FACTORS
Exercise
Until the age of 30, regular exercise helps women get a head start on building peak bone mass. In fact, studies have found that children who spend the most time being physically active have stronger bones than those who are sedentary. But the effect of exercise doesn't stop once you've achieved your peak mass. Bone cells are constantly active, tearing up old bone and laying down new bone. Participating in weight-bearing activities like brisk walking or stair climbing stimulates bones to increase in strength and density during the premenopausal and post-menopausal years. One study found that post-menopausal women who worked out three times a week for nine months actually increased their bone mass by 5.2 percent.[31] Another report revealed that, compared to women who didn't exercise, those who worked out with weights for one hour three times a week gained bone mass, to the tune of 1.6 percent. The non-exercisers actually lost 3.6 percent of the bone mass in their spine over the course of the study.[32]

If you have osteoporosis, a safe exercise program can help you slow bone loss, improve posture and balance, and build muscle strength and tone. The benefits of exercise can reduce your risk of falling and fracturing a bone.

Your best bet is to incorporate a mix of activities in your week. Aim to get four weight-bearing, cardiovascular activities each week (e.g., brisk walking) and two or three weight workouts. If you've never used weights before, be sure to consult a certified personal trainer. Personal trainers work in fitness clubs and many will come to your home. They'll design a safe and effective program for you. And don't worry—you don't need a basement full of exercise equipment. Some of the best trainers I know teach women creative ways of building muscle strength without using weights.

THE BOTTOM LINE...
Leslie's recommendations for preventing osteoporosis and bone fracture

1. If you're approaching menopause, get your bone density measured to determine the health of your bones. This will help you and your doctor determine the need for medication.
2. If you're already a fan of soy foods, consider boosting your intake to achieve a daily intake of 90 milligrams of isoflavones.
3. To strengthen your bones, make sure you're eating enough protein-rich foods like fish, poultry, lean meat, legumes, tofu and dairy products. But don't go overboard—some studies suggest that very high intakes of animal protein cause your kidneys to excrete calcium.
4. Limit your intake of alcoholic beverages to at most one per day.
5. To prevent too much calcium from being lost from your body, keep your caffeine intake to a daily maximum of 450 milligrams (no more than three small 8 ounce/250 ml cups of coffee). If you have osteoporosis, keep this to no more than 200 milligrams. And be sure you're meeting your calcium requirements.
6. Depending on your age and your risk for osteoporosis, get 1000 or 1500 milligrams of calcium each day.
   - If you're using a calcium carbonate supplement, be sure to take it with food since it needs plenty of stomach acid to make it ready for absorption.
   - If you produce less stomach acid because of a medication, buy a supplement made from calcium citrate.

7. To help you absorb the calcium in your diet, supplement with 1000 international units (IU) of vitamin D each day.

8. Other nutrients that help build bone density include vitamin A, vitamin C, vitamin K, magnesium, phosphorus, boron, manganese, zinc and copper. Take a look at the food sources I've outlined to see if your diet is lacking any of these. Avoid taking single vitamin A supplements since excess vitamin A can increase the risk of bone fracture.

9. Go easy on sodium from processed foods, restaurant meals and the salt shaker. Consume no more than 2300 milligrams of sodium per day.

10. If you don't work out now, add regular weight-bearing exercise to your life.

12

Heart disease and high LDL cholesterol

Heart disease is a serious health problem faced by post-menopausal women. Once seen as a man's disease, the gap between the number of men and the number of women with heart disease has narrowed. In fact, today in Canada, women are more likely than men to die of a heart attack or stroke. With the loss of estrogen, a woman's risk of getting heart disease increases with age and rises significantly after menopause.

Compared to men, women are more likely to die in the year following their heart attack. This is largely because women are older when they get heart disease and have more advanced heart disease by the time they're diagnosed. Symptoms like chest pain tend to be ignored or overlooked in women. Both women and their doctors may attribute these symptoms to indigestion, stress or gallbladder problems. As well, after having a heart attack, women tend to get to a hospital much later than do men, and they also tend to receive less aggressive therapy.

What causes heart disease?

Heart disease is a general term that includes coronary heart disease, congenital heart disease (which you're born with), congestive heart failure and malfunctioning heart valves. This chapter discusses only coronary heart disease, which affects the blood vessels that feed the heart. It's caused by atherosclerosis, a gradual process that narrows the heart's arteries and leads to a heart attack. Simply put, atherosclerosis is the buildup of fatty plaques (collections) on the inner lining of the arteries, like the accumulation of rust in a water pipe. These cholesterol-rich plaques cause hardening of the arteries and narrowing of the inner channel (called the lumen) of the artery. Narrowed coronary arteries can't deliver enough blood and oxygen to maintain normal function of the heart. Reduced blood flow to the heart can cause angina, heart attack, sudden death, abnormal heart rhythms and heart failure.

Atherosclerosis can begin in adolescence when fatty streaks, which may one day cause heart disease, can appear on the lining of arteries as cholesterol sticks to the arteries. The next stage of atherosclerosis is an injury to the lining of an artery. An infection or virus, high blood pressure, cigarette smoke or diabetes may cause this damage. Your body attempts to heal itself, just like it would with any wound. Immune cells are attracted to the injured artery wall and accumulate. Over time, the fatty streaks enlarge and become hardened with minerals, tissue, fat and cells, forming plaques. As plaques form beneath the artery wall, they stiffen arteries and narrow the passage through them. Most people have well-developed plaques by the time they are 30 years old. If atherosclerosis progresses, it can restrict blood flow to the heart.

Blood cells called platelets respond to damaged spots on blood vessels by forming clots. A clot may stick to a plaque and gradually enlarge until it blocks blood flow to an area of the heart; that portion of the heart may die slowly and form scar tissue. But a clot can also break loose and circulate in the blood until it reaches an artery too small for it to pass through. When a clot that's wedged in a vessel cuts off the supply of oxygen and nutrients to a part of the heart muscle, a heart attack results.

Who's at risk?

Risk factors for heart disease are usually classified as either modifiable or non-modifiable. Non-modifiable factors—like getting older or having a strong family history of early heart attacks—are risk factors that you can't change. But you can reduce your risk by changing modifiable risk factors. You can change your diet, exercise more or quit smoking. You can even control risk factors such as high blood pressure or diabetes. Here's a glance at the factors that put you at risk for heart disease (the more risk factors you have, the greater your risk):

NON-MODIFIABLE RISK FACTORS
- **Aging.** As you get older, the heart's function tends to weaken, your arteries get stiffer and the artery walls become thicker. As well, other known risk factors for heart disease—high blood pressure, elevated

cholesterol and diabetes—become more prevalent with increasing age.

- **Family history.** If a male member of your immediate family developed heart disease before the age of 55 or a female relative was diagnosed before age 65, you then have a higher risk of developing the disease.
- **Gender.** It's true that men are more likely than women to have heart attacks and to have them at a younger age. However, a women's risk of heart disease increases as she ages and rises significantly after menopause. During a woman's reproductive lifecycle, the naturally occurring hormone estrogen provides built-in protection from heart disease. By the time a woman is 65 years old, her risk of heart attack equals that of a man because she no longer produces estrogen.

MODIFIABLE RISK FACTORS

- You have high LDL (bad) blood cholesterol.
- You have high blood triglycerides (fats).
- You have low HDL (good) cholesterol.
- You have high blood pressure.
- You smoke cigarettes. Smokers are two to four times more likely to develop heart disease than non-smokers. Smoking damages the lining of the arteries, increasing the likelihood of plaque formation. Inhaling cigarette smoke also produces free radicals in the body, which then damage LDL cholesterol, making it stick to the artery walls. Finally, smoking increases blood pressure and makes blood-clot formation more likely.
- You don't exercise regularly. Regular exercise helps you maintain a healthy weight. It lowers LDL cholesterol, raises HDL cholesterol, helps keep blood pressure in check and strengthens the heart and blood vessels.
- You have diabetes or prediabetes. In diabetes, fatty plaques develop and progress much more rapidly. In the 35 to 64 age group, people with diabetes are six times more likely to have heart disease or stroke than those without the condition.
- You're overweight or obese. Carrying extra weight puts stress on your heart and circulatory system. Being overweight can also cause high blood pressure and elevated blood cholesterol. Excess weight around the waist, called abdominal obesity, is much more dangerous to your heart than excess lower body fat.
- You have a poor diet. The foods and nutrients you consume—or don't consume—can increase the likelihood of developing risk factors such

as high cholesterol and triglycerides, elevated blood pressure, type 2 diabetes and obesity.

- The way in which you cope with stress can contribute to your risk of developing heart disease.

CHOLESTEROL LEVELS: YOUR LIPID PROFILE

The lipid profile is a group of blood tests, often ordered together, that measure the amount of lipids (fats) in your bloodstream. The profile includes total cholesterol, HDL cholesterol, LDL cholesterol and triglycerides. It can also include a calculated value for the total cholesterol/HDL ratio or a risk score based on lipid profile results, age, sex and other risk factors. Women who are post-menopausal or 50 years of age or older should have a lipid profile every one to three years. Younger women should have a lipid profile at least once every five years.

LDL cholesterol

Cholesterol is a waxy substance that can't dissolve in your blood. That means it needs to piggyback on carriers called lipoproteins in order to circulate in your bloodstream. Low-density lipoprotein (LDL) cholesterol is referred to as "bad" cholesterol because too much of it in your bloodstream causes the buildup of fatty plaques on artery walls. The higher your LDL cholesterol, the greater your risk for heart disease.

What's a desirable LDL cholesterol level? That all depends on your risk for developing heart disease over the next ten years. Your doctor will add up points for your age, LDL cholesterol, HDL cholesterol, blood pressure and whether or not you smoke to calculate what's called the Framingham Risk Score. The points used to determine this ten-year risk for heart disease are weighted differently for men and women. Your risk is determined as a percentage based on the following:

Framingham Risk Score

	Risk factors	10-year risk
High	Those who have had a cardiac event or have been diagnosed with heart disease or diabetes	≥20%
Moderate	2 or more risk factors	10–19%
Low	Zero to one risk factor	<10%

Your Framingham Risk Score determines the target value for your LDL cholesterol. As you'll see in the chart below, if you're "low risk" for developing heart disease, your target LDL cholesterol should be less than 5.0 millimoles per litre (mmol/L). If you're at high risk for heart disease (e.g., you have diabetes), your doctor will want your LDL cholesterol level to be less than 1.8 mmol/L. If your LDL value is higher than the desirable level, your doctor will recommend treatment with lifestyle changes such as diet and exercise, and possibly medication.

Risk ratio

The ratio of your total cholesterol to HDL cholesterol is helpful in predicting the risk of developing atherosclerosis. The risk ratio is simply the number obtained by dividing your total cholesterol value by the value of the HDL cholesterol. A high ratio indicates a higher risk of heart attack, whereas a low ratio denotes a lower risk. Having a high total cholesterol and low HDL cholesterol increases the ratio and is undesirable. Conversely, low total cholesterol and high HDL cholesterol lowers the ratio and is desirable.

The following chart outlines the relationship between the Framingham Risk Score and these factors.

LDL Cholesterol and Risk Ratio Targets Based on Framingham Risk Score

Framingham Risk Score	10-year risk of heart disease	LDL cholesterol target	Risk ratio target (Total cholesterol/HDL)
High	≥20%	<1.8 mmol/L	<4.0
Moderate	10–19%	<3.5 mmol/L	<5.0
Low	<10%	<5.0 mmol/L	<6.0

HDL cholesterol

High-density lipoprotein (HDL) carries cholesterol away from the arteries towards the liver where it's broken down. HDL cholesterol keeps the arteries open and blood flowing through them. The higher your HDL level, the lower the risk for heart disease. That's why HDL cholesterol is called the "good" cholesterol.

Reference Ranges for HDL Cholesterol

	Desired	Increased risk
Females to age 19	0.90–2.40 mmol/L	<0.90 mmol/L
Females, 20+ years	≥1.30 mmol/L	<1.30 mmol/L
Males to age 19	0.90–1.60 mmol/L	<0.90 mmol/L
Males, 20+ years	≥1.0 mmol/L	<1.0 mmol/L

Total cholesterol

This is a sum of your blood's cholesterol content. A high level can put you at increased risk of heart disease. Desired total cholesterol is <5.2 mmol/L.

Triglycerides

Triglycerides are fat that's made in the liver from the food you eat. They're transported in your blood on very low-density lipoproteins (VLDL). High triglyceride levels usually mean you eat more calories than you burn or you drink too much alcohol. High triglyceride levels increase your risk of heart disease. Desired triglycerides is <1.7 mmol/L.

HIGH BLOOD PRESSURE

The higher your blood pressure is above normal, the greater your risk for heart disease. Blood pressure is the force on your artery walls that's generated by your heart as it pushes blood through your arteries. When your heart beats, blood pressure in your arteries rises. Between beats, when your heart relaxes, blood pressure falls. Your blood pressure rises and falls throughout the day, but when it remains elevated over time it's called high blood pressure, or *hypertension.*

Blood pressure is recorded in millimetres of mercury (written as mmHg). It's composed of two measurements: systolic blood pressure and diastolic blood pressure. You may have heard someone say their blood pressure is 115 over 75. The first (top) number is the systolic pressure, created when your heart is pumping out blood. The second (bottom) number is the diastolic pressure, created when your heart is relaxing and filling with blood.

Adults should have a blood pressure of less than 120/80. Hypertension is defined as a systolic pressure of ≥140 mmHg or a diastolic pressure of

≥90 mmHg. One in five Canadians fall into the category between, called prehypertension (130–139/85–89 mmHg). Unless lifestyle changes are made to bring blood pressure down, 60 percent of people with prehypertension will develop hypertension within four years.

Do You Have High Blood Pressure?

	Millilitres of mercury (mmHg)
Normal blood pressure	≤120 / ≤80
Prehypertension	130–139 / 85–89
Hypertension	≥140 / ≥90

Because prehypertension and hypertension usually don't cause symptoms, it's important to have your blood pressure checked regularly—at least once every two years, and more often if your blood pressure is high. If you have prehypertension you should have your blood pressure monitored once a year. High blood pressure is treated by weight loss, dietary modifications and, often, medication.

HOMOCYSTEINE

Homocysteine is an amino acid normally produced by the body to help build and maintain tissues. However, although the body needs homocysteine to function properly, too much is not a good thing. An elevated level of homocysteine in the bloodstream is linked with a greater risk of atherosclerosis, heart attack and stroke. High homocysteine damages artery walls and promotes the buildup of fatty plaques.

Homocysteine is transformed into harmless compounds with the help of folic acid (a B vitamin also called folate), vitamin B12 and vitamin B6. A lack of these vitamins in the body can hamper the natural breakdown of homocysteine, causing it to accumulate in the bloodstream. Studies show that higher intakes of folic acid and higher blood levels of the B vitamin are associated with lower blood-homocysteine levels. Although it's well established that B vitamins can lower elevated homocysteine, it's not clear if doing so can actually ward off a heart attack. Even so, your doctor may order a homocysteine blood test if you've had heart problems or if you have a family member who developed heart disease at a young age. The normal range for homocysteine is 5 to 15 micromoles per litre (umol/L).

Preventing heart disease

Many of the risk factors for heart disease are influenced by what you eat. Here are a few strategies that can reduce your chances of getting heart disease. My nutrition recommendations will (1) keep your blood lipids at a healthy level, (2) prevent damage or oxidation to your LDL cholesterol, (3) lower blood pressure and (4) promote weight loss.

DIETARY STRATEGIES
Saturated fat
When it comes to heart health, the evidence is pretty clear that what's most important is the type of fat you eat, rather than the total amount. Dietary fats are named according to their chemical structure. Saturated fats are solid at room temperature. This is the type of fat found in animal foods—meat, poultry, eggs and dairy products. Studies have consistently demonstrated that excess saturated fat in the diet raises total and LDL cholesterol levels, a major risk factor for heart disease. What's more, there's clear evidence that reducing your intake of these so-called bad fats can lower blood cholesterol, helping to guard against heart attack. Saturated fat seems to inhibit the activity of LDL receptors on cells so that this type of cholesterol accumulates in the bloodstream.

Foods contain many types of saturated fats, and not all of them influence blood-cholesterol levels to the same degree. For instance, the saturated fat in dairy products is more cholesterol raising than the saturated fat in meat. What's most important is to eat less saturated fat, period. Saturated fat should account for less than 10 percent of your daily calories. Make a habit of choosing animal foods that are lower in fat. Lean cuts of meat (sirloin, tenderloin, flank steak, eye of round), skinless poultry breast, 1% or skim milk, 1% or non-fat yogurt, and part-skim or skim milk cheese are examples of animal foods lower in saturated fat.

Use the chart on the next page to help you choose foods lower in saturated fat.

Total and Saturated Fat Content of Selected Foods

Food	Total fat (grams)	Sat. fat (grams)
Dairy products		
Mozzarella cheese, part-skim, 16.5% MF, 1 oz (30 g)	4.6 g	2.9 g
Cheddar cheese, low-fat, 7% MF, 1 oz (30 g)	2.0 g	1.2 g
Cottage cheese, 1% MF, 1/2 cup (125 ml)	1.1 g	0.8 g
Cottage cheese, fat free, 1/2 cup (125 ml)	0.5 g	0.3 g
Frozen yogurt, vanilla, 5.6% MF, 1/2 cup (125 ml)	4.0 g	2.5 g
Milk, 1% MF, 1 cup (250 ml)	2.5 g	1.7 g
Milk, skim, 0.1% MF, 1 cup (250 ml)	0.5 g	0.3 g
Meat & Poultry		
Beef, steak, strip loin, broiled, 3 oz (90 g)	9.2 g	3.5 g
Beef, steak, eye of round, grilled, 3 oz (90 g)	7.7 g	2.7 g
Beef, steak, top sirloin, grilled, 3 oz (90 g)	6.8 g	2.6 g
Beef, tenderloin, roasted, 3 oz (90 g)	7.3 g	2.3 g
Beef, patty, ground extra lean, broiled, 3 oz (90 g)	7.8 g	2.1 g
Beef, steak, inside round, grilled, 3 oz (90 g)	3.9 g	1.4 g
Pork, back (peameal) bacon, grilled, 3 oz (90 g)	7.5 g	2.5 g
Pork, ham, lean (5% fat), 3 oz (90 g)	4.8 g	1.6 g
Pork, tenderloin, roasted, 3 oz (90 g)	3.2 g	1.0 g
Veal, patty, ground, broiled, 3 oz (90 g)	6.8 g	2.7 g
Veal, loin chop, grain fed, lean, broiled, 3 oz (90 g)	5.7 g	2.4 g
Veal, sirloin, roasted, 3 oz (90 g)	5.6 g	2.2 g
Veal, cutlet, grain fed, pan-fried, 3 oz (90 g)	2.5 g	0.8 g
Chicken, dark meat, roasted, skinless, 3 oz (90 g)	8.7 g	2.4 g
Chicken, white meat, roasted, skinless, 3 oz (90 g)	4.0 g	1.1 g
Chicken breast, roasted, skinless, 3 oz (90 g)	1.9 g	0.6 g
Turkey, dark meat, roasted, skinless, 3 oz (90 g)	2.7 g	0.9 g
Turkey, white meat, roasted, skinless, 3 oz (90 g)	0.9 g	0.2 g

Food	Total fat (grams)	Sat. fat (grams)
Eggs		
Egg, whole, 1 large	5.3 g	1.6 g
Egg, whites only, 2 large	0 g	0 g

Source: Data adapted from the *Canadian Nutrient File*, Health Canada (2006). Available at: http://webprod.hc-sc.gc.ca/cnf-fce/index-eng.jsp.

Trans fat

Trans fats are formed during partial hydrogenation, a process used by the food industry to harden and stabilize liquid vegetable oils. The vegetable oil becomes saturated *and* it forms a new type of fat called trans fat. Roughly 90 percent of the trans fat in our food supply is found in commercial snack foods and baked goods, including cookies, cakes, pastries and doughnuts, as well as fried fast foods and some brands of margarines.

Compared to saturated fats, trans fats are linked with a 2.5- to 10-fold higher risk of heart disease. Trans fats increase levels of LDL (bad) cholesterol and decrease levels of HDL (good) cholesterol, both of which are strongly linked to a greater risk of heart disease. Studies also indicate that a steady intake of trans fats can trigger inflammation in the body, disrupt the normal functioning of blood vessel walls and impair the body's use of insulin. When it comes to the development of heart disease itself, researchers have found that higher intakes of trans fat are linked with a greater risk of developing coronary heart disease.[1-3]

To help reduce your intake of trans fat, read nutrition labels. You'll find the grams of trans fat listed per one serving of the food. More useful, however, is the Daily Value (DV) for saturated plus trans fat combined, which is written as a percentage. This value tells you whether there's a little or a lot of these cholesterol-raising fats in a food. The daily value for saturated plus trans fat is set at 20 grams, 10% of the calories in a standard 2000-calorie diet. Foods with a DV for saturated plus trans fat of 5% or less are very low in these fats.

If a packaged food doesn't have a Nutrition Facts box, as may be the case for foods prepared in-store, read the ingredient list. Avoid buying foods that list partially hydrogenated vegetable oil, hydrogenated vegetable oil and shortening. When buying margarine, choose one that's made from non-hydrogenated vegetable oil since it will be trans fat free.

Cut down on your consumption of processed foods such as crackers, cookies, snack foods and toaster pastries; these foods supply most of the trans fat we consume. Trans fats also occur naturally at low levels in foods from ruminant animals, such as beef, lamb, goat and dairy products. However, unlike industry-produced trans fat, naturally occurring trans fats are not considered harmful.

Polyunsaturated fat and omega-3 fatty acids

This type of dietary fat is liquid at room temperature. Omega-6 polyunsaturated fats are found in all plant oils (such as corn, soybean, canola, grapeseed, sunflower, safflower, sesame and flaxseed oils). Omega-3 polyunsaturated fats are found in fish and seafood. Replacing foods that provide mostly saturated fat with those rich in polyunsaturated fat can help you lower your cholesterol level.

Omega-3 fatty acids, called DHA and EPA, found in fish and fish oil also help lower high levels of blood triglycerides and reduce the stickiness of platelets, the cells that form blood clots in arteries. As well, they may increase the flexibility of red blood cells, enabling them to pass more readily through tiny blood vessels. Many studies have found that populations that consume fish a few times each week have lower rates of heart disease than those that rarely or never eat fish.

To increase your intake of DHA and EPA, eat fish two times per week. Choose oilier fish such as salmon, trout, Arctic char, sardines, herring, mackerel and sea bass.

Consuming foods rich in alpha-linolenic acid (ALA) is an alternative way to ensure that you're consuming omega-3 fatty acids. ALA is an omega-3 fatty acid plentiful in flax, canola and walnut oils as well as soybeans. Although the evidence for ALA's cardio-protective properties isn't nearly as abundant or compelling as it is for DHA and EPA, numerous studies do suggest this omega-3 fat may offer some protection. A large study of healthy women revealed that after eighteen years of follow up, a greater ALA intake was linked with significant protection from sudden cardiac death. Women who consumed 1.16 grams of ALA per day were 40 percent less likely to suddenly die of cardiac arrest than women whose diets provided only 0.66 grams per day. In this study, a greater intake of ALA didn't reduce the risk of non-fatal heart attacks.[4]

Women require 1.1 grams (1100 milligrams) of ALA per day. The richest sources of ALA are flaxseed, walnut and canola oil as well as ground flaxseed and salba. For instance, 1 teaspoon (5 ml) of flaxseed oil contains 2400 milligrams of ALA as does 2 tablespoons (30 ml) of ground flaxseed or ground salba. ALA is also found to a lesser extent in soybean oil, tofu and food products fortified with flaxseed oil such as yogurt and juice. Flaxseed oil capsules sold in drugstores and health food stores supply 500 milligrams of ALA per capsule.

Monounsaturated fats

These fats, which are liquid at room temperature but become semi-solid when stored in the fridge, are abundant in olive, canola and peanut oils as well as in avocados and almonds. Many studies have demonstrated that replacing saturated and trans fats with monounsaturated fats helps to lower the risk of heart disease. Higher intakes of monounsaturated fat are linked with lower death rates from heart disease. Research suggests that extra-virgin olive oil helps prevent blood clots from forming and has anti-inflammatory properties in the body. (Extra-virgin olive oil is extracted from olives using minimal heat and no chemicals, resulting in a higher concentration of protective plant compounds.) As a general guideline, one-third to two-thirds of your daily fat (10 percent to 20 percent of calories) should come from monounsaturated fats.

Dietary cholesterol

This wax-like fatty substance is found in meat, poultry, eggs, dairy products, fish and seafood. It's particularly plentiful in shrimp, liver and egg yolks. Although there's compelling evidence that high cholesterol intakes can cause hardening of the arteries in rabbits, pigs and mice, there's little evidence that this is so in humans. For most people, only a small amount of cholesterol in food passes into the bloodstream. A number of short-term studies have demonstrated that feeding healthy people as many as three whole eggs per day doesn't raise LDL cholesterol. In fact, some research has even found that an egg-rich diet increases HDL cholesterol. What's more, so far, thirty years of research have not turned up a connection between eating eggs and heart disease risk. Studies have determined that healthy people who eat one egg per day don't have an increased risk of coronary heart disease or stroke.[5-9]

Too much dietary cholesterol can raise levels of LDL cholesterol in some people, especially those with hereditary forms of high cholesterol. There's also evidence that people with diabetes are more efficient at absorbing cholesterol from foods, which may increase their risk of heart disease. Health Canada recommends that we consume no more than 300 milligrams of cholesterol each day. If you have high blood cholesterol, it's wise to limit your daily intake to 200 milligrams. As you'll see from the chart below, choosing animal foods low in saturated fat will also help you reduce your cholesterol intake.

Cholesterol Content of Selected Foods

Food	Cholesterol (milligrams)
Dairy products	
Cheese, cheddar, 31% MF, 1 oz (30 g)	31 mg
Cheese, mozzarella, part skim, 1 oz (30 g)	18 mg
Yogurt, 1.5% MF, 3/4 cup (175 ml)	11 mg
Milk, 2% MF, 1 cup (250 ml)	19 mg
Milk, skim, 1 cup (250 ml)	5 mg
Cream, half and half, 12% MF, 2 tbsp (30 ml)	12 mg
Butter, 1 tsp (5 ml)	10 mg
Meat & Poultry	
Beef, steak, sirloin, lean, 3 oz (90 g)	64 mg
Calf liver, fried, 3 oz (90 g)	416 mg
Chicken breast, skinless, 3 oz (90 g)	73 mg
Pork, from the loin, lean, 3 oz (90 g)	71 mg
Fish & Seafood	
Salmon, 3 oz (90 g)	54 mg
Shrimp, 3 oz (90 g)	135 mg
Eggs	
Egg, whole, 1 large	190 mg
Egg, white only, 1 large	0 mg

Source: Data adapted from the *Canadian Nutrient File*, Health Canada (2006). Available at: http://webprod.hc-sc.gc.ca/cnf-fce/index-eng.jsp.

Legumes and soy foods

Numerous studies have demonstrated the cardio-protective properties of legumes and foods made from soybeans. A regular intake of these foods has been shown to help lower LDL cholesterol and elevated blood pressure as well as guard against type 2 diabetes. Researchers attribute the cardio-protective properties of legumes to their vegetarian protein, B vitamin, potassium, calcium, magnesium, potassium and phytochemical content. Rather than just one nutrient, it's the unique package of nutrients and phytochemicals in legumes and soy that works synergistically to reduce the risk of heart disease.

To increase your intake of legumes and soy, include at least 3 servings in your diet each week. One serving is equivalent to 3/4 cup (175 ml) of cooked legumes or tofu or 1 soy-based veggie burger. The following tips will help you add these heart healthy foods to your family's meals:

- Enjoy a mixed bean salad in a pita pocket for a high-protein vegetarian sandwich.
- Add black beans to tacos and burritos. Use half the amount of lean ground meat you usually would and make up the difference with beans.
- Make a vegetarian chili with kidney beans, black beans and chickpeas.
- Sauté chickpeas with spinach and tomatoes and serve over pasta.
- Add white kidney beans to tomato-based pasta sauce.
- Toss chickpeas or lentils into your next salad or soup.
- Try a soy-based veggie burger for a change from beef burgers. Most veggie burgers require only three minutes' grilling per side. Overcooking causes veggie burgers to dry out.
- Substitute soy ground round for ground beef or chicken in pasta sauce and chili recipes.
- Try an unflavoured soy beverage on cereal or in smoothies. Sample a few different brands to find the one you like best.
- Snack on roasted soy nuts with dried fruit for an afternoon energy boost.
- Replace up to one-half of the all-purpose flour with soy flour in baked good recipes.

Nuts

There's compelling evidence that eating nuts on a regular basis can lower your risk of developing heart disease and dying from it. To date, four large studies involving 172,000 men and women have found that those who eat nuts at least four times per week are almost 40 percent less likely to succumb to heart disease than those who eat nuts less than once per week.[10-13] Nuts—all types—can help control certain risk factors for heart attack such as high cholesterol and high blood pressure. For women, a regular intake of nuts has also been found to reduce the risk of developing type 2 diabetes, a strong risk factor for heart disease.

Nuts are rich sources of unsaturated fat, vitamin E, folate, B vitamins, magnesium, potassium and fibre, nutrients demonstrated to have cardio-protective properties. Add a 1/4 cup (60 ml) portion of nuts to your diet five times a week. Try the following:

- Add peanuts to an Asian-style stir-fry.
- Stir-fry collard greens with cashews and a teaspoon (5 ml) of sesame oil.
- Add walnuts to your tossed green salad.
- Try walnut oil in your next salad dressing (use half olive oil and half walnut oil).
- Mix sunflower or pumpkin seeds into a bowl of yogurt or hot cereal.
- Snack on a mix of almonds and dried apricots.
- Sprinkle your casserole with a handful of mixed nuts.

Whole grains

In general, studies have revealed that people with the highest intake of whole grains (about 3 servings per day) have a risk of heart disease or stroke that's 20 percent to 40 percent lower than those whose diets contained little or no whole-grain foods. Some research even hints that a steady intake of whole grains may delay the progression of heart disease by slowing the buildup of plaque in the arteries.

Whole grains such as 100% whole-grain breads and cereals, whole rye, oats, brown rice, quinoa and millet have many protective ingredients that might help lower the risk of heart disease. Whole grains are important sources of fibre, vitamin E, magnesium, zinc, selenium, copper, iron, manganese and phytochemicals. Many of these natural compounds have antioxidant properties and may offer protection from heart disease by keeping LDL cholesterol levels in check, maintaining the health of blood vessels and reducing the risk of type 2 diabetes.

A food made from whole grains means that it contains *all* parts of the grain—the outer bran layer where most of the fibre is, the germ layer that's rich in nutrients like vitamin E and the endosperm that contains the starch. When whole grains are processed into flakes, puffs or white flour, all that's left is the starchy endosperm. Refined grains offer significantly less vitamin E, B6, magnesium, potassium, zinc and fibre. Include at least 3 servings of whole grains in your daily diet. One serving is equivalent to 1 slice of bread, 1/2 cup (125 ml) of cooked oatmeal, 1 ounce (30 g) of cold cereal or 1/2 cup (125 ml) of cooked brown rice or whole-wheat pasta.

Use the following guide to help you get more whole grains in your diet.

Whole grain	Refined grain
Barley	Cornmeal
Brown rice	Pasta
Bulgur	Pearled barley
Flaxseed	White rice
Kamut	Unbleached flour
Oat bran	
Oatmeal	
Quinoa	
Whole spelt	
Whole-rye bread	
Whole-wheat bread*	
Wild rice	

*When buying bread, look for the words "whole-grain whole-wheat flour" on the list of ingredients. "Wheat flour" and "unbleached wheat flour" mean it's refined.

Soluble fibre

Plant foods contain a mix of two types of fibre, soluble and insoluble, but will have more of one than the other. Soluble fibre, which dissolves in water, has been shown to lower high LDL blood-cholesterol levels.

Numerous studies have demonstrated the ability of foods rich in soluble fibre, such as legumes, oats and oat bran, and psyllium, to lower elevated LDL blood cholesterol in adults and children. Most of the research suggests that including a good source of soluble fibre in your daily diet can lower LDL cholesterol by 9 percent. A combined analysis of eight clinical trials involving people with high blood cholesterol concluded that, in conjunction with a low-fat diet, consuming 10.2 grams of psyllium per day lowered total cholesterol by 4 percent and LDL cholesterol by 7 percent.[14-16]

When soluble fibre reaches the intestine, it attaches to bile, causing it to be excreted in the stool. Bile is a digestive aid that's released into the intestine after you eat. The liver makes bile from cholesterol and sends it to your gallbladder for storage until it's needed. Since soluble fibre causes your body to excrete bile, your liver has to make more of it from cholesterol in the bloodstream. The end result is a lower blood-cholesterol level. When unabsorbed fibre reaches your colon, bacteria degrade it and form compounds called short-chain fatty acids. These fatty acids may also hamper the liver's ability to produce cholesterol.

To lower elevated LDL cholesterol, consume at least 3 grams of soluble fibre each day. You'll find this amount in the following foods:

Sources of Soluble Fibre

Food	Total fibre (grams)	Soluble fibre (grams)
Barley, cooked, 1-1/2 cups (375 ml)	12 g	3 g
Flaxseed, ground, 1/4 cup (60 ml)	8 g	2.6 g
All-Bran Buds cereal with Psyllium, Kellogg's, 1/3 cup (75 ml)	12 g	3 g
Guardian cereal, Kellogg's, 1 cup (250 ml)	6 g	4 g
SmartBran cereal, Nature's Path, 2/3 cup (150 ml)	13 g	3 g
Oatmeal, cooked, 1-1/2 cups (375 ml)	6 g	3 g
Oatmeal, instant, unflavoured, 3 packs	8.4 g	3 g
Oat bran, cooked, 1 cup (250 ml)	6 g	3 g
Baked beans, cooked, 1/2 cup (125 ml)	6 g	3 g
Black beans, cooked 3/4 cup (175 ml)	8.2 g	3 g
Kidney beans, cooked, 1/2 cup (125 ml)	6 g	3 g
Lentils, cooked, 1-1/2 cups (375 ml)	24 g	3 g

Tea

Many studies have shown clear evidence that drinking at least 3 cups (750 ml) of tea per day reduces the risk of developing coronary heart disease. In a combined analysis of seventeen studies, the researchers found that a 3 cup (750 ml) increase in daily tea consumption was associated with an 11 per-cent lower risk of heart attack. A seven-year study of U.S. women found the risk of heart attack and stroke and death from heart disease was significantly lower in women who drank at least 4 cups (1000 ml) of black tea per day. In a study of 4807 Dutch men and women aged 55 and older, those who drank more than 1-1/2 cups (375 ml) of black tea per day were 43 percent less likely to suffer a heart attack than non-tea drinkers. Drinking black tea on a regular basis might also safeguard people with existing heart disease.[17-20]

Tea leaves contain antioxidants called catechins. Studies in the lab have demonstrated the ability of catechins in tea to reduce blood clotting, shield LDL cholesterol from oxidation, reduce inflammation and improve blood vessel function. Catechins are found in green tea, black tea and oolong tea, but not in herbal teas. To incorporate tea into your diet, replace coffee and soft drinks with your favourite type of tea, be it green or black. Tea brewed from loose leaves will have a higher concentration of antioxidants than that brewed from tea bags.

Alcoholic beverages

Moderate alcohol consumption—one to two drinks per day—is linked with 20 percent to 30 percent reductions in heart disease risk. Alcohol is thought to protect against heart disease by increasing the level of HDL (good) cholesterol in the bloodstream and by reducing the ability of blood cells called platelets to clump together and form clots. However, alcohol's protective effects are limited to middle-aged and older adults. Alcohol's protective effects are attributed to all types of alcoholic beverages, including wine, beer and spirits.

The Heart and Stroke Foundation of Canada doesn't recommend that you drink alcohol for the purpose of reducing your risk for heart attack and stroke. Drinking more than two drinks per day boosts blood pressure and increases the long-term risk of developing hypertension. Drinking alcoholic beverages can also increase blood triglycerides. Even just one drink a day can increase these blood fats in susceptible people. If you have elevated triglycerides, limiting or avoiding alcohol is strongly advised.

A moderate alcohol intake also increases the risk for several cancers, including breast and colon cancers.

If you drink alcohol, limit yourself to one drink per day for women and two for men. Avoid binge drinking, which can elevate blood pressure. (For elderly people, two drinks per day may be too much to be considered a low-risk intake.)

VITAMINS AND MINERALS
B vitamins
The theory that these nutrients help ward off heart disease and heart attack stems from the fact that three B vitamins in particular—folic acid, B6 and B12—lower homocysteine levels in the blood. Homocysteine is an amino acid made by the body during normal metabolism. A high homocysteine level in the blood is considered by many experts to be a risk factor for heart disease and stroke. Many studies have suggested that excess homocysteine in the bloodstream increases the likelihood of developing heart disease by damaging the lining of the arteries. Studies in the lab have demonstrated the ability of homocysteine to cause oxidative stress, inflammation, blood clotting and blood vessel dysfunction.

Folic acid and vitamins B6 and B12 help break down homocysteine in the body so it doesn't accumulate. Even marginal deficiencies of these nutrients—the result of poor dietary intake or the inability of the body to absorb the vitamins—can lead to a high homocysteine level. Numerous studies have clearly shown that taking a supplement of folic acid, alone or in combination with vitamins B6 and B12, lowers homocysteine levels. Studies have used daily doses of folic acid ranging from 0.5 to 5 milligrams, although 0.8 to 1 milligram appears to provide maximal homocysteine lowering. (The recommended daily intake for folate for men and women is 0.4 milligrams. The word *folate* is often used to describe folic acid. Folate refers to the B vitamin found naturally in foods; folic acid is the synthetic version added to vitamin pills and fortified foods.)

Although consuming adequate amounts of these B vitamins can help keep blood homocysteine in the normal range, large randomized controlled trials have failed to show that taking a B vitamin supplement actually prevents heart attack. It's unclear why the B vitamin homocysteine-lowering trials conducted to date have not demonstrated any benefit. One possibility is that since the introduction of mandatory folic acid food fortification in 1998, B vitamin supplements have a lesser effect on homocysteine levels than expected. It's also possible that B vitamins simply have no effect on your risk of heart disease. Keep in mind that all trials have been conducted in high-risk individuals—people with documented heart disease or kidney disease. The effect of long-term folic acid supplementation on the risk of heart disease in healthy people is unknown.

The Heart and Stroke Foundation of Canada doesn't feel there's enough evidence to recommend an amount of folic acid, B6 or B12 for the prevention of heart disease. It's important, however, that you increase your intake of B vitamins from food sources to help meet your recommended daily intakes.

The best food sources of folate include cooked spinach, broccoli, lentils, orange juice, asparagus, artichokes and whole-grain breads and cereals. Foods rich in vitamin B6 include meat, poultry, fish, liver, legumes, nuts, seeds, whole grains, green leafy vegetables, bananas and avocados. Vitamin B12 is found in animal foods such as meat, poultry, fish, eggs and dairy products, and also in fortified soy and rice beverages.

If you have difficulty eating a varied diet, take a multivitamin and mineral supplement to ensure that you're meeting your B vitamin requirements (see Chapter 1, pages 32–33).

Vitamin C

Many studies have reported a link between high dietary intakes and high blood levels of vitamin C and a lower risk of heart disease. American researchers observed that rates of heart disease were 27 percent lower in the men and women with the highest vitamin C levels compared to those with the lowest.[21] The level of vitamin C in your bloodstream is a good indicator of the amount of vitamin C in your diet. A Portuguese study conducted among 194 adults determined that, compared with those individuals with marginal vitamin C intakes, those who consumed the most vitamin C had an 80 percent lower risk of heart attack.[22] Vitamin C supplements have not been shown to reduce the risk of heart disease.

Dietary vitamin C may protect from heart disease by acting as an antioxidant; it neutralizes harmful free radical molecules that damage your LDL cholesterol. Studies also suggest vitamin C may inhibit the formation of blood clots by reducing the stickiness of platelets.

Include two vitamin C–rich foods in your daily diet. The best sources of vitamin C include citrus fruit, citrus juices, cantaloupe, kiwi, mango, strawberries, broccoli, Brussels sprouts, cauliflower, red pepper and tomato juice. See Chapter 1, page 33, to learn about your daily vitamin C requirements.

Vitamin D

There's growing evidence that vitamin D guards against heart disease. In most populations studied, death rates from cardiovascular disease rise at higher latitudes (e.g., Canada and the northern United States), increase during the winter months and are lower at high altitudes. This pattern fits with the observation that vitamin D deficiency is more common at higher latitudes, during long, dark winters and at lower altitudes. (Our main source of vitamin D comes from sunshine. Vitamin D is synthesized in the skin when it's exposed to the sun's UVB rays for short periods of time.) Although vitamin D is found in foods such as fortified milk, oily fish and egg yolks, the amount we consume from diet is considered insufficient to maintain good health.

Recent studies have revealed that people who are deficient in vitamin D have a higher risk of heart attack and coronary heart disease. In a study of 18,255 healthy men aged 40 to 75 who were followed for ten years, men who were vitamin D deficient were twice as likely to suffer a heart attack as those with sufficient vitamin D levels, even after controlling for other risk factors such as blood cholesterol, body weight and family history of heart disease. Even men with intermediate blood–vitamin D levels were at increased risk of a heart attack.[23] Although this research was conducted in men, there's no reason to think that vitamin D doesn't protect women from heart disease.

Vitamin D helps maintain normal immune function and reduces inflammation in the body. It also assists in keeping heart cells healthy and in maintaining normal blood pressure. Studies have linked low blood–vitamin D levels to greater inflammation, impaired fasting glucose, metabolic syndrome and hypertension—all risk factors for heart disease.

At this time, there's no evidence that taking a daily vitamin D pill will lower the odds of developing heart disease. We'll have to wait for the results of randomized controlled trials to give us this answer. In the meantime, there are other reasons why you should be taking a daily vitamin D supplement. First, foods don't supply much vitamin D to aid in maintaining adequate blood levels of the nutrient. Second, Canadians don't produce enough vitamin D from sunlight from October through March.

Third, there's now strong evidence that vitamin D helps reduce the risk of certain cancers, which prompted the Canadian Cancer Society to recommend in 2007 that adults consider taking 1000 international units (IU) of vitamin D each day in the fall and winter. Older adults, people with dark skin, those who don't go outdoors often and those who wear clothing that covers most of their skin should take the supplement year-round.

To determine the extra dose of vitamin D you need to take, add up how much you're already getting from your multivitamin and calcium supplements, subtract that from your RDA and make up the difference. Choose a vitamin D supplement that contains vitamin D3 instead of vitamin D2, which is less potent. Vitamin D is typically sold in 400 IU and 1000 IU doses, which can make it difficult to hit the 1000 IU dose on the nose. There's no need to be concerned if your vitamin D intake from supplements is slightly over 1000 IU. Consuming up to 2000 IU per day is considered safe.

Vitamin E

Studies conducted in the 1990s hinted that taking a vitamin E supplement can help lower the odds of developing heart disease. More recently the Women's Health Study, a long-term randomized trial, investigated the effect of a 600 IU vitamin E supplement, taken every other day, on the prevention of heart disease in almost 40,000 healthy American women aged 45 or older. Overall, vitamin E had no effect on dying from any cause. But among women 65 and older, those taking vitamin E were 26 percent less likely to have a heart attack or die from heart disease than women not taking the vitamin supplement.[24]

There's little evidence, however, that vitamin E is effective in preventing heart attacks in people with existing heart disease. Two large trials conducted in individuals with a previous heart attack or stroke or evidence of heart disease found that a daily vitamin E supplement didn't change the risk of a subsequent heart attack or stroke.[25,26]

Some trials have found that high-dose vitamin E supplements may actually cause health problems in people with existing heart disease or diabetes.[27,28] Instead of reducing oxidative stress, high doses of vitamin E might possibly cause it. Excess vitamin E might also displace other fat-soluble nutrients, disrupting the body's natural balance of antioxidants. Some researchers believe that other forms of vitamin E, such as gamma-tocopherol found in walnuts, pecans and sesame oil, may be more important for cancer prevention than alpha-tocopherol (the main type of vitamin E found in supplements).

To meet your daily vitamin E requirements, add vitamin E–rich foods such as vegetable oils, avocado, nuts, seeds, wheat germ, whole grains and leafy greens to your daily diet. If you're a healthy post-menopausal woman, consider taking a 400 IU vitamin E supplement. However, if you have existing cardiovascular disease or diabetes, avoid high-dose vitamin E supplements. If you have heart disease or diabetes and still want to take a supplement, take no more than 100 IU per day.

Magnesium

Among its many important roles, magnesium keeps your heart rhythm steady, maintains normal blood pressure and helps regulate blood sugar— all of which influence your heart health. Studies have revealed that higher magnesium intakes and higher body stores of the mineral are linked with protection from type 2 diabetes and heart disease. Consuming more magnesium may improve the prognosis of heart disease by helping to maintain the normal functioning of blood vessels during exercise by allowing vessels to dilate, or relax.[29-34]

Many Canadian women don't consume the recommended amount of magnesium (see Chapter 1, page 23). Although symptoms of magnesium deficiency are rarely seen in Canada, many experts have expressed concern about the prevalence of marginal, or suboptimal, magnesium stores in the body. The best way to increase your intake of magnesium and to maintain normal body stores is to boost your intake of magnesium-rich foods, including whole grains, nuts, legumes, leafy green vegetables and dried fruit.

If a blood test indicates you have very low magnesium stores, increasing your intake of heart healthy foods may not be enough to restore normal magnesium levels. In this case, a daily magnesium supplement will be necessary. Older adults are at risk for magnesium deficiency because they tend to consume less of the mineral in their diets than younger adults and, as well, magnesium absorption decreases with age. If you feel your magnesium intake is below par despite your best efforts to eat more heart healthy foods, consider taking a magnesium supplement. Take 200 to 250 milligrams of magnesium citrate once daily. Magnesium supplements can cause diarrhea and abdominal cramping if taken in high doses. Don't exceed the safe upper limit of 350 milligrams of supplemental magnesium per day.

And keep in mind, when it comes to promoting healthy blood pressure, studies show that magnesium-rich foods do the trick, not supplements. What's more, magnesium-rich foods also supply other nutrients and antioxidants linked to heart health.

HERBAL REMEDIES
Garlic *(Allium sativum)*
Interest in garlic's potential to guard against heart disease began when researchers noticed that people living near the Mediterranean Sea—where garlic is a common ingredient in meals—had lower rates of death from cardiovascular disease. Since then, many studies have investigated garlic's effect on such risk factors for heart disease as blood cholesterol, blood pressure and blood clot formation. Some, but not all, trials suggest that garlic supplements modestly lower total cholesterol, LDL (bad) cholesterol and blood triglycerides over the short term (one to three months). However, similar cholesterol-lowering effects haven't been found in studies lasting six months.

The heart disease–fighting property of garlic is attributed to a variety of powerful sulphur-containing chemicals, in particular allicin and allyl sulphides. Many of these sulphur compounds are responsible for garlic's distinctive smell. In addition to sulphur compounds, fresh and cooked garlic also adds vitamins C and B6, manganese and selenium to your diet.

Many studies show garlic and garlic supplements can significantly impede the ability of platelets in the blood to clump together (aggregate). Platelet aggregation is one of the first steps in the formation of blood clots, which can lead to a heart attack or stroke. A few studies also suggest that garlic might help lower blood pressure. Furthermore, in test tube studies, garlic's sulphur compounds have been shown to have antioxidant powers and reduce the oxidation of LDL cholesterol. In addition, garlic may help reduce inflammation, a process thought to play an important role in the development of heart disease.

If you have high blood cholesterol, a garlic supplement might help— at least in the short term. Several types of garlic supplements are available, each providing differing amounts and types of sulphur compounds, depending on how they are manufactured.

- **Supplements of powdered or dehydrated garlic** are made from garlic cloves that are sliced and dried at a low temperature to preserve an enzyme that triggers the production of allicin, which in turn stimulates the production of other active sulphur compounds. The most commonly used doses range from 600 to 900 milligrams per day.
- **Supplements of aged garlic extract** are made by aging garlic cloves for up to twenty months in a water and ethanol solution. This aging process reduces the content of allicin and sulphur compounds that cause garlic's strong odour. Aged garlic extract is usually standard-ized to contain a guaranteed amount of S-allyl-L-cysteine, a powerful sulphur compound believed to lower LDL cholesterol and inhibit blood clotting. Doses typically used in studies range from 2.4 to 7.2 grams per day.
- When it comes to **fresh garlic**, 4 grams (roughly one clove) per day has been used in cholesterol-lowering studies.

Consuming high amounts of garlic—from supplements or raw—can have side effects, most commonly breath and body odour. More uncom-fortable and potentially serious adverse effects include irritation of the digestive tract, heartburn, flatulence, nausea, vomiting and diarrhea. As well, a high dose of garlic may increase the risk of bleeding. If you're planning to have surgery, avoid using fresh garlic and garlic supplements for the seven days prior to the procedure. There's also potential for garlic to enhance the blood-thinning effects of some prescription drugs (e.g., warfarin [Coumadin]) and of other supplements (e.g., fish oil, vitamin E, ginkgo biloba). Be sure to inform your health care provider if you're taking a garlic supplement, especially if you're taking an anticoagulant medication.

OTHER NATURAL HEALTH PRODUCTS
Coenzyme Q10 (CoQ10)

Coenzyme Q10 (CoQ10) is a fat-soluble, vitamin-like substance made by every cell in the body and stored in cell membranes. The highest concen-trations are in heart, liver, kidney and pancreas cells, but CoQ10 is also found in lipoproteins that transport cholesterol and fat in the bloodstream.

CoQ10's role in producing energy in cells and its antioxidant powers have led researchers to study its effectiveness in preventing and treating heart disease. Studies conducted in test tubes have demonstrated the ability of CoQ10 to inhibit the oxidation of LDL cholesterol. It's also thought that CoQ10 works with vitamin E in the fight against oxidation.

Research hints that CoQ10 supplements may help improve heart health in people with heart disease. Studies have examined the effect of CoQ10 in addition to conventional medical therapy in patients with chronic stable angina (chest pain) and have found that the supplement (60 to 600 milligrams per day) improved exercise tolerance during an exercise stress test and reduced or delayed electrocardiographic changes associated with angina.[35] Several small studies also suggest that taking a CoQ10 supplement could be beneficial in treating hypertension. Some, but not all, research suggests that a daily 200 milligram CoQ10 supplement can improve the functioning of the inner lining of blood vessels (the endothelium) in patients who have both diabetes and high blood cholesterol.[36-38]

A number of studies have shown statins, a class of drugs prescribed to lower LDL cholesterol, decrease blood levels of CoQ10. There's also preliminary research that supports a role for CoQ10 in decreasing muscle pain caused by statins. Despite the fact that more research is needed to confirm if CoQ10 supplements might be beneficial for those taking cholesterol-lowering statins, many people take the supplement as a safeguard. Supplements might also offset the natural decline of CoQ10 in the body due to aging.

There's no consensus on how much CoQ10 is beneficial for heart health. In clinical studies that have reported beneficial effects among participants, the following amounts of CoQ10 were used:

- for angina, a dose of 50 milligrams three times per day
- for reducing the risk of future heart problems in patients who suffered a recent heart attack, a dose of 60 milligrams twice daily
- to prevent statin-induced muscle pain, 100 to 200 milligrams per day
- for treating high blood pressure, 120 to 200 milligrams per day, in divided doses (e.g., 60 milligrams twice per day)

There have been no reports of adverse effects from taking CoQ10 supplements. However, there have been reports that concurrent use of warfarin (Coumadin) and CoQ10 reduced the blood-thinning effect of warfarin. If you take warfarin, don't take CoQ10 supplements without first consulting your doctor.

Fish oil supplements

If you don't eat fatty fish twice per week, consider taking a fish oil capsule to get your DHA and EPA. Experts advise a daily intake of at least 500 milligrams of DHA + EPA combined to help prevent heart disease. The American Heart Association recommends that people who have coronary heart disease consume 1000 milligrams of DHA + EPA combined each day, an amount that requires taking a daily supplement.

Randomized controlled trials have found fish oil reduces the risk of heart attack, stroke, sudden cardiac death and dying from all causes. Findings from studies conducted in people without documented heart disease also suggest that fish oil supplements benefit the heart. One study conducted in overweight men who had high blood pressure and high cholesterol or elevated triglycerides found that a daily fish oil supplement and regular exercise resulted in lower triglycerides, increased HDL cholesterol and a loss of body fat.[39,40] In addition, it's well documented that taking fish oil lowers elevated triglycerides by 20 percent to 50 percent.

Fish oil supplements are made from salmon, anchovies, sardines, herring and mackerel, species of fish rich in omega-3 fatty acids. Most fish oil capsules (1 gram each) provide 300, 500 or 600 milligrams of DHA + EPA combined (check the label to be sure).

For triglyceride lowering, studies have used 1 to 4 grams (1 to 4 capsules) per day. Because fish oil thins the blood, taking high doses may increase the risk of bleeding in people taking prescription anticoagulants such as heparin or warfarin (Coumadin). If you take such a medication, check with your doctor before taking a fish oil supplement.

THE BOTTOM LINE...

Leslie's recommendations for preventing heart disease

1. To keep your LDL cholesterol level in the healthy range, reduce your intake of saturated fat by choosing lower-fat meat, poultry and dairy products.
2. To eat less trans fat, avoid foods that contain partially hydrogenated vegetable oils. If you use margarine, choose one labelled "non-hydrogenated." Read nutrition labels and choose packaged foods that contain no trans fat.
3. Be sure to include the heart healthy omega-3 fats in your diet. Aim to eat fish two times a week. If you don't eat fish, take a fish oil capsule

that provides 500 to 600 milligrams of DHA + EPA combined each day. (DHA supplements made from algae are available for vegetarians and people who are allergic to fish.)

4. To increase your intake of alpha-linolenic acid, a member of the omega-3 family, use flaxseed oil, walnut oil and/or canola oil. Or add ground flaxseed or salba to meals. Include 1/4 cup (60 ml) of nuts in your diet up to five times a week.

5. If you use olive oil, buy the extra-virgin form. It's been processed the least and contains the most antioxidant compounds.

6. If your cholesterol level is in the normal range and you don't have diabetes, feel free to enjoy one whole egg up to six times a week.

7. Plan meals around legumes and soy three times per week.

8. Enjoy a small serving of plain, unsalted nuts five times per week.

9. Include at least 3 grams of soluble fibre in your daily diet. In conjunction with a low-fat diet, foods like psyllium-enriched breakfast cereals, oatmeal and oat bran can lower elevated LDL cholesterol levels.

10. When it comes to buying breads, cereals, rice and pasta, always choose those made from 100% whole grain.

11. Drink a cup or more of tea each day as a source of catechins, antioxidant compounds that protect your LDL cholesterol.

12. If you drink alcohol, limit your intake to no more than one alcoholic beverage per day.

13. Boost your intake of foods rich in B vitamins, especially folate, to help keep your homocysteine levels down. To ensure you're meeting your needs, take a daily multivitamin and mineral supplement.

14. Eat at least one vitamin C–rich food in your diet each day.

15. For even more antioxidant protection, add vitamin E–rich foods to your daily diet. To get the amount of vitamin E that research has found to be protective, take a daily vitamin E supplement (100 to 400 IU).

16. Supplement with 1000 IU of vitamin D each day.

17. Increase your intake of magnesium-rich foods. Consider taking a 200 to 250 milligram magnesium supplement to ensure you're meeting your daily requirements.

18. To get heart-protective sulphur compounds, increase your intake of garlic, both raw and cooked. Use 1/2 to 1 clove a day in cooking. If your cholesterol levels are high, consider taking aged garlic extract (it's odourless). Take one to two capsules up to three times daily with

meals. If you're on blood-thinning medication, check with your physician or pharmacist for possible side effects or interactions.

19. For additional protection from heart disease, consider taking a daily supplement of coenzyme Q10 (CoQ10).

PART 4

EMOTIONAL HEALTH

13
Depression

It's estimated that as many as three million Canadians suffer from serious depression.[1] In fact, at some point in their lives, one in every ten Canadians will experience a degree of depression serious enough to require treatment. What's more, study after study has indicated that women suffer depression twice as often as men.

Rates of depression have been increasing in every generation since 1915. Ongoing scientific research continues to explore the causes of this pervasive condition. However, much of the research on mental illness has been conducted on men, using male standards. As a result, women suffering from mood disorders often don't receive the diagnosis or treatment that's appropriate to their needs. Researchers are only just beginning to understand the factors that contribute to gender-based differences in mental illness.

What causes depression?

When faced with the stresses and losses of life, the natural response is sadness and grief. Everyone experiences emotional highs and lows in life and it's very normal to suffer through a bout of the blues once in a while. But depressive illness goes beyond these reactions. Depression is a prolonged emotional response that significantly interferes with the ability to cope with daily living. It may cause profound lifestyle changes and, without treatment, symptoms may linger for months or even years.

Depression becomes an illness, or clinical depression, when feelings of sadness, emptiness and worthlessness are severe, last for several weeks and begin to interfere with one's work and personal and social life. Depressive illness changes the way a person thinks and behaves, and how his or her body functions. There are three types of depression:

1. **Major depression (clinical or unipolar depression).** This diagnosis is made if symptoms of deep despair persist and consistently interfere with normal functioning during a two-week period.
2. **Dysthymia.** This milder form of depression is a chronic mood disorder that lasts for at least two years. Those who suffer from dysthymia are usually able to function adequately but might seem consistently unhappy.
3. **Manic depression (bipolar disorder).** Less common than the other forms of depression, this condition involves disruptive cycles of elation or euphoria alternating with depressive episodes, irritable excitement and mania.

It's thought that several factors—including a genetic or family history of depression; psychological or emotional vulnerability to depression; body chemistry, such as hormone levels; and major life stress—may play a part in the onset of depression. Modern brain imaging technologies reveal that specific neural circuits in the brain don't function properly during depression, impairing the performance of crucial brain chemicals called neurotransmitters. Another theory holds that depression is caused by an imbalance in the body's response to stress, which results in an overactive hormonal system. Some studies also suggest that low levels of certain brain chemicals, known as amines, may slow down the nervous system and impair brain function enough to cause depression.

In women, there's evidence that the hormonal fluctuations of menstruation and pregnancy can trigger mental disorders.

Symptoms and diagnosis

Symptoms of depression develop gradually, over a period of days or weeks. People with depression often appear slow and sad or irritable and anxious. They may be preoccupied with intense feelings of guilt and may have difficulty sleeping, concentrating or experiencing normal emotions. As the depression progresses, they may feel more and more helpless and hopeless and may even have thoughts of suicide and death.

Not everyone with depression experiences a full range of symptoms, and their severity can vary from person to person. To be diagnosed with depression, you must be experiencing at least four of the following indicators consistently over a period of at least two weeks:

- general sluggishness or agitation
- loss of interest in daily activities
- withdrawal
- acute sadness or feeling of emptiness
- demoralization, despair, feelings of worthlessness and hopelessness
- anxiety
- frequent outbursts of anger and rage
- difficulty concentrating, memory loss, unusual indecisiveness
- self-criticism, self-deprecation
- changes in eating habits
- sleep disorders (insomnia, frequent awakening)
- chronic fatigue, lack of energy
- physical discomfort, such as constipation, headaches

In dysthymia, these symptoms are present in a milder form. This illness begins early in life and may last for years, even decades. People with dysthymic depression are pessimistic, humourless, introverted, lethargic and often self-critical. They're preoccupied with inadequacy, failure and negative events.

People with manic depression often appear elated, uncontrollably enthusiastic and intrusively friendly. But they may just as easily become irritable or hostile. As the condition progresses, mental activity speeds up and the need for sleep decreases. A manic person is easily distracted, shifting constantly from one task or project to another, may indulge in inappropriate sexual or personal behaviours or may have delusions of power and wealth. People suffering from mania often don't recognize their own condition and may put themselves at risk in many ways, without ever realizing they're in danger.

A typical depression can last for six to nine months and episodes may recur several times over a lifetime. Symptoms rarely go away on their own, but with professional diagnosis and treatment, depression can be managed and controlled very successfully.

Who's at risk?

Depression can affect anyone, at any time. The illness is a complicated process and is rarely due to a single event or condition. Some of the main risk factors associated with depression include the following:

- **Family history.** If you have an immediate family member with depression, your risk is much higher. Family environment may also play a role, as children growing up with a depressed person may learn inappropriate ways of handling stress.
- **Traumatic life events.** Early childhood events such as the loss of a parent, sexual abuse or divorce increase the risk of adult depression.
- **Stress.** Work-related pressures or negative life events such as the loss of a loved one, a divorce, financial problems or a move to a new location might trigger depression.
- **Marital and work status.** Depression is highest among divorced, separated or widowed people and among those living alone. Unemployment lasting more than six months is also a factor.
- **Physical illness.** Cancer, heart disease, AIDS/HIV, hormonal disorders and thyroid conditions are associated with depression.
- **Medications.** Many medications, including sedatives and pain medications, produce mood disorders as a side effect.
- **Gender and age.** Women suffer from depression and attempt suicide more often than men. Children, adolescents and the elderly experience stressful life events that may predispose them to depression.
- **Ethnicity.** Depression occurs in every culture and ethnic group. However, cultural and ethnic differences do affect the symptoms and treatment of this condition.
- **Alcohol, drugs and tobacco.** Many people who are depressed suffer from alcoholism too. Alcohol is a depressive drug and will aggravate the symptoms of depression. Some people turn to mood-altering drugs for relief of symptoms, but this type of drug tends to complicate depression and interfere with its treatment. Depression is also associated with an increased frequency of cigarette smoking.

WOMEN AND DEPRESSION

The higher incidence of depression in women begins in adolescence. Teenage girls react to the stresses of forming an identity, confronting sexuality and pursuing independence much differently from boys, and it's here that the seeds of depressive tendencies are sown.

There appears to be a strong relationship between the biology of a woman's body and the incidence of mood disorders. Fluctuations in the level of estrogen can create mood changes shortly before menstruation and after pregnancy. These hormonal fluctuations are also associated with the use of oral contraceptives and with hormone replacement therapy during menopause. Research has confirmed that hormones do indeed affect the brain chemistry that controls our emotions and mood.

The fact that women suffer depression more often than men may be related to the fact that women synthesize serotonin, a brain chemical that carries messages between brain cells, at a lower rate than men. Melatonin, a chemical involved in regulating certain bodily functions, is also produced at different levels in women and men. Both differences may predispose women to become depressed with a lack of sunlight, a condition known as seasonal affective disorder (SAD).

Because of our unique biology, women also suffer from different forms of depression. Between 20 percent and 40 percent of women experience premenstrual syndrome (PMS). PMS can cause mood swings that may interfere with family life and work performance. It's an abnormal response to normal hormone changes and may be associated with malfunctions in brain-serotonin levels.

Postpartum depression is a condition experienced by women shortly after pregnancy. Once the baby is born, women may have a bout of the "baby blues," which is a fairly typical reaction to normal hormonal shifts and the pressures of a new role in life. However, in some women, the reaction is more extreme and may involve many of the symptoms of a major depression. If a woman has one episode of postpartum depression, she has a 50 percent chance of developing it again during subsequent pregnancies.

Eating disorders, anxiety disorders and perimenopausal depression are other depressive illnesses that affect women more seriously than men. Women also seem to be more vulnerable to stress, often as a result of poverty, single parenthood, caring for aging parents or exposure to domestic violence and sexual abuse.

Conventional treatment

Depression is one of the most common and treatable mental disorders. It's usually treated without hospitalization, using a combination of medications and psychotherapy. Even severe depression can be highly responsive to treatment. The earlier treatment begins, the more effective it is and the more likely it will prevent serious recurrences. However, even when treatment is successful, depression may recur. Results of any treatment should be apparent within two to three months.

Several different types of antidepressant drugs are available today and they all provide effective treatment for depression. They work by influencing the activity of brain neurotransmitters, primarily serotonin, norepinephrine and dopamine, and must be taken for several weeks before they begin to work.

- **Selective serotonin reuptake inhibitors (SSRIs)**—Prozac (fluoxetine), Paxil (paroxetine), Zoloft (sertaline). These drugs raise serotonin levels in the brain. (It's thought that reduced serotonin levels in the brain play a role in depression.) SSRIs have fewer side effects than other antidepressant drugs and are often the first choice of treatment for depression. They may cause mild nausea, diarrhea and headaches that usually subside over time. SSRIs commonly cause sexual dysfunction as a side effect.
- **Monoamine oxidase inhibitors (MAOIs)**—Nardil (phenelzine), Parnate (tranylcypromine). Monoamine oxidase is an enzyme that normally breaks down neurotransmitters. Monoamine oxidase inhibitors inactivate this enzyme, leaving more of the neurotransmitter to produce an antidepressant effect. This medication may be helpful for people with atypical symptoms such as overeating, excessive sleeping and anxiety, panic attacks and phobias, or for those who failed to improve on other types of medication. People who take MAOIs must avoid foods and beverages that contain tyramine (such as red wine, beer, aged cheeses, soy sauce and yeast extracts). Combining MAOIs with tyramine can lead to rare but severe high blood pressure or even a stroke or heart attack.
- **Tricyclic antidepressants**—Elavil (amitriptyline), Tofranil (imipramine), Pamelor (nortipyline). These drugs inhibit the reabsorption of two neurotransmitters, norepinephrine and serotonin, into brain cells (neurons). As a result, the receiving neurons get extra stimulation. Although useful in treating depression, these drugs bring with them a host of unpleasant side effects such as weight gain, drowsiness, dizziness and an increased heart rate. They're not usually used to treat mild to moderate depression because the side effects are often worse than the disorder.

Psychotherapy—individual and group—can help to gradually change negative attitudes and feelings of hopelessness and can provide guidance in adjusting to the normal pressures of life. It's often used in conjunction with antidepressant drugs. Electroconvulsive therapy (ECT) is used for severe cases of depression. An electric current is applied to the head to induce a seizure in the brain. For reasons not completely understood, the seizure will quickly and very effectively alleviate depression.

Managing depression

DIETARY STRATEGIES
Carbohydrate-rich foods
Carbohydrate has been one of the most widely studied nutrients with respect to mood. High-carbohydrate meals have been associated with a calming, relaxing effect and even drowsiness. A meal like pasta allows an amino acid called tryptophan to get into the brain, which is then used to make the neurotransmitter serotonin. Numerous studies have linked high serotonin levels with happier moods and low levels with mild depression. Most of this research has been done in women with PMS. These studies find that mood can be improved within 30 to 90 minutes of consuming a carbohydrate-rich food or beverage.

If you're feeling depressed, try a high-carbohydrate meal that contains very little protein. Protein foods like chicken, meat or fish provide many different amino acids that compete with tryptophan for entry into the brain. That means that less serotonin will be produced. Try pasta with tomato sauce, a slice of whole-grain toast with jam or a bowl of whole-grain cereal with low-fat milk. You might also try high-carbohydrate beverages like unsweetened fruit juice, a sports drink or even a glass of low-fat milk.

Omega-3 fats
Low blood levels of two omega-3 fatty acids—DHA and EPA—are common in people who are depressed. It has been established that DHA plays a fundamental role in brain structure and function: As an important component of nerve and brain cell membranes, it helps cells communicate messages effectively. DHA may work to ease depression by altering the structure of cell membranes in the brain, making them more responsive to the effects of serotonin, and by acting as an anti-inflammatory in the brain, which can also influence mood. Many studies have found omega-3

supplementation—alone or in combination with other medication—effective in treating clinical depression. Omega-3 fatty acids also seem to improve a person's response to conventional antidepressants. As well, one study of omega-3 fatty acids combined with medication showed positive effects in treating depression in patients with bipolar disorder.[2-7]

The best food sources of DHA are cold-water fish such as salmon, trout, Arctic char, mackerel, herring, sardines and fresh tuna. Aim to eat fish at least two times a week. (Women of childbearing age and young children should avoid tuna steaks, as they're high in mercury.)

If you have clinical depression, you'll need to take a fish oil supplement to get the required amount of DHA and EPA. The doses used in clinical research are as follows:

- For treating depression: Along with conventional antidepressants, 9.6 grams of fish oil have been used. Take three fish oil capsules three times per day or 1 teaspoon (5 ml) of liquid fish oil two to three times per day.
- For treating bipolar disorder–related depression: Daily supplementation of 6.2 grams of EPA and 3.4 grams of DHA has been used.

Buy an omega-3 fatty acid supplement that contains both EPA and DHA. A good-quality fish oil supplement should also contain vitamin E, which is added to help stabilize the oils. Avoid fish *liver* oil capsules. Fish liver oil supplements often contain only small doses of DHA and EPA. Furthermore, supplements made from fish livers are a concentrated source of vitamin A: Too much vitamin A can be toxic when taken in large amounts for long periods of time.

High doses of fish oil can have side effects, such as leaving an unpleasant taste in the mouth. Fish oil also has a blood-thinning effect. If you take medication that thins the blood, consult your physician before taking any supplements. Fish oil supplements should never replace your medication. Always discuss any alternative or complementary treatment with your doctor first.

VITAMINS AND MINERALS
Vitamin B6
Even marginal deficiencies of the B vitamins have been associated with irritability, depression and mood changes. And if you've suffered from

PMS, chances are you've already heard about vitamin B6 (Chapter 18, Premenstrual Syndrome [PMS], has more on this subject). This B vitamin has been the focus of study in more than 900 women suffering from PMS.[8] Based on the evidence available, a daily supplement of B6 seems likely to balance emotions in women suffering from PMS-related depression.

The body uses B6 to form an important enzyme that's needed to convert tryptophan to serotonin, a brain chemical that has a calming and relaxing effect. Healthy women need 1.6 milligrams of the vitamin each day. The best sources of B6 are high-protein foods like meat, fish and poultry. Other good sources include whole grains, bananas and potatoes. To see how common foods stack up for vitamin B6, see Chapter 1, page 32.

To supplement, a daily dose of 50 to 100 milligrams has been used to treat PMS-related depression. Don't exceed 100 milligrams per day, as too much vitamin B6 taken for an extended period of time can cause irreversible nerve damage.

Folate (folic acid)

People with depression have consistently been found to have lower blood levels of folate than those who don't have depression. Reduced folate levels have been associated with poorer response rates to serotonin reuptake inhibitor drugs (Prozac, Paxil, Zoloft). A number of studies have shown that taking a daily supplement of folic acid (the synthetic version of folate) improves medication response, which may help patients keep the condition in remission.[9-16]

A folate deficiency can contribute to depression by lowering levels of serotonin. In most, but not all, studies of patients with depression, folate deficiency is accompanied by low levels of serotonin in the central nervous system. Research has also shown that supplementing with folic acid restored serotonin levels. The link between low folate and low serotonin is not fully understood but researchers speculate that a compound called S-adenosyl-methionine (SAMe) is involved (see below). Folate deficiency reduces SAMe, which has known antidepressant effects because it increases serotonin in the brain.

The best food sources of folate include cooked spinach, artichokes, asparagus, lentils, dried peas and beans, chicken liver, orange juice and wheat germ. Folic acid is added to white flour, white pasta and enriched cornmeal in Canada. To enhance the response to antidepressant medications, a daily folic acid supplement of 200 to 500 micrograms (0.2 to

0.5 milligrams) has been used in studies. If you take a single supplement of folic acid, ensure that it has B12 added.

Chromium

In patients with atypical depression who are overweight or obese and who also have severe carbohydrate cravings, supplementing with chromium may be beneficial. Research has found that a daily supplement can help reduce appetite, overeating and carbohydrate cravings.[17,18] There's also preliminary evidence that chromium might improve the response to antidepressants in people with dysthymia by maintaining brain levels of serotonin and improving how the body uses the hormone insulin to regulate blood sugar.

Chromium-rich foods include calf liver, chicken breast, oysters, refried beans, brewer's yeast, wheat germ, wheat bran, whole grains, blackstrap molasses, mushrooms, broccoli, green peas, grape juice and apples (with skin). To reduce carbohydrate cravings in depressed patients, studies have used a supplemental dose of 600 micrograms of chromium picolinate. To improve mood in patients with dysthymia, take 200 micrograms of chromium picolinate or chromium nicotinate once or twice daily. A daily dose of 600 micrograms or more of chromium picol-inate has been associated with adverse effects, so use cautiously. Be sure to inform your doctor if you decide to take chromium in addition to your medication.

Zinc

More than three hundred enzymes in the body require zinc and the highest amounts of this trace mineral are found in the brain. Low blood levels of zinc have been linked to major and minor depression. Furthermore, supplementing with zinc has been shown to have an antidepressant effect. Studies conducted in healthy older adults suggest that getting adequate zinc from a variety of foods or a supplement may help reduce the likeli-hood of depression.[19,20] Research has also found that adding a daily zinc supplement to standard antidepressant therapy significantly improves symptoms of depression.[21,22]

To ensure an adequate intake of zinc, include the following foods in your diet: seafood (especially oysters and crab), red meat, poultry (dark meat), yogurt, nuts, legumes, wheat bran, wheat germ, whole grains and enriched breakfast cereals. A daily multivitamin and mineral supplement will also supply 10 to 20 milligrams of zinc. (See Chapter 1, page 34, to determine your daily zinc requirement.) To augment the effects of standard antidepressant medication in people with unipolar depression, a daily zinc supplement of 25 milligrams has been used. Don't take more than 40 milligrams of zinc per day.

HERBAL REMEDIES
St. John's wort *(Hypericum perforatum)*

For years, this herb has been used in Europe to treat both mild depression and seasonal affective disorder. Findings from numerous clinical trials have concluded that St. John's wort is an effective treatment for mild depression.[23,24] Studies clearly suggest that St. John's wort is likely as effective as low-dose tricyclic antidepressants (e.g., Amitriptyline, Nortriptyline) and selective serotonin reuptake inhibitors (e.g., Prozac, Zoloft, Paxil) in treating depression. Taking St. John's wort improves mood, decreases anxiety and reduces insomnia caused by mild to severe major depression.

Clinical guidelines from the American College of Physicians–American Society of Internal Medicine suggest that St. John's wort can be considered an option along with conventional antidepressants for short-term treatment of mild depression. However, because the herbal remedy interacts with so many different medications (see below), this might not be a viable option for people who take other conventional medications.

Experts believe that St. John's wort keeps brain serotonin levels high for a longer period, just like the popular antidepressant drugs Paxil, Zoloft and Prozac. St. John's wort also appears to alter levels of dopamine and norepinephrine in the brain, two other neurotransmitters involved in mood.

Buy a St. John's wort supplement that is standardized to 0.3 percent hyperforin content, the extract used in most clinical studies of mild and moderate depression. The recommended dose is 300 milligrams taken three times daily.

When taken in high doses for a long period, the herb may cause sensitivity to sunlight in very light-skinned individuals. St. John's wort has the potential to interact with a number of medications including anti-cancer agents (e.g., imatinib and irinotecan), anti-HIV agents (e.g., indinavir, lamivudine and nevirapine), anti-inflammatory agents (e.g., ibuprofen and fexofenadine), anti-microbial agents (e.g., erythromycin and voriconazole), heart drugs (e.g., digoxin, ivabradine, warfarin, verapamil, nifedipine and talinolol), and certain antidepressants, oral contraceptives and statins (e.g., atorvastatin and pravastatin). If you take medication, be sure to consult with your pharmacist and doctor before taking St. John's wort.

The herb is not recommended for use during pregnancy and breast-feeding. If you're currently taking a prescription antidepressant drug, don't take it concurrently with St. John's wort. Always consult your physician before stopping any medication.

OTHER NATURAL HEALTH PRODUCTS
SAMe (S-adenosyl-methionine)
SAMe is a compound the body makes naturally from certain amino acids found in high-protein foods like fish and meat. The production of SAMe is closely linked with folate and vitamin B12, and deficiencies of these two nutrients can lead to depressed levels of SAMe in the brain and nervous system.

The results of recent well-controlled studies show that SAMe is significantly better than a placebo in treating depression, and it may even be more effective than tricyclic antidepressant medication.[25-32] In patients taking SAMe, symptoms improve in as few as four to five days. Exactly how SAMe works to treat depressive symptoms is not entirely clear. It's associated with higher levels of brain neurotransmitters, but it may also work by favourably changing the composition of cell membranes in the brain, enabling neurotransmitters and cell receptors to function more efficiently.

SAMe is sold as a dietary supplement in the United States, but it hasn't been approved for sale in Canada. If you're shopping on the Internet or visiting the United States, look for an enteric-coated supplement to help SAMe withstand the acidity of your stomach. There are several forms of SAMe available: sulphate, sulphate-p-toluenesulphonate (tosylate) and butanedisulphonate. Some experts believe butanedisulphonate is more stable than tosylate.

For depression, take 800 to 1600 milligrams per day, in divided doses. Start with one 400 milligram tablet twice daily, working up to two tablets three times daily. Take SAMe on an empty stomach. It may take thirty days of treatment to notice significant improvements in mood. If you're currently taking medication for depression and you're thinking about trying SAMe, don't discontinue your medication without first speaking to your doctor. When taken with antidepressant drugs, SAMe may have an additive effect that causes potentially dangerous side effects.

THE BOTTOM LINE...
Leslie's recommendations for managing depression

1. Eat three meals each day plus one or two midday snacks to avoid wide fluctuations in blood sugar and neurotransmitter levels.
2. Ensure your diet includes 6 to 7 servings of grain foods, and 7 to 10 servings of fruit and vegetables each day to ensure you get enough carbohydrates in your diet.
3. Get more omega-3 fats in your diet. Eat oily fish such as salmon, trout, sardines and herring twice per week. Consider taking a fish oil capsule; buy a product that offers both EPA and DHA, the two omega-3 fatty acids found in fish oil.
4. Eliminate alcoholic beverages, which can worsen feelings of depression.
5. Make sure you're getting enough vitamin B6 in your diet. If you suffer from PMS-related depression, supplement your diet with 50 to 100 milligrams of B6 each day.
6. Make sure your daily diet includes folate-rich foods. To ensure you're meeting your daily requirement, take a multivitamin and mineral supplement each day.
7. Increase your intake of chromium-rich foods; consider taking a 200 microgram supplement of chromium each day.
8. In addition to your daily multivitamin and mineral supplement, include foods rich in zinc in your daily diet.
9. If altering your diet and nutrient intake doesn't ease symptoms of depression, try a standardized extract of St. John's wort. Take 300 milligrams three times a day. Buy a product that's standardized for 0.3 percent hyperforin.
10. Consider taking 400 milligrams of SAMe, a dietary supplement used to treat depression, two to three times daily. Buy an enteric-coated product and take it on an empty stomach.
11. If your mood swings don't improve with dietary changes or the recommended supplements, consult your doctor. Serious emotional problems may require medication.

14
Eating Disorders

We live in a society that's dominated by the cult of thinness. Everywhere we look, we're bombarded with the message that thin is beautiful. The waifish looks of ultra-thin models and entertainers have become our ideal—establishing standards of beauty that are not only unattainable but also unhealthy. It's no wonder that so many North American women struggle with their body image. By the time they reach adulthood, nearly half of all females have concerns about their weight and many have already begun the vicious cycle of dieting and weight gain. Recent studies show that girls as young as 9 years old are preoccupied with their weight.

Some women, especially during their vulnerable teenage years, carry their struggle with body image to the extreme. They become the victims of the complex, chronic illnesses known as eating disorders. Women suffer from these illnesses far more often than men, representing nearly 90 percent of all cases. Among teenage girls, the statistics are even more dramatic. In this age group, eating disorders rank as the third most common cause of chronic illness. An increasing number of older women are also seeking treatment for eating disorders.

Anorexia nervosa, *bulimia nervosa* and *binge eating disorder* are the three main types of eating disorders. Women who suffer from these conditions experience physical, psychological and social symptoms that eventually threaten their well-being, their overall health and even their lives. Eating disorders can be treated with long-term therapy but usually require the intervention of a variety of health professionals, including registered dietitians, physicians and mental-health specialists.

Because the treatment for each type of eating disorder is unique and involves a multidisciplinary approach, it's beyond the scope of this chapter to outline all possible nutrition recommendations. Rather, I have presented important information about each condition to help you better understand the causes, risk factors and symptoms. If your eating disorder is not serious enough to warrant a treatment program, I strongly recommend that you seek the advice of a registered dietitian (www.dietitians.ca) to help you develop a plan that will normalize your eating patterns and correct any nutritional deficiencies. This is imperative to prevent long-term health problems associated with eating disorders.

Anorexia nervosa

This eating disorder is characterized by an extreme fear of gaining weight. People with anorexia nervosa are obsessed with being thin and have an unrealistic concept of their body image. Even though they are noticeably underweight, anorexics always believe they're fat. To achieve their goal of weight loss, they eat very little and may exercise excessively. Sometimes they even engage in self-induced vomiting or misuse laxatives or diuretics as part of a binge-purge cycle. Anorexia nervosa is an extremely dangerous and potentially life-threatening condition. People suffering from this eating disorder can literally starve themselves to death.

Anorexia means loss of appetite. Ironically, anorexics are very often hungry. They become obsessive about food, frequently collecting recipes and making elaborate meals for other people that they themselves will not eat. They ritualize food preparation and sometimes hide food in special places, but never eat it. They get pleasure from controlling their eating and, as they begin to starve, they may even achieve a sense of euphoria from being so disciplined and successful in achieving their goals.

There's no precise cause of anorexia nervosa but it's thought to be an illness of psychological origin. What begins as a normal desire to lose a few pounds rapidly becomes a compulsive obsession with body image. Anorexia nervosa primarily affects women, particularly young women. Research indicates that these women are responding to societal and cultural pressures that may predispose them to developing an eating disorder.

Often, women with anorexia nervosa have very low self-esteem. They may not feel good about themselves or the way they look. In an attempt to change their self-image, these women may take their interest in dieting and weight loss to an extreme. For some women, anorexia is not an issue of self-confidence but rather a means of taking control of their lives. They may have feelings of powerlessness and of being dominated by outside forces. By taking rigid control of their eating, these women are able to maintain a sense of control over some aspect of their lives. This response is frequently triggered by stress, anxiety or anger towards family members or in other personal relationships.

In many cases, women who suffer from anorexia are perfectionists and over-achievers. In constantly striving to reach perfection, they lay the foundation for failure. They are overly critical of themselves, set unreasonable standards of performance and have a compulsive need to please others. Having low self-confidence and setting unrealistic goals often results in feelings of ineffectiveness that may lead to abnormal eating behaviours.

Studies indicate that there may also be a biochemical explanation behind the psychology of eating disorders. Certain brain chemicals, known as neurotransmitters, are at lower levels in people with anorexia. Reduced levels of serotonin, a powerful neurotransmitter, are known to be associated with depression. There may be a link between anorexia and depression, but further research is needed to confirm the theory. Higher levels of cortisol, a brain hormone released in response to stress, and vasopressin, a brain chemical associated with obsessive-compulsive disorders, have also been identified with anorexia.

SYMPTOMS

The warning signs of anorexia nervosa include:

- a preoccupation with food and weight: excessive dieting, counting calories, checking body weight several times a day
- feeling fat, even when weight is below normal; distorted body image
- significant weight loss, with no evidence of related illness
- depression
- denial of hunger, despite an extreme reduction in eating
- strange eating habits: cutting food into small pieces, preferring food of specific texture or colour, refusing to eat in front of others
- complaints of feeling cold: loss of body fat leads to dropping body temperatures
- appearance of long, fine hair on the body: a way of conserving body heat after loss of body fat
- brittle hair and nails
- dry, yellow skin
- loss of sex drive
- cessation of menstrual periods

As anorexia progresses, the symptoms of starvation become increasingly evident. Eventually, every major organ in the body will be affected. The heart becomes weaker and pumps less blood through the body. Dehydration sets in and fainting spells are common. Electrolyte imbalances develop as the body loses potassium, sodium and chloride; this results in fatigue, muscle weakness, irritability, muscle spasms and depression. In severe cases, these physical changes cause irregular heartbeat, convulsions and death due to kidney or heart failure. Approximately one in ten women suffering from anorexia will die—a death rate that is among the highest for a psychiatric disease.

WHO'S AT RISK?

In Canada, it's estimated that 200,000 to 300,000 women between the ages of 13 and 40 suffer from anorexia nervosa. It's a condition that usually surfaces during the teenage years, when girls are between 14 and 18. Unfortunately, anxiety about weight and body image is beginning at younger and younger ages, with girls as young as 9 years old reporting weight concerns. Because adolescence is a time of growth and development, the nutritional disturbances caused by disordered eating can have devastating implications for teenage girls. Adequate energy, protein, vitamins and minerals are all necessary for proper growth. Young girls with eating disorders may lose essential muscle mass, body fat and bone minerals at a crucial point in their development, leaving them at greater risk for osteoporosis, diabetes and high blood pressure in later life.

In many cases, the incidence of anorexia is influenced by social environment. Girls with a peer group or family network that emphasizes physical attractiveness and thinness are more likely to acquire eating disorders. Girls and women with low self-esteem or depressive tendencies are also very susceptible to the condition, especially if they're dealing with high levels of stress or traumatic events such as rape or abuse. There are also indications that anorexia nervosa may run in families.

In our society, there are certain professions or activities that emphasize thinness and appearance to an exceptional degree. People who participate in dancing, gymnastics, wrestling, modelling, acting and long-distance running are likely to be very aware of their weight or body image. They may be particularly susceptible to an eating disorder such as anorexia nervosa.

DIAGNOSIS

Because the eating habits of people with anorexia nervosa are very secretive, the condition can be hard to diagnose. Anorexics typically refuse to admit anything is wrong and may become angry or defensive when family or friends express concern. For this reason, the disorder may go undiagnosed for a long time.

Anorexia is usually diagnosed by the appearance of specific symptoms. When a girl loses at least 15 percent of her body weight, there's a good chance that she is anorexic. If she demonstrates a compulsive drive for thinness, coupled with an excessive fear of becoming fat, unhealthy weight-control practices or obsessive thinking about food, weight, body image or exercise, the diagnosis of anorexia is appropriate. In females, anorexia also lowers estrogen production, which causes menstrual cycles to stop. A failure to menstruate for at least three months is another crucial part of the diagnostic puzzle of anorexia.

CONVENTIONAL TREATMENT

Treatment is usually complicated by the fact that most people with the condition deny that they have a problem. They refuse therapy, yet they clearly need help to manage their disorder. Anorexia nervosa rarely goes away on its own.

The goal of therapy for most eating disorders is to restore a normal weight, develop normal eating patterns, overcome unhealthy attitudes about body image and self-worth, and provide support to family and friends who may be helping with the recovery process. Because anorexia nervosa has such a widespread influence and affects so many aspects of daily life, effective treatment requires a collaborative effort from a team of health professionals. Often, the team consists of a family physician to manage physical symptoms, a psychiatrist or psychologist to introduce behavioural modification and a nutritionist to establish a healthy diet for recovery.

The sooner anorexia nervosa is identified and treated, the better the eventual outcome. In the early stages, the disorder may be treated without hospitalization. But when weight loss is severe, hospitalization is necessary to restore weight and prevent further physical deterioration. A structured approach that involves careful observation of all eating and elimination— urinating, bowel movements and vomiting—is the first stage of treatment.

When weight is restored and symptoms are stabilized, some type of psychotherapy is required to deal with the underlying emotional issues that trigger the abnormal eating patterns. Family therapy is especially helpful for younger girls, and behavioural or cognitive therapy is also effective in helping replace destructive attitudes with positive ones. A nutritionist will add support by providing advice on proper diet and eating regimens. In some cases, antidepressant medications may be prescribed, but they shouldn't be used as a substitute for appropriate psychological treatment.

Unfortunately, many people with anorexia nervosa have a tendency to relapse and return to dysfunctional eating habits. Long-term therapy and regular health monitoring are essential for a successful result. A strong network of love and support from family and friends is also crucial to the recovery process.

Bulimia nervosa

Bulimia nervosa is the most common type of eating disorder. You may also hear it referred to as bingeing and purging. A person with this condition eats large amounts of high-calorie food in a very short period of time, and then uses vomiting, diuretics or laxatives to eliminate the food before the body can absorb it. Fasting or excessive exercising are other methods that bulimics may use to counteract the weight gain caused by binge eating.

People suffering from bulimia binge as often as several times a day, sometimes consuming 10,000 calories or more in a matter of minutes or hours. Comfort foods that are sweet, soft and high in calories, such as ice cream, cake or pastry, are favourite choices for bingeing. Immediately after the binge comes the purge, when some bulimics use as many as twenty or more laxatives a day to rid their bodies of these huge quantities of food.

Just like people with anorexia nervosa, bulimics are extremely afraid of becoming fat and are obsessed with body image. They fear food, and yet they consume vast amounts of it. With anorexia nervosa, the extreme weight loss becomes an obvious signal of the disorder. But people with bulimia usually look quite normal and often show few signs of their condition. Their weight may fluctuate wildly, but usually stays within normal ranges. They may even be slightly heavy. Because bulimics are often very secretive about their abnormal behaviour, the presence of bulimia can be hard to identify.

As with most eating disorders, bulimia nervosa is a psychological condition. It may be triggered by elevated stress levels and often affects women who are intelligent and high achievers. In many cases, these women are striving to conform to unrealistic ideals of thinness and beauty, and are using food and weight as a means of controlling their underlying emotional problems. People with bulimia nervosa are very aware of their behaviour and feel guilty or remorseful. In this way, they're quite unlike anorexics, who deny the existence of their condition. Nearly half of all people with anorexia go on to develop some symptoms of bulimia.

Studies have shown that bulimics are particularly prone to impulsive behaviour. They have difficulty dealing with anxiety, have little self-control and often indulge in drug or alcohol abuse or sexual promiscuity. They're also susceptible to depression, anxiety disorders and social phobias. As with anorexia nervosa, people with bulimia have lower levels of brain neurotransmitters, such as serotonin, which may predispose them to developing these psychological disturbances.

SYMPTOMS
In addition to the preoccupation with food and weight that's characteristic of most eating disorders, symptoms of bulimia may include:

- evidence of binge eating, large amounts of food going missing, stealing money or food
- food cravings
- frequent weight fluctuations
- evidence of purging, vomiting, abuse of laxatives or diuretics, frequent fasting or excessive exercising
- swelling of glands under the jaw caused by vomiting
- erosion of tooth enamel and other dental problems caused by vomiting
- feelings of shame, self-reproach and guilt
- emotional changes, depression, irritability, social withdrawal

The purging behaviour associated with bulimia can also cause physical complications that are very dangerous to long-term health. Vomiting and purging can lead to imbalances in fluids and electrolytes. When potassium levels fall too low, abnormal heart rhythms develop. Some bulimics use a medication called ipecac to induce vomiting; overuse of this substance has been known to cause sudden death.

WHO'S AT RISK?
Like anorexia, bulimia is primarily a women's disorder. Nearly twice as many women suffer from bulimia as anorexia and, in Canada, estimates run as high as 600,000 women affected by this eating disorder. Bulimia

tends to develop in later adolescence, often striking young women between the ages of 18 and 20; however, it can appear in earlier adolescence.

As with other eating disorders, bulimia surfaces most often in people who have low self-confidence and are insecure about their appearance. They may be very self-critical and may set unreasonable goals of perfection for themselves. Often, bulimia becomes an issue of control and may be a response to stressful events. Girls reporting sexual or physical abuse are very susceptible to developing an eating disorder such as bulimia. Studies also indicate that the disorder may have a genetic element and may run in families.

DIAGNOSIS
Bulimia is usually suspected in people who are obsessed about weight gain and have wide fluctuations in weight, especially if there's evidence of excessive use of laxatives. Swollen salivary glands and tooth decay are also recognizable signs of the disorder. Blood tests may be necessary to identify dehydration, electrolyte imbalances and nutrient deficiencies.

CONVENTIONAL TREATMENT
In most cases, people with bulimia are treated without hospitalization. Because it's a psychological condition, cognitive and behavioural therapy are necessary to deal with the emotional issues underlying the symptoms of this disorder. As with anorexia nervosa, a multidisciplinary approach to treatment works best. Physicians, nutritionists and mental health professionals will work together to address the many different facets of this eating disorder. In particular, long-term psychotherapy is needed to help reduce destructive tendencies and develop better coping strategies. Antidepressant medication has proven to be an effective psychological intervention.

Binge eating disorder (BED)

Binge eating disorder (BED) is a condition that has many similarities to bulimia nervosa. People with BED frequently eat huge quantities of food and feel that they have no control over their eating. Unlike bulimics, however, they don't purge afterwards with vomiting or laxatives.

Although most of us are guilty of overeating at some time or other, binge eaters have much more serious problems. In most cases, the disorder causes considerable distress to the people who suffer from it and is often accompanied by depression. At this time, scientists are not sure whether depression is a symptom or an underlying cause of BED. People do report that emotions such as anger, sadness, anxiety or boredom trigger episodes of binge eating. Studies are currently being done on neurotransmitters and other brain chemicals to determine if they're linked to binge eating disorder.

SYMPTOMS
The symptoms of BED include:

- frequently eating an abnormally large amount of food
- feeling unable to control what or how much food is eaten
- eating more rapidly than usual
- eating until uncomfortably full
- eating large amounts of food, even when not hungry
- experiencing feelings of disgust, guilt or depression after overeating
- eating alone because of embarrassment at the quantity of food being eaten

WHO'S AT RISK?
Binge eating disorder occurs most often in people who are obese—with a body mass index (BMI) of 30 or greater—and becomes more prevalent as body weight increases. Obese people with BED become overweight at an earlier age than those without the disorder and may suffer more frequent bouts of losing and regaining weight. However, it's not uncommon for people with normal, healthy weight to suffer from BED. It occurs slightly more often in women than in men and tends to appear in later years, affecting an older population than either anorexia or bulimia nervosa.

DIAGNOSIS
BED can be very difficult to distinguish from other causes of obesity. Because people with the disorder are embarrassed about their behaviour, they work very hard to conceal their bingeing tendencies. Right now, there are probably thousands of people suffering from BED who aren't properly diagnosed.

Perhaps the most distinctive diagnostic feature of the condition is the depression that accompanies it. Doctors look for overeating habits that establish an "out-of-control" pattern and that are followed by feelings of anxiety, guilt and depression.

CONVENTIONAL TREATMENT

Many of the medical problems associated with obesity also apply to binge eating disorder. Treatment may be necessary for conditions such as high cholesterol, high blood pressure, type 2 diabetes, gall bladder disease and heart disease. Other than the appropriate therapies for obesity-related disorders, there are no standard treatments for BED. As with most eating disorders, an approach that involves psychotherapy and antidepressant drugs seems to be most effective. In striving for a successful result, it's essential to deal with the emotional issues of the illness. Because people with BED find it very difficult to stay on a treatment regimen and frequently return to inappropriate behaviour, long-term therapy is always recommended.

Getting help for eating disorders

The following organizations can provide information, literature and qualified referrals for the treatment of eating disorders:

National Association of Anorexia Nervosa and
Associated Disorders (ANAD)
www.anad.org
P.O. Box 7
Highland Park, IL, USA 60035
Tel: 847-831-3438
Fax: 847-433-4632

National Eating Disorder Information Centre
www.nedic.ca
200 Elizabeth Street
ES 7-421
Toronto, ON, Canada M5G 2C4
Tel: 416-340-4156
Fax: 416-340-4736
Email: nedic@uhn.on.ca

www.something-fishy.org
The Something Fishy website, an extensive resource on eating disorders, is posted by a recovering sufferer of anorexia nervosa.

PART 5

CONCEPTION, PREGNANCY AND MOTHERHOOD

15
Infertility

Infertility is a condition fraught with disappointment, frustration and heartbreak for couples. Defined as the inability to conceive after one year of frequent, unprotected intercourse, infertility affects approximately one in six couples. Throughout North America, infertility is on the rise, possibly due to the increase in sexually transmitted diseases and the decision of a growing number of women to delay having children until later in life.

Once thought to be solely a woman's problem, failure to conceive can be caused by reproductive difficulties in both men and women. Thirty percent of all cases of infertility originate with the woman, 30 percent originate with the man, 30 percent are the result of combined factors and the remaining cases are unexplained.[1]

For women, infertility is often associated with ovarian disorders; for men, it's usually linked to problems with sperm production. Treatment for infertility varies, depending on the reproductive problems involved. Over 80 percent of all infertility cases are treated with either drugs or surgery. As well, assisted reproductive technologies (ART), such as in vitro fertilization, have been providing effective solutions for many couples struggling with the emotional distress of infertility.

What causes infertility?

The discovery of infertility usually comes as an unexpected shock, and both partners suffer from the tension, disappointment, anger and grief that accompany a failure to conceive.

CONCEPTION

For a woman, the basis of her future conception is established while she's still in the womb. By the fifth month of her development before birth, a woman's lifetime supply of more than seven million eggs, or ova, has been created and stored in her tiny fetal ovaries. As she grows and matures, millions of these eggs disintegrate, leaving her with about 300,000 eggs available for fertilization by the time she reaches puberty. A woman becomes fertile once her menstrual cycle begins, usually sometime between the ages of 9 and 16. From this point onwards, an egg will ripen inside her ovaries once every month until she reaches menopause.

Stimulated by a sequence of hormones, the egg matures inside a tiny, saclike structure called a follicle and is released into one of the two Fallopian tubes. For conception to take place, a sperm must fertilize the egg as it travels from the ovaries and through the Fallopian tubes to reach the uterus.

A man produces sperm in his testicles on a continuous basis throughout his lifetime. Sperm are shaped like tadpoles, carrying genetic material in their "heads" and lashing their "tails" to move in a swimming motion. During intercourse, a man ejaculates millions of sperm into a woman's vagina. Ideally, because both sperm and egg deteriorate fairly quickly, the sperm will fertilize the egg within twenty-four hours of ovulation. To reach the egg, the sperm must travel through the acidic environment of the vagina into the uterus and up the Fallopian tubes. Although millions of sperm make this difficult journey, only one will penetrate the tough outer membrane of the egg.

Once the first sperm has entered the egg, a chemical reaction makes the egg impenetrable to other sperm. The genetic material in the head of the sperm then combines with the genetic material in the egg, completing the process of conception. The fertilized egg travels down through the Fallopian tube into the uterus, where it implants on the thickened lining of the uterine wall, called the endometrium. The woman's body nurtures this tiny collection of cells for nine months as it grows and develops within the protective environment of the uterus into a fully formed fetus.

FEMALE INFERTILITY

At any stage along the way, from the development of a woman's eggs and ovaries before birth to the migration of a fertilized egg into her uterus, this intricate reproductive process can go astray. Infertility has been linked to many different factors, all of which influence the normal course of conception.

Approximately one-third of female infertility is caused by a failure to ovulate, a condition known as anovulation. Unless ovulation takes place, there's no egg available for the sperm to fertilize. A balance of hormones is necessary for ovulation to occur successfully. Two small glands located in your brain, the hypothalamus and the pituitary gland, regulate most of these hormonal responses.

The hypothalamus secretes gonadotropin-releasing hormone (GnRH), which stimulates the pituitary gland to relay hormonal messages to the ovaries. In response to these messages, the ovaries nurture an egg to maturity and release it into the Fallopian tubes, ready to be fertilized. Many factors can interfere with the performance of your hypothalamus, preventing it from sending the correct signals to the pituitary gland. Emotional stress, extreme exercise, dieting, poor nutrition, low body fat, anorexia, medications and environmental toxins can all affect the hypothalamus. When the hypothalamus and the pituitary gland are unable to communicate effectively, conception is disrupted.

The pituitary gland contributes to conception by producing two hormones, follicle-stimulating hormone (FSH) and luteinizing hormone (LH). These hormones stimulate the follicles in the ovaries to grow and release mature eggs. They also tell the ovaries to produce estrogen and progesterone. The pituitary gland may malfunction because of a tumour, an injury, surgical complications or various medical disorders. A defective pituitary gland can over- or under-produce FSH and LH, resulting in ovulation failure.

The pituitary gland also produces prolactin, a hormone involved in the production of breast milk. Prolactin suppresses ovulation, acting as a natural form of birth control during pregnancy and breastfeeding. The pituitary gland may secrete too much prolactin due to severe kidney disease, adrenal gland disorders, hypothyroidism and the effect of certain medications. Ten percent to 20 percent of infertile women have elevated levels of prolactin.

Other glands also affect hormones involved in conception. The thyroid gland, for example, establishes your metabolic rate by circulating hormones to control the speed and efficiency of your internal functions. If the thyroid gland becomes overactive (hyperthyroid) or underactive (hypothyroid), it can speed up or slow down your body's ability to use hormones, causing problems with fertility.

Although you may not realize it, every woman has small amounts of male sex hormones, called androgens, circulating through her bloodstream. These hormones are secreted by the adrenal glands and are necessary for normal sexual development. If your adrenal glands malfunction, the elevated levels of male hormones will suppress ovulation. Excessive androgen production is a sign that you may be suffering from a very common disorder known as polycystic ovary syndrome (read Chapter 20 for more information), one of the leading causes of female infertility.

There are a variety of ovarian disorders, including cysts, tumours, infections and medical conditions, that can cause infertility. For some women, their ovaries simply fail to function: Due to surgery, injury, radiation or chromosomal problems, their ovaries run out of eggs too early, sending them into premature menopause. In rare instances, women are born without ovaries or without a normal supply of eggs, making ovulation impossible.

Several disorders of the uterus can also hamper conception. During the normal reproductive process, progesterone and luteinizing hormone stimulate the uterine lining to thicken into a nourishing bed for the fertilized egg. If the uterus is unable to respond to these hormones, the egg cannot implant properly, and spontaneous abortion or miscarriage usually results. Some women find it difficult to carry a fetus to full term because their uterus is structurally abnormal. Others discover that they're infertile because they were born without a uterus.

Infections that affect the reproductive tract are another cause of infertility. Sexually transmitted diseases (STDs) such as gonorrhea, chlamydia and pelvic inflammatory disease are on the rise in North America, and are destroying the fertility of thousands of women every year. These insidious infections can go undetected for long periods of time and, if left untreated, can scar your uterus, block your Fallopian tubes and cause the formation of pelvic adhesions. Even frequent yeast infections (vaginitis) can cause tubal damage that's severe enough to prevent the sperm from intercepting the egg. Abdominal or pelvic surgery, appendicitis, endometriosis, ectopic pregnancies or the use of an IUD contraceptive device may also cause uterine or tubal damage. Occasionally, the use of oral contraceptives may delay ovulation for as long as six months, causing temporary infertility.

Many women fail to realize that diet, nutrition and lifestyle can also influence fertility. Excessive exercise, low-calorie diets, eating disorders, obesity, certain medications, elevated stress levels—even the use of vaginal lubricants—are all factors that affect the reproductive process. Fortunately, these are among the easiest fertility problems to correct.

MALE INFERTILITY

Men are considered to be infertile when they don't produce enough sperm or when their sperm are of poor quality. Each time a man ejaculates, he releases approximately 50 million sperm in each millilitre of seminal fluid. If his sperm count drops below 20 million sperm per millilitre of ejaculate, his fertility will be impaired. The quality of the sperm is also important. Normal sperm have oval heads and long tails. Poor-quality sperm have large heads and deformed tails. These abnormalities interfere with the motility of the sperm, which means that they're unable to swim to the egg in a vigorous, forward motion. If the sperm cannot reach or penetrate the egg, it's impossible for conception to take place.

Problems with sperm production can result from:

- medical illnesses, including mumps and sexually transmitted diseases
- injury to the testicles, an undescended testicle or testicular cancer
- certain drugs, including recreational drugs such as marijuana
- lifestyle factors, such as cigarette smoking or drinking alcohol
- antibodies that are produced by the immune system to attack or disable the sperm
- vasectomy (surgical sterilization)
- overheating the sperm by wearing tight clothes, taking too many long baths or using saunas
- environmental toxins
- defects in the sperm-producing cells

COMBINED INFERTILITY FACTORS

One of the main factors behind the increased rate of infertility in North America is age. Many couples are waiting until they're well into their thirties or forties before attempting to have children. However, the quality and numbers of both sperm and eggs deteriorate as men and women grow older. By leaving their plans for parenthood until later in life, many couples are putting their chances of conception at risk.

Sometimes infertility arises because the man's sperm is incompatible with the woman's cervical mucus. Normally, the cervix secretes a thick mucus to protect the vagina from foreign invaders, such as bacteria. During ovulation, chemical changes take place to thin out the mucous consistency, allowing the sperm to enter the reproductive tract. For some couples, the chemistry between the sperm and the cervix just isn't right. The mucus remains thick, creating an environment that can block or damage the sperm, thereby preventing conception.

Approximately 10 percent of all infertile couples discover that their infertility has no apparent cause. Both partners appear to be normal, healthy and able to reproduce; however, they simply cannot conceive together. This can be the most frustrating situation of all, as there's no obvious solution.

Symptoms

The main symptom of infertility is the inability to conceive a child after one year of unprotected, frequent intercourse. Each specific medical disorder, hormonal disruption or anatomical abnormality produces additional symptoms in the woman that may indicate infertility. These symptoms may include:

- history of recent weight loss or gain
- irregular menstrual periods
- absent menstrual periods (amenorrhea)
- prolonged or heavy periods
- spotting between periods
- abnormal vaginal discharge
- discomfort in the lower abdomen
- pain during sexual intercourse

Who's at risk?

One in six couples experiences infertility problems. Many of the risk factors for female and male infertility are the same. You may be at increased risk of developing fertility problems if you:

- are a female over 32 years of age or a male over 35
- are a smoker
- are a female who is overweight or underweight

- are a male who is obese
- have irregular or absent periods
- have a history or have a partner with a history of sexually transmitted diseases (STDs), pelvic infections or genital infections
- have polycystic ovary syndrome (PCOS)
- have a history of using an intrauterine device (IUD) for birth control
- have had a surgical sterilization reversed or if your partner has undergone this procedure
- have had abdominal surgery or your partner has undergone this type of surgery
- have endometriosis
- have a history of emotional stress

Diagnosis

Because there are so many causes of infertility, an accurate diagnosis requires an extensive period of evaluation. The process begins with a thorough physical and gynecological examination. Additional tests that may be necessary include the following:

1. **Basal temperature records.** There's a slight rise in the body's basal temperature when ovulation occurs. Recording your temperature each morning will help to pinpoint this crucial time in your menstrual cycle. You'll be asked to chart your body temperature as soon as you wake up, before you get out of bed.
2. **Cervical mucous tests.** The cervical mucus can reveal a great deal of information about the conditions that may be causing your infertility. The *ferning test* determines if your estrogen levels are normal. The *postcoital test* determines if the sperm entering your reproductive tract are healthy and mobile.
3. **Blood tests.** Levels of estrogen, progesterone, luteinizing hormone, follicle-stimulating hormone and prolactin are usually measured. Abnormalities in these hormone levels can help explain ovulation difficulties.
4. **X-ray examinations.** Called a hysterosalpingogram, this test is used to identify structural abnormalities to your uterus and Fallopian tubes, or certain medical conditions that may interfere with fertility.

5. **Laparoscopic surgery.** A laparoscope, a fibre-optic telescope, is inserted into your abdomen to examine your uterus, Fallopian tubes and ovaries to detect conditions such as scarring in your Fallopian tubes, endometriosis and polycystic ovary syndrome.
6. **Semen analysis.** The quality, quantity and motility of the sperm, plus the sperm concentration and volume, are determined.

Conventional treatment

Most healthy couples under 35 years of age have a 25 percent chance of becoming pregnant in the first month of trying to conceive. That rate rises to 60 percent after three to six months and reaches 85 percent after one year. For the majority of couples, giving nature enough time is usually the only treatment required for successful conception. That's why most physicians won't evaluate you for infertility until you've tried to become pregnant for at least one year.

In many cases, mistimed intercourse is the only reason for infertility. Detecting the changes in your body that signal the beginning of ovulation is often the first step towards solving your fertility problems. Your basal temperature chart will help you to pinpoint your most fertile days. A urine test, indicating the presence of luteinizing hormones, is another method of establishing ovulation. By planning intercourse to maximize the chances of a mature egg meeting a viable sperm, your likelihood of conception may improve considerably.

Since the primary cause of infertility is anovulation, the major objective of most fertility treatments is to stimulate ovulation. The fertility drug Clomid (clomiphene citrate) triggers ovulation by affecting the release of luteinizing hormone. It has a high success rate but often leads to multiple births. In some women, this drug can cause painful ovarian cysts and may increase the risk of ovarian cancer.

If you're not having success with Clomid, you may benefit from supplements of the hormones FSH, LH or GnRH. The addition of these hormones should restore a normal menstrual cycle and improve fertility by stimulating egg production.

In some instances, surgery may be necessary to repair damaged reproductive organs. Laparoscopy is performed to open up damaged Fallopian tubes or to remove scar tissue resulting from infections or endometriosis.

Surgery is also helpful in correcting certain uterine abnormalities and removing polyps and fibroids.

Assisted reproductive technologies (ART) have been available for many years and are proving to be very successful in treating a wide variety of infertility problems. The most well-known ART is in vitro fertilization. This process begins with prescribing fertility drugs to stimulate your ovaries to produce many eggs. When they're mature, several eggs are retrieved from your ovaries and fertilized in a laboratory. Between three and five embryos are then implanted into your uterus in the hope of establishing a successful pregnancy. In vitro fertilization is used most frequently for women who have Fallopian tube damage, endometriosis, anti-sperm antibodies or unexplained infertility. This technique has a success rate of approximately 25 percent per attempt. There are many other ART techniques that can be discussed with your doctor.

Dealing with infertility is a highly emotional experience for most couples. Fortunately, there's a great deal of research underway in the field of infertility, and treatments are becoming increasingly effective. Continual advances, especially in the area of ART, are offering new hope for couples who dream of the joys of parenthood.

Enhancing fertility

DIETARY STRATEGIES
Weight control
There's no question that a woman's body weight can affect her chances of becoming pregnant. If you're obese, fat cells can produce enough estrogen to interfere with your ability to conceive. High estrogen levels tell your brain to stop stimulating the development of follicles and, as a result, ovulation doesn't occur. This is common in women with polycystic ovary syndrome (see Chapter 20 for more on this disorder). Studies show that losing weight can lead to pregnancy. When obese women lose excess body weight, ovulation resumes, making conception possible.

Weighing too little is not healthy either. Menstruation occurs at a critical level of "fatness." If you lose too much weight, or you're already thin, your body fat diminishes and hormone levels are affected; this, in turn, can lead to an inability to ovulate.

In Chapter 2, Strategies for Weight Control, I give you tools to assess your body weight. Figure out if you're at a healthy weight. If you're overweight and have polycystic ovary syndrome (PCOS), follow my weight-loss recommendations and meal plans in that chapter. Even if you don't have PCOS, these are healthy strategies for any overweight woman.

Obesity also contributes to male infertility. Studies have shown that obese men tend to have lower testosterone levels, which can result in reduced sperm count and sperm density.[2]

If you're underweight, read my guidelines for a healthy diet in Chapter 1. Incorporate some of these suggestions to make sure you're getting enough calories and nutrients in your daily diet. If you recognize that your low body weight is caused by an eating disorder, read Chapter 14, Eating Disorders, for information on how to begin your recovery process.

Caffeine and alcohol

If you and your partner have difficulty conceiving, I strongly recommend that you avoid caffeine and alcohol while you try to get pregnant (and, of course, during your pregnancy too). A handful of studies have found that consuming more than 300 milligrams of caffeine per day (about 2 cups/ 500 ml of coffee) is associated with a delay in conception. A large study from Johns Hopkins University revealed that, compared to women who consumed less than 300 milligrams of caffeine per day, those who consumed more caffeine reduced their chances of conceiving each month by 25 percent.[3] Another American study of 104 healthy women found that women who consumed more than the equivalent of 1 cup/250 ml of coffee per day were half as likely to become pregnant as women who drank less.[4] Other studies find that the relationship between caffeine and fertility is even stronger in women who smoke.[5]

Studies also support the notion that drinking alcoholic beverages reduces fertility in women. Women who drink heavily are more likely than non-drinkers to experience infertility problems and spontaneous abortion. A study from the Harvard School of Public Health looked at the effect of alcohol in more than 4000 women. The researchers found that even moderate drinking (two drinks per day) affected the ability to conceive by interfering with ovulation. And the more alcohol consumed, the higher the risk of not conceiving.[6]

VITAMINS AND MINERALS

B Vitamins: Folate and Vitamin B12

There's a growing body of evidence demonstrating a relationship between B vitamin deficiencies and impaired sperm production, reduced ovarian reserve and male and female infertility. A deficiency of B vitamins, especially folate and B12, can lead to elevated blood levels of an amino acid called homocysteine. High homocysteine levels are thought to contribute to infertility. (B vitamins are needed to break down homocysteine into other harmless amino acids.) Two case reports also revealed that when women with a B12 deficiency who were having trouble conceiving were given supplemental B12, pregnancy occurred.[7-9]

One study looked at the effects of B12 supplements among infertile men. Supplementing the diet with extra B12 helped only those men with low sperm counts and impaired sperm motility.[10]

The best food sources of folate include cooked spinach, broccoli, lentils, orange juice, asparagus, artichokes and whole-grain breads and cereals. Vitamin B12 is found in animal foods such as meat, poultry, fish, eggs and dairy products and also in fortified soy and rice beverages.

If you have difficulty eating a varied diet, take a multivitamin and mineral supplement to ensure that you're meeting your B vitamin requirements (see Chapter 1, page 32, for RDAs for folate and B12). It's vital that women of childbearing age take a multivitamin that contains 0.4 milligrams (400 micrograms) of folic acid to help reduce the risk of neural defects in their newborns. (Folic acid is the synthetic form of folate that's added to vitamins and fortified foods.)

Antioxidants (male infertility)

It appears that certain vitamins and minerals affect the health and motility of sperm. Most research attention has been paid to the antioxidant nutrients, in particular vitamin E, vitamin C and selenium. It's widely accepted that oxidative stress caused by free radicals is involved in male infertility. Free radicals are unstable oxygen molecules produced in the body that damage cells. Cigarette smoking increases the formation of free radical compounds, which can damage sperm as well as decrease their motility and ability to fuse with a woman's egg. Oxidative stress can also alter the DNA of sperm, resulting in defective sperm. Antioxidant nutrients neutralize these harmful chemicals, rendering them inactive in the body.

Studies have found that the vitamin C level of seminal fluid is significantly lower in infertile men than in those who are fertile. Cigarette smokers also have lower levels of vitamin C in seminal fluid.[11,12] Furthermore, studies have found that compared with fertile men, infertile men have significantly lower levels of selenium in their semen.[13,14] In addition to its role as an antioxidant, selenium is required for sperm maturation and motility.

Some research has shown that vitamin E supplements, taken in doses of 100 and 200 international units (IU), improved sperm activity in infertile men and increased the rate of pregnancy in their partners. Preliminary research suggests that vitamin C may improve sperm count and sperm motility.[15,16] Although studies are not conclusive, consuming adequate dietary antioxidants may help prevent male infertility that's caused by oxidative stress.

VITAMIN C. The recommended dietary allowance (RDA) for men is 90 milligrams (smokers need 125 milligrams). Best food sources include citrus fruit, citrus juice, cantaloupe, kiwi, mango, strawberries, broccoli, Brussels sprouts, cauliflower, red pepper and tomato juice. To supplement, take 500 milligrams of vitamin C once daily. The daily upper limit is 2000 milligrams.

VITAMIN E. The RDA is 22 IU. Best food sources include wheat germ, nuts, seeds, vegetable oils, whole grains and kale. To supplement, take 200 to 400 IU of natural source vitamin E. Buy a "mixed" vitamin E supplement if possible. The daily upper limit is 1500 IU.

SELENIUM. The RDA is 55 micrograms. Best food sources are fish, seafood, chicken, organ meats, whole grains, nuts, onions, garlic and mushrooms. To supplement, take 200 micrograms per day. Check how much your multivitamin and mineral formula gives you before you buy a separate selenium pill. The daily upper limit is 400 micrograms.

Zinc (male infertility)

This mineral is essential for growth, sexual development and sperm production. Many studies have found a link between infertility in men and a low zinc concentration in seminal fluid. A zinc deficiency may also lead to low testosterone levels. One study found that a daily zinc supplement improved sperm motility. Another small study conducted in men with low testosterone levels found that zinc supplements increased their sperm count and the rate of pregnancy in their partners.[17,18]

Zinc-rich foods include oysters, dark turkey meat, lentils, ricotta cheese, tofu, yogurt, lean beef, wheat germ, spinach, broccoli, green beans and tomato juice. If supplements are used, take 15 to 30 milligrams (many multivitamin and mineral formulas offer 15 milligrams). A zinc supplement should have 1 milligram of copper for every 10 milligrams of zinc. Don't exceed 40 milligrams of zinc per day.

HERBAL REMEDIES
Chasteberry *(Vitex agnus-castus)* (female infertility)

If irregular menstrual periods caused by an imbalance of hormones are interfering with your ability to become pregnant, you might consider trying this herbal remedy. European physicians have used chasteberry since the 1950s to treat menstrual irregularities in women. Preliminary research suggests that taking chasteberry can increase the chances of getting pregnant in women who are infertile due to a progesterone deficiency. The herb is believed to increase your pituitary gland's production of luteinizing hormone (LH), which, in turn, boosts the secretion of progesterone during the last fourteen days of your menstrual cycle. But it appears that chasteberry also works to keep prolactin levels in check. Its ability to lower excessive levels of prolactin has made it a potential treatment for infertility in some women.

European studies suggest that when taken daily, chasteberry can restore progesterone and prolactin levels to normal and result in pregnancy. Researchers from Stanford University in California found that a nutritional supplement containing chasteberry, green tea, L-arginine, vitamins and minerals increased progesterone levels and increased the rate of pregnancy in women taking the supplement.[19] (The supplement used in the study is called FertilityBlend, manufactured by the Daily Wellness Company Honolulu, Hawaii.)

If you decide to try chasteberry, buy a product that's standardized to 6 percent agnuside, one of the plant's active ingredients. The recommended dose varies and will depend on the formulation of chasteberry. Research and clinical experience suggest that it takes five to seven months to restore regular menstrual periods. In women who haven't had a period for more than two years, it can take up to eighteen months to have an effect.

To date, the herb has a good safety record. In rare cases it may cause gastrointestinal upset and skin rashes. If you become pregnant, stop taking chasteberry, as it may stimulate the uterus.

OTHER NATURAL HEALTH PRODUCTS
L-carnitine (male infertility)

This compound isn't an essential nutrient because the body makes it in sufficient quantities. Carnitine helps the body generate energy by transporting fat into cells. Most of the body's carnitine is located in muscles and in the heart, but some is also found in sperm and seminal fluid. A number of studies have found a positive relationship between sperm count and motility and the concentration of L-carnitine: The higher the concentration of L-carnitine, the higher the sperm count. Researchers have also found that infertile men have much lower levels of L-carnitine in their semen than fertile men.[20]

An Italian study revealed that 3 grams per day of supplemental L-carnitine taken for three months increased sperm count and sperm motility in 37 out of 47 men.[21] A recent review of randomized clinical trials found that, compared with taking placebo, taking L-carnitine for six months improved sperm motility and pregnancy rate.[22]

L-carnitine is found in meat and dairy products, but to get 3 grams a day, you'll need to take supplements. To supplement, take 1 to 3 grams per day. L-carnitine is available in the United States but isn't legally available in Canada. Avoid products that contain D-carnitine or DL-carnitine, as they compete with L-carnitine in the body and may lead to a deficiency. Occasional side effects of gastrointestinal upset have been reported.

LIFESTYLE FACTORS
Cigarette smoking

It's quite clear that smoking can negatively affect sperm. Study after study has shown that the harmful chemicals inhaled from cigarettes reduce sperm count, impair the health of sperm and decrease sexual performance. There's little doubt that cigarette smoking increases a man's odds of being infertile. If your spouse smokes, suggest a visit to his family doctor to learn options available to help him quit.

Scientists have also learned that smoking can affect female fertility. According to a recent study from researchers in the U.K., the pregnancy rate among women attending a fertility clinic was significantly lower in smokers compared to non-smokers.[23] Other studies have found that women who smoke while trying to get pregnant experience delayed time to conception compared to both non-smokers and past smokers.[24] Scientists believe that smoking impairs the healthy functioning of a woman's ovaries; it also causes damage to a woman's eggs and the female sex hormone estrogen. If you're planning to start a family and you're a smoker (even a social smoker), I strongly urge you to quit for the benefit of your and your baby's health.

THE BOTTOM LINE...
Leslie's recommendations for enhancing fertility

1. To ensure an optimal intake of calories, protein, carbohydrates, fat, vitamins and minerals, both you and your partner should follow the healthiest diet possible. Consider consulting a registered dietitian who can assess your diet and develop a customized eating and supplement plan for both of you. Check out www.dietitians.ca to find a private-practice nutritionist in your community.
2. Avoid caffeine and alcohol, two beverages that may affect female fertility.
3. Achieve and maintain a healthy body weight.
4. Both you and your partner should make sure you're getting proper amounts of vitamin B12.
5. If you've been experiencing irregular periods, consider the herbal remedy chasteberry (*Vitex agnus-castus*). Once daily, take an extract standardized to contain 6 percent agnuside.
6. Make sure your male partner consumes plenty of antioxidant nutri-ents. The ones to pay attention to are vitamin C, vitamin E and selenium.
7. Have your male partner assess his intake of zinc from foods.
8. L-carnitine is a natural compound found in animal food and made by the body that may be important for male fertility. If you want to give this a try, your partner should take 1 to 3 grams of L-carnitine daily. Avoid products that contain D-carnitine or DL-carnitine.

16
Pregnancy

Pregnancy is a nine-month continuum that begins with conception and ends with the birth of your new baby. It's a time of tremendous change in your life, often accompanied by feelings of anticipation and fear. It's also a time when maintaining good health is vitally important. From the moment of conception—and even before—the choices that you make about diet, exercise and medical care will have a profound effect on the growth and development of your baby. There's no greater gift you can give your child than to live a healthy lifestyle every single day of your pregnancy.

Before you delve into this chapter, I want to let you know that it's not formatted in my usual style. My recommendations aren't categorized by diet, vitamins/minerals, herbal remedies and other natural health products; nor do I conclude this chapter with my Bottom Line summary of nutrition recommendations. Due to the heftiness of this topic, and the fact that nutrition needs and concerns change with each trimester, nutrition strategies are provided throughout the text. In the latter part of this chapter I sum up your nutrient and food requirements during *all* stages of your pregnancy. Therefore, anyone concerned with this topic should read this chapter in its entirety. Enjoy the journey to motherhood!

Confirming your pregnancy

The first sign of pregnancy is usually a missed menstrual period. If you're sexually active and your menstrual cycles are quite regular, there's a good chance that you're pregnant if your period is more than a week late. Menstrual cycles usually stop during pregnancy, although some women have been known to have light periods during the entire nine months.

To confirm your pregnancy, you can take a urine test that will detect the presence of pregnancy hormones—HCG (human chorionic gonadotropin)—in your system. You can choose to have the urine test done at your doctor's office or you can do it yourself, using one of the many home pregnancy test kits available in most drugstores. By the second week after conception, home pregnancy tests are 90 percent accurate. As an alternative to the urine test, you can have a blood sample taken at your doctor's office and tested at a laboratory. A blood test can detect pregnancy hormones as early as eight days after conception.

If you wait to confirm your diagnosis until you are four weeks past conception, your doctor will perform an internal examination and physically check for signs of pregnancy. He or she will look for a slight enlargement of your uterus and colour changes in your vagina and cervix caused by increased blood flow. This examination is very accurate in determining pregnancy.

A typical pregnancy lasts thirty-nine weeks or nine months from conception. Your expected date of delivery is usually 280 days from the first day of your last menstrual period. However, less than 5 percent of all babies arrive on their due date, so you should anticipate that your baby might arrive earlier or later than expected. Traditionally, pregnancies are divided into three stages or trimesters, each lasting roughly three months. Your body undergoes many changes during these stages and each trimester represents important growth and development milestones. By following a healthy lifestyle and arranging for good prenatal care throughout all the stages of your pregnancy, you can give your baby the very best start in life.

The first trimester

Every pregnancy is unique and the symptoms that you experience may be different from those of other women. By understanding what these symptoms mean and how they affect your body and your baby, you'll be better prepared for the many physical and emotional adjustments that lie ahead.

SYMPTOMS

Fatigue

During the early stages of pregnancy, there are profound changes taking place in your body. Your baby, or fetus, is growing rapidly in your uterus and requires many nutrients to build essential structures and systems. Your body produces up to 50 percent more blood to carry these nutrients to the fetus. To handle the increased blood flow, your heart rate speeds up and you breathe faster, which sends more oxygen to the fetus. Your metabolic rate increases and all of your bodily functions are accelerated.

In addition to these physical changes, it's quite natural to feel some emotional stress at this time, even if you're very happy to be pregnant. You may have fears about your baby's health or your ability to be a good mother, or you may worry about work, finances or lifestyle changes. As you adapt to these physical and emotional symptoms, you may find that your energy level drops and you feel much more tired than usual.

Fatigue is a common symptom in the first trimester. This is a time in your pregnancy when you may need to slow down a little, because your body is working hard. Rest as often as you can, take a nap when time allows and go to bed early. Incorporating moderate exercise, such as a 30-minute walk, into your daily routine will increase your energy level and help you combat your fatigue. Making sure you eat a healthy diet that includes three meals and a midday snack will also help you feel more energetic.

Urinary frequency

It's quite likely that you'll suffer from an increasing need to urinate during these early days of pregnancy. Laughing, sneezing or coughing may cause embarrassing leakage of urine, and you may have to get up more often during the night to use the bathroom. Because of the demands of pregnancy, your kidneys are working overtime to filter the larger volume of blood in your system, and this stimulates your body to produce more urine. At the same time, your uterus is growing and putting extra pressure on your bladder. The result is a reduced bladder capacity that keeps you from straying too far from a bathroom.

Although you shouldn't be restricting your fluid intake during pregnancy, you may find that avoiding beverages for a few hours before bedtime helps to minimize nighttime interruptions. Wearing panty liners during the day will also help protect you against unexpected leaking.

Morning sickness

Many women are troubled by nausea and sometimes vomiting during the first fourteen to sixteen weeks of their pregnancies. This is one of the most uncomfortable symptoms of the first trimester and affects nearly 70 percent of all pregnant women. Although it's commonly referred to as morning sickness, nausea isn't limited to the morning hours—it can and does occur at any time of the day. Normally, these symptoms come to an end after the first three to four months but, in some cases, morning sickness lasts beyond the first trimester and may even persist throughout the entire pregnancy. Rarely, the vomiting may be so severe that hospitalization is necessary to maintain adequate nutrition and fluid intake.

Nausea and vomiting may be caused by the hormone changes produced by the placenta and the uterus. Increases in the hormone progesterone tend to slow down the gastrointestinal system, allowing food to remain in your stomach for a longer time. This extra digestion time is good for your baby because it helps your body extract additional nutrients from the food you eat. Unfortunately, it may also upset your stomach and add to your feelings of nausea.

The majority of pregnant women are at risk of developing morning sickness, but experts believe that the following may be more susceptible:

- women pregnant with twins or higher multiples
- women who have suffered nausea taking birth control pills
- women who have suffered motion sickness
- women who have a mother or sister who experienced morning sickness
- women with a history of migraine headache

As long as you can keep some food down and drink plenty of fluids, morning sickness shouldn't harm your baby. However, morning sickness can become more of a problem if you can't keep any foods or fluids down and begin to lose a lot of weight. Luckily, only 1 percent of Canadian women suffer symptoms severe enough to endanger their health and the health of their babies.[1]

Strategies to manage morning sickness

These tips have helped many of my clients manage morning sickness during the first trimester:

- **Eat plain, bland carbohydrate-rich foods before rising each morning, to avoid hunger.** Keep soda crackers or rice cakes by your bed and nibble on a few before you get up. Then wait for 20 to 30 minutes before you rise. Eat a snack before bedtime.

- **Avoid foods and smells that trigger your nausea.** Ask your partner to cook the meals while you're not feeling well. You may find you tolerate cold foods, like a sandwich, better than a hot meal. If you don't know what makes you feel nauseous, evaluate your surroundings. It could be the smell of coffee brewing, the sight of raw food, your perfume, patterned carpets, camera angles on television programs and so on. It might not always be the obvious.

- **Eat several small meals during the day** (every two to three hours is a good target) so that you're never too full or too hungry. This helps to keep your blood-sugar level more stable, which may prevent episodes of morning sickness. Drink a small amount of unsweetened fruit juice every one to two hours. And don't lie down after you eat.

- **Choose lower-fat protein foods** such as lean meat, canned light tuna, chicken breast, egg whites and legumes, and easily digestible carbohydrates such as fruit, rice, pasta, sweet potato, toast and dry cereals.

- **Avoid fried foods and other high-fat foods.** Fatty foods take longer to digest—particularly when you're pregnant—so they remain in your stomach longer and increase the likelihood of feeling queasy. Spicy and acidic foods may irritate your stomach and should also be avoided.

- **Drink fluids between rather than with your meals.** This prevents you from feeling too full. Sip beverages slowly throughout the day. If your morning sickness includes vomiting, sip a sports drink like Gatorade or Powerade. These beverages provide a little carbohydrate along with sodium, potassium and chloride, electrolytes that are lost through vomiting.

- **Reach for foods and beverages that calm an upset stomach**—gelatin desserts, Popsicles, chicken broth, herbal teas, sports drinks and ginger ale (let the ginger ale sit on the counter for 30 minutes to allow some of the gases to escape).

- **Take your prenatal vitamin with food or at bedtime.** Sometimes the iron prenatal supplements can upset your stomach. If changing the time you take your supplement doesn't help, try another brand. If you have to stop taking your prenatal supplement all together, there's no need to worry. Your iron requirements begin to rise around the end of the first trimester, which is when morning sickness typically subsides. At that point, you should have no difficulty finding a brand you can tolerate.

- **Consider taking extra vitamin B6.** A few studies suggest that vitamin B6 supplements ease pregnancy-related nausea and vomiting, especially severe forms or morning sickness.[2] One study found that low-dose B6 supplements improved nausea, but not vomiting, in early pregnancy.[3] The dose of vitamin B6 used in the studies was 10 or 25 milligrams three times per day. Look for a low-dose B6 supplement (10 or 25 milligrams) or, alternatively, a low-dose B complex supplement that provides all the B vitamins. Choose a product that supplies 25 milligrams of B6. Don't exceed a daily dose of 100 milligrams.

- **Cook with ginger.** Ginger has been scientifically shown to help reduce morning sickness. It's believed that the active ingredients in ginger root, called gingerols and shogaols, speed the movement of food through the intestinal tract. Gingerol compounds may also improve appetite and digestion by reducing stomach acid secretions and increasing the release of important digestive aids. Add fresh ginger root to stir-fries and marinades. If you have a juicer, add a thick slice of ginger root to your juice blend.

- **Use ginger supplements cautiously.** A few studies have found that ginger supplements reduce feelings of nausea in pregnant women.[4,5] Although the use of ginger during pregnancy is controversial, so far, there's no conclusive evidence that ginger is harmful during pregnancy. You can buy ginger extract supplements in health food stores or pharmacies. The dose used in clinical studies is 250 milligrams taken four times per day. If you take ginger supplements, use them for only a short period of time and don't exceed 1 gram (1000 milligrams) per day. The effects of long-term high doses of ginger on the growing fetus are not known. Adding fresh ginger root to your meals is safe throughout your pregnancy.

Other symptoms

Your breasts rapidly increase in size and weight, new milk ducts grow and breast veins become more noticeable. You may find that your breasts are tender and sore because of the increased production of estrogen and progesterone hormones. These hormonal changes, as well as the increased blood flow in early pregnancy, may also trigger headaches and dizziness. Stress, fatigue and hunger can make the headaches worse. Warm compresses and relaxation exercises should help ease these mild aches and pains. Painkillers and other medications should be avoided, unless recommended by your doctor.

Weight gain

How much weight you need to gain during your entire pregnancy will depend upon how much you weighed—your body mass index (BMI)—before you became pregnant. If you were a healthy weight at the time you conceived, you should expect to gain 25 to 35 pounds (11 to 16 kg) in total. (See Chapter 2, page 37, to calculate your pre-pregnancy BMI.) If you don't know how much you weighed before you became pregnant, determine your BMI based on your weight as early in your pregnancy as possible. The recommended weight gain guidelines below are associated with the lowest risk for a single pregnancy and delivery complications.

Weight Gain Guidelines for a Single Pregnancy

Pre-pregnancy BMI less than 20	28 to 40 lbs (12.5 to 18 kg)
Pre-pregnancy BMI between 20 and 27	25 to 35 lbs (11.5 to 16 kg)
Pre-pregnancy BMI over 27	15 to 25 lbs (7 to 11.5 kg)

Throughout the first trimester, you should expect to gain only a small amount of extra weight, normally not more than 6 to 8 pounds (2.7 to 3.6 kg). Even though your body requires extra nutrients, during the first trimester you don't require additional calories in your daily diet to maintain good fetal development.

Gaining too little or too much weight during your pregnancy can be harmful to you and your baby. Women who gain the right amount of weight are less likely to have *low-birthweight babies* (less than 5.5 pounds/ 2500 g). There are two types of low-birthweight babies. *Preterm*, or premature babies, are born before the end of the 37th week of pregnancy. The earlier a baby is born, the less developed its organs will be and the less it's likely to weigh. *Small-for-date* babies are born full term but are underweight. These babies are born small, in part, from a slowing or temporary halting of growth in the womb.

Low-birthweight babies are more likely than normal-birthweight babies to have health problems, for example, with breathing, digestion and vision, when they're newborns. Some of these medical problems are mild and resolve themselves with no or few lasting effects. Serious medical problems are more common in very low-birthweight babies—weighing less than 3 pounds, 5 ounces (1500 g)—and such complications can have lasting effects such as mental retardation or vision or hearing loss.

Women who are overweight and have a high BMI before pregnancy are more likely to develop gestational diabetes and to give birth to *high-birthweight* babies (more than 8.8 pounds/4000 g). Studies suggest that heavy babies have a higher risk for adult weight problems. Giving birth to a large baby also increases the risk of complications at delivery.

If you're expecting twins or triplets, you will, of course, need to gain more weight than the recommendations stated above. Based on the evidence to date, here's a general guide used for weight gain goals during a multiple pregnancy.

Weight Gain Guidelines for Multiple Pregnancies

	Twins	Triplets
Total gain	35 to 45 lbs (16 to 20 kg)	45 to 55 lbs (20 to 25 kg)
First trimester	4 to 6 lbs (2 to 3 kg)	1.5 lbs (0.7 kg) per week
Second & third trimesters	1.5 lbs (0.7 kg) per week	1.5 lbs (0.7 kg) per week

Keep in mind that these targets serve as a guide. How much weight your doctor wants you to gain also depends on your pre-pregnancy weight. And in a multiple pregnancy, beyond how much weight you gain, it's when you gain it that's important. Studies indicate that gaining adequate weight at critical periods during pregnancy can reduce the chance that multiples will be born weighing less than 5-1/2 pounds (2500 grams).

Early weight gain is important since multiple pregnancies have a shorter term. Research in twin pregnancies shows that it's especially important for underweight and normal-weight women to gain adequate weight before twenty weeks to reduce the risk of delivering low-birthweight babies.[6] A higher rate of weight gain after twenty weeks to delivery can improve the birthweight of twins born to normal-weight and overweight women.[7]

FETAL DEVELOPMENT

The first trimester is a very crucial time in your baby's development. During these few weeks, all the essential organs, structures and systems necessary to sustain life are formed. The heart begins beating and the digestive system is developing. The brain, backbone and spinal cord are all growing. Limbs are taking shape and facial features can be seen. Reproductive organs are in place, although they're still too small to indicate the baby's sex. The circulatory and respiratory systems are functioning and so are the liver and kidneys. By the end of the first trimester, the fetus is usually about 3 inches (7 cm) long and weighs about 1 ounce (30 g).

CARE

Once your pregnancy has been confirmed, you should visit your doctor for a complete physical examination. This is usually done during the first six to eight weeks of pregnancy. Your doctor will take a detailed medical history, including chronic medical problems and complications of earlier pregnancies. You'll also be given pelvic and rectal exams to determine the size and position of your uterus. At this stage, routine lab tests include blood tests for rubella (German measles), hepatitis B, syphilis and other sexually transmitted diseases. Your blood will also be typed and screened for Rh antibodies. HIV testing is recommended, as well as urine tests and a Pap test for cervical cancer. During this appointment, your doctor will also determine the expected date for the delivery of your baby.

After your first visit, unless there's a medical reason for more frequent appointments, you'll normally see your doctor once a month for routine examinations until the 28th week of pregnancy. At that time, your appointments will increase to once every two weeks. As you approach the end of your pregnancy, you'll be scheduled for weekly medical visits.

If your doctor suspects that your pregnancy is high risk for certain medical disorders, he or she may send you for chorionic villus sampling. This special test identifies abnormalities in your fetus that could result in conditions such as cystic fibrosis or Down syndrome. The chorionic villi are located on the edge of the placenta and are genetically identical to your baby. A small probe is inserted through your vagina and into your uterus to gather cell samples from the surface of the placenta. By analyzing these cells, a great deal of information can be gathered about the overall health of your baby. The test is usually performed at ten to twelve weeks and results are available within one or two days. Chorionic villus sampling is similar to amniocentesis in that both tests identify fetal abnormalities. Chorionic villus sampling gives results much earlier; however, it carries a slightly higher risk of miscarriage.

The second trimester

The second trimester lasts from the 13th to the 28th week of pregnancy. Most women feel their best at this stage, because the discomforts of early pregnancy have subsided and the uncomfortable symptoms of the last trimester are still ahead. At this point, you're probably sleeping better and your energy levels are returning to normal.

SYMPTOMS
Aches and pains

During the second trimester, every organ in your body is busy adapting to the changes of pregnancy. Your growing uterus is the most obvious sign of change, as it begins to protrude out of the abdominal cavity, giving you a much more rounded shape. As the uterus enlarges, it pushes other internal organs out of the way and causes tension in surrounding muscles and ligaments. You may feel pain in your lower abdomen because the structures that support the uterus are stretching and thickening. This type of pain isn't severe and doesn't pose a threat to your pregnancy. If you're bothered by abdominal pain, try lying down and resting for a short time. Relaxation exercises help and a warm bath may soothe the aches away.

Back pain

To allow your baby to pass through your pelvis during birth, the joints in your pelvic area begin to soften and loosen. Sometimes, the panels of muscle running along the front of your abdomen separate under pressure from your expanding uterus. As well, the growing weight of your fetus changes your centre of gravity, causing you to compensate by adjusting your posture. All of these factors may result in back pain during your last two trimesters.

To minimize the discomfort, try to maintain a correct posture, with your pelvis tucked in and your shoulders back. Sit with your feet slightly elevated, try not to stand for long periods and sleep on your side with one pillow between your knees and another under your abdomen. Exercises to strengthen your abdominal muscles will also reduce the tension in your back.

Other symptoms

The hormones that loosen your pelvic joints also affect your intestinal tract, slowing down digestion and causing food to remain longer in your stomach. This allows more time for nutrients to be absorbed into your bloodstream for use by the fetus. Unfortunately, it can also result in nausea, indigestion and bloating. Heartburn is another symptom of this slowdown in digestion. Heartburn develops when the contents of your stomach flow backwards into your esophagus. The stomach acids irritate the esophagus, creating the burning sensation that gives heartburn its name. Eating small meals more often throughout the day can help minimize heartburn. You should also avoid drinking fluids with your meals; instead, have them between meals. Because your intestinal muscles are more relaxed, you may also become constipated, a condition that's aggravated by the pressure of the growing uterus on your rectum.

As you progress through your second trimester, your heart is working twice as fast as it was before you were pregnant, your blood volumes are 50 percent higher and your kidney functions are still accelerated. Skin darkening is a very common symptom at this stage, especially among dark-skinned women. The skin around your nipples, navel and vulva become a deeper colour and you may notice the appearance of a dark vertical line between your navel and your pubic bone. This darkening of the skin usually disappears after pregnancy.

WEIGHT GAIN

Weight gain tends to vary during the second trimester. On average, for a single pregnancy, you should expect to gain about 1 pound (0.5 kg) a week after the first three months. You should be striving for a steady, gradual weight gain, without sudden increases or decreases. For a multiple pregnancy, women should gain 1-1/2 pounds (0.7 kg) per week during the second trimester.

FETAL DEVELOPMENT

This is a very exciting time, because you will begin to feel your baby move. The kicking and fluttering movements of your growing baby make the pregnancy feel more emotionally involving and real to you. You can expect to detect some fetal activity by the 20th week of pregnancy.

As you enter your fourth month, most of your baby's bones are formed, facial features are becoming more defined and external genitalia are evident. The brain is growing and the baby's head proportions are more balanced. By the end of the second trimester, your baby's eyes are opening and closing, there's some fat accumulating under the skin and regular intervals of sleeping and waking are beginning. At this stage, the baby has grown to 9 inches (23 cm) and weighs just over 1 pound (nearly 670 g). After twenty-four to twenty-six weeks, there's a strong possibility that the baby could survive outside the womb.

CARE

Medical visits during the second trimester focus primarily on tracking the development of the fetus, establishing an accurate due date and monitoring your general health. Your doctor checks your blood pressure and weight, and discusses any symptoms that you may be experiencing. He or she also measures the size of your uterus to help determine your baby's true age.

Special tests may be suggested for you during this stage of pregnancy:

1. **Ultrasound exam.** This is the safest form of imaging during pregnancy. High-frequency sound waves create images of the fetus that you can see on a monitor. The images are high quality and often show the baby in motion. Experts recommend that an ultrasound be performed, ideally between 18 and 22 weeks of pregnancy, to make sure that you and your baby are progressing well. Ultrasounds are used to
   - record fetal heartbeats and breathing movements
   - measure fetal growth
   - determine if you're carrying more than one fetus
   - find the location of the placenta
   - date the pregnancy through fetal measurements
   - assess the amount of amniotic fluid

   Ultrasound scanning may also be used during the first trimester to confirm evidence of pregnancy and fetal growth. Later in your pregnancy, it may be used to monitor the baby's health or to identify conditions that may cause problems during the pregnancy or delivery.

2. **Maternal serum screen** (MSS). Also called a single screen test, MSS is usually done at fifteen to sixteen weeks. It's a blood test that identifies the level of alpha fetoprotein (AFP) in your bloodstream. AFP is a protein produced by the fetus. Normally, a small amount of this protein passes through the placenta to enter your bloodstream. If the AFP level in your bloodstream is higher than normal, it could indicate

that your baby has spina bifida. A low level of AFP may mean that your baby has Down syndrome; the single screen test identifies approximately 30 percent of such babies.

Only two or three out of one hundred women with an abnormal MSS will have a child with a birth defect.[8] A common cause of misleading or false results is an incorrectly estimated due date, which will make your hormone levels appear abnormal.

3. **Amniocentesis.** Most often used to diagnose prenatal chromosome problems, this test can detect genetic abnormalities (e.g., Down syndrome), genetic disorders (e.g., cystic fibrosis) and neural tube defects (e.g., spina bifida). At a later stage of pregnancy, amniocentesis can determine if lungs are developed enough for the baby to breathe on its own.

During amniocentesis, a small sample of the amniotic fluid that surrounds the baby is removed from your uterus. Before the sampling procedure begins, an ultrasound is used to determine the location of the placenta and the baby. A long, thin needle is inserted through your abdomen into the amniotic sac to gather the fluid. The fluid sample, which contains cells that the baby has shed from its skin and bladder, is analyzed in a laboratory. The procedure may sound a little frightening but I've heard from many of my clients that, although it can be slightly uncomfortable, it really isn't as bad as it sounds. After amniocentesis you may have some slight cramping or spotting, so you should go home and rest for a few hours before returning to normal activities.

According to the Society of Obstetricians and Gynaecologists of Canada, amniocentesis increases your risk of miscarriage to 1 in 200 or approximately 0.5 percent. It's usually conducted between your 15th and 16th week of pregnancy and results are available about two or three weeks later.

Amniocentesis is recommended for women at increased risk for having a baby with a birth defect, especially women who are over 35 years old or who have a family history of birth defects. Amniocentesis is also used to find out if your baby's lungs are mature enough for an early delivery or to follow up on an AFP test that's positive for abnormalities. The procedure is usually performed between the 16th and 18th week, when there's enough amniotic fluid for an effective sample.

4. **Glucose testing**. Gestational diabetes is a pregnancy-related condition that affects approximately 3 percent of pregnant women. Unfortunately, gestational diabetes doesn't always cause obvious symptoms, so it may be difficult to detect. As a result, the Canadian Medical Association recommends that all pregnant women be screened for the condition with a random blood-glucose blood test. Your doctor will usually suggest that you take it between the 26th and 28th week of pregnancy, near the end of your second trimester. If you're at greater risk for getting gestational diabetes, your doctor may send you for testing earlier, at the 16th week.

   Approximately 15 percent of women tested have high blood-glucose levels, but only a few of them will actually develop gestational diabetes during their pregnancy. If your glucose levels are elevated, your doctor will recommend a glucose tolerance test to determine if you do indeed have gestational diabetes. During this test, you drink a sugary solution that contains a specified amount of glucose. Your blood-glucose level is then tested one hour and two hours after drinking the solution. High sugar readings indicate you have a problem with glucose control.

5. **Rh-factor testing**. The Rhesus (Rh) factor is a type of protein that's sometimes present in your blood. If you have it, you're Rh positive; if you don't, you're Rh negative. If you and your baby have incompatible Rh factors, your body produces antibodies that will cause damage or death to your fetus. A sample of your blood will be tested at a laboratory to determine your Rh factor.

6. **Hemoglobin testing**. By measuring your hemoglobin levels, your doctor can determine if you have iron-deficiency anemia. Most pregnant women don't absorb enough iron from their food to meet the demands of pregnancy. The condition can be improved with dietary changes and iron supplementation.

The third trimester

The third trimester is a time of conflicting emotions. You'll be excited at the prospect of your baby's upcoming birth, yet worried about your baby's health and safety during these crucial last weeks. You'll probably be very tired of being pregnant, yet fear the pain and uncertainty of giving birth.

For most women, the final three months of pregnancy is a time of decision-making, planning and great anticipation. This stage lasts from the 28th week of pregnancy until the delivery of your baby.

SYMPTOMS
Sleeping problems
At the end of your pregnancy, you may have trouble sleeping through the night. By this time, your uterus has undergone enormous change, stretching your abdomen to accommodate your constantly growing baby, the amniotic fluid and the placenta. As you try to cope with this additional weight and size, it's more and more difficult for you to find a comfortable sleeping position. To make sleeping easier, try to lie on your side, rather than your back, with your legs bent. This takes pressure off the large vein that carries blood from your legs and feet back to your heart, thereby reducing swelling, discomfort and back pain. You may also want to read my recommended dietary approaches for Insomnia, in Chapter 6.

Shortness of breath
In late pregnancy, it's very common for you to feel breathless and tired. Your expanding uterus pushes the diaphragm, a band of muscle under-neath your lungs, up higher into your chest. This decreases the capacity of your lungs by only a few centimetres, but that's enough to make you feel short of breath. At the same time, the action of the progesterone in your system causes you to breathe more deeply, increasing the volume of air that you take in with every breath. The result is an enriched oxygen supply that circulates through your bloodstream to meet the demands of your growing fetus. Just before delivery, the pressure on your diaphragm is relieved when your baby drops farther down into your pelvis. By improving your posture and maintaining a routine of gentle aerobic exercise throughout your pregnancy, you should be able to breathe a little better and increase your lung capacity.

Aches and pains
You'll find that your rapidly growing uterus puts pressure on numerous nerves, muscles and joints, causing you a variety of aches and pains. You can expect to experience at least a few of the following symptoms:

- **Sciatica.** This type of low back pain results from pressure on the sciatic nerves that run from your lower back down to your feet.
- **Hip pain.** Hormones cause your joints and connective tissue to loosen in preparation for delivery.
- **Stretching of the ligaments of your hips and pelvis.** Caused by hormones that loosen connective tissue, this can make walking difficult.
- **Vaginal pain.** This may indicate the early stages of dilation in your cervix.
- **Fluid retention.** Your hands and feet swell as you retain fluids.
- **Frequent urination.** The discomfort that plagued you in the first trimester returns with a vengeance as the growing fetus squeezes your bladder.
- **Itchy skin.** Your skin is stretching and tightening across your abdomen, making it feel dry and itchy.
- **Stretch marks.** Reddish or white streaks develop on your breasts, abdomen and upper thighs.
- **Urine leakage.** This is the result of increased pressure on the bladder.
- **Varicose veins.** These appear frequently in pregnancy, caused by the pressure of the uterus on the veins in your legs.

Throughout the last trimester of your pregnancy, you feel uncomfortable and tired much of the time. But your due date is approaching quickly and most of these normal symptoms subside after delivery. During these last few weeks, rest, gentle exercise and a balanced diet are essential to prepare you for the rigours of delivery and the demands of your newborn infant.

WEIGHT GAIN

In the second trimester, your expanding tissues—the placenta, your body fat, your breasts—caused most of your weight gain. But now, during the last few months of pregnancy, it's your growing baby that accounts for most of your weight gain. During the third trimester, your baby doubles in size—and your breasts are gearing up for nursing, so that's also behind some of your weight gain.

Just like in the second trimester, women who had a healthy pre-pregnancy weight can expect to gain about 1 pound (0.5 kg) each week. If you were overweight before pregnancy, aim for 1/2 pound (0.25 kg) per week. Conversely, if you were underweight and had a body mass index below 20, aim for a weekly weight gain of 1-1/2 pounds (0.7 kg). For a multiple pregnancy, women should gain 1-1/2 pounds (0.7 kg) per week during the third trimester.

Healthy weight gain is critical during this last trimester. Evidence suggests that maternal weight during this time is the most important indicator of the baby's birthweight.

FETAL DEVELOPMENT

In these last weeks of pregnancy, your baby is steadily gaining weight. Fat is building up on your baby's body and a slick, fatty substance called vernix caseosa covers the skin. Thumb sucking may begin and your baby's eyes open and close. Bones and limbs elongate and the lungs are maturing. You may notice increased activity as the baby's movements become more vigorous. When you reach the end of your term, the baby drops farther down into your abdomen, settling into a position for delivery. By the 39th week, your baby will weigh approximately 7 pounds (3 kg) and have grown to 18 inches (46 cm) or more in length.

CARE

Routine examinations are very important during your last stage of pregnancy. Your doctor will expect to see you every two weeks between your 28th and 36th week, then weekly until delivery. Your weight and blood pressure are measured regularly and the activity levels of your fetus are monitored. As your due date approaches, your doctor checks to see if the baby has moved into the proper position for delivery. The baby should be head-down in the uterus, with the head at the top of the birth canal. Some babies are positioned with their feet or buttocks down in a breech presentation.

You can expect to have regular vaginal exams to evaluate the state of your cervix. Your doctor determines how much the cervix has softened and whether it has begun to efface (thin out) or dilate (open), in preparation for delivery. If there are concerns about your baby's health or you're having a high-risk pregnancy, your doctor may perform a non-stress test (NST), which measures the baby's heart rate when it moves. Using ultrasound techniques, your baby's heart rate is recorded for 20 minutes. The heartbeat should accelerate as the baby moves. If the acceleration rate is not normal, further tests may be necessary.

Concerns and complications of pregnancy

Although most women have normal pregnancies and healthy babies, there are some conditions and complications that can create problems for you and your baby. By understanding the concerns and recognizing the symptoms, you'll know when to contact your doctor and what the impact will be on the outcome of your pregnancy.

SPOTTING AND BLEEDING

It's not unusual for you to have slight bleeding or spotting during early pregnancy. You may notice a small amount of bleeding about a week or ten days after conception. This is implantation bleeding and it occurs when the fertilized egg attaches itself to the wall of the uterus. The episode of bleeding should be quite brief. Some women may also have light bleeding at the time of their regular menstrual period throughout the first six months of their pregnancy, or even longer. Most episodes of bleeding are caused by normal events of pregnancy. However, you should always notify your doctor if you have spotting because it can be a warning sign of other problems with your pregnancy.

MISCARRIAGE

If your bleeding is heavy and is accompanied by pain, cramping or fever, or if you notice that you have passed some tissue, you may be experiencing a miscarriage. Also known as a spontaneous abortion, a miscarriage is the loss of a fetus that's less than twenty-eight weeks past conception. It occurs in 15 percent to 30 percent of all pregnancies, although it often happens so early that many women may not even realize they're pregnant. More than 80 percent of all miscarriages happen in the first twelve weeks of pregnancy.

The most common cause of miscarriage is an abnormality in the fetus's chromosomes. This is an error that occurs as the fertilized egg begins to divide and grow. The abnormality prevents the fetus from implanting or developing properly. Chromosome errors that result in miscarriage don't usually indicate a genetic problem. Other causes of miscarriage include defects in the uterus, hormonal imbalances, viral or bacterial infections, or chronic diseases, such as diabetes or high blood pressure. You should be aware that the normal activities of daily life, including exercising, lifting heavy objects or having sex will *not* cause you to miscarry. Nor will a fall or an injury, unless it's very severe.

The main warning sign of a miscarriage is vaginal bleeding. Any type of bleeding may indicate a miscarriage, even if it's quite light, so you should contact your doctor immediately if you begin spotting. Your doctor may suggest bedrest in an attempt to stabilize the pregnancy. However, the miscarriage may continue, despite your best efforts, simply because the fetus doesn't have the proper chromosomes to survive. During a miscarriage, you eliminate fetal tissue through your vagina. In some cases, you may need to have a surgical procedure to gently scrape or suction the tissue out of the uterus. If you have a miscarriage, there's very little need to worry about future pregnancies. You have an excellent chance of successfully completing full-term pregnancies, even if you have repeated—i.e., more than three—miscarriages.

ECTOPIC PREGNANCY

Vaginal bleeding may also indicate that you're experiencing an ectopic or tubal pregnancy, which occurs when the fertilized egg attaches itself somewhere other than the wall of the uterus. In 95 percent of these cases, the fertilized egg becomes stuck inside one of your Fallopian tubes on its way from the ovary to the uterus. This usually happens because an infection or inflammation causes the Fallopian tube to become partially or completely blocked by scar tissue. In most cases, this type of scarring is the result of pelvic inflammatory disease, a fairly common type of sexually transmitted disease. Because the Fallopian tube isn't designed to accommodate a growing fetus, the fertilized egg won't develop properly. Eventually, the tube wall stretches and bursts, resulting in a life-threatening loss of blood for you.

At first, you may not be aware that you have an ectopic pregnancy. The first signs are usually sharp, stabbing pain in the pelvis, abdomen, shoulder or neck. Vaginal bleeding and dizziness are other symptoms of this condition. Once your doctor has diagnosed the ectopic pregnancy by sending you for a blood test or ultrasound exam, you'll probably require surgery to remove the fetus. Through a small incision in your abdomen, the doctor inserts a long instrument, called a laparoscope, and removes the fetal tissue. Depending on the degree of damage, the Fallopian tube is either repaired or removed. Your chances for a successful pregnancy after an ectopic pregnancy depend on whether the condition was detected early enough to save the Fallopian tube. Once you've had one ectopic pregnancy, you're at increased risk of having another one.

VAGINAL YEAST INFECTIONS

It's quite common to have increased vaginal discharge during pregnancy. A normal discharge consists of thin, white mucus and is caused by hormones that stimulate glands in the cervix. However, if you notice a discharge that's green or yellow, strong smelling and accompanied by irritation and itching in your vaginal area, then you may have vaginitis, or a vaginal infection.

A yeast organism called *Candida albicans* often causes vaginal infections. This irritating condition is known as a yeast infection or candidiasis and can be a recurring problem during pregnancy. The candida organism is found in nearly one-quarter of all pregnant women as they approach their due date. Symptoms of a yeast infection include a burning sensation and thick curd-like discharge. It's treated with an antifungal drug that's applied in a topical cream or suppository. To prevent these and other vaginal infections, you should keep your vaginal area clean and dry, wear loose-fitting clothing, avoid synthetic materials next to your skin, wear underwear with a cotton insert gusset and avoid douches or feminine hygiene sprays.

Try the following dietary strategies to prevent and treat vaginal yeast infections.

1. **Include probiotics in your daily diet.** Foods such as yogurt, kefir and sweet acidophilus milk that contain friendly bacteria, known collectively as lactic acid bacteria, are called probiotics. Lactic acid bacteria such as *Lactobacillus acidophilus* and bifidobacteria normally live in your intestine, where they prevent the growth of infection-causing bacteria and fungi; they also prevent the overgrowth of *Candida albicans*. A number of studies have shown that women who consume yogurt or fermented milk beverages each day have a significant reduction in vaginal yeast infections. In fact, two studies found that 3/4 to 1 cup (175 to 250 ml) of yogurt eaten daily for six months resulted in a threefold decrease in infection among women experiencing recurrent candida infections.[9,10] Some studies have found a yogurt douche to be effective against vaginal yeast infections.

Probiotic bacteria are also available in supplement form. The strength of a probiotic supplement is usually quantified by the number of living organisms, or colony-forming units (CFUs), per capsule. Typical doses usually range from 1 billion to 10 billion viable organisms taken daily, in three to four divided doses. Probiotic supplements may cause flatulence, which usually subsides as you continue treatment. There are no safety issues associated with taking these supplements. If possible, take your probiotic supplement with food. After a meal, stomach contents become less acidic because of the presence of food, allowing live bacteria to withstand stomach acid and reach their final destination in the intestinal tract.

2. **Add garlic to your meals.** You may want to use cooked garlic more often than raw, since some women report being sensitive to fresh uncooked garlic during their pregnancy. A daily intake of garlic, with its accompanying sulphur compounds, enhances the body's immune system and kills many types of bacteria and fungi. A half to whole clove a day is recommended. Garlic has been used alone or in combination with yogurt to treat candida infections.

HEMORRHOIDS

Hemorrhoids are a type of varicose vein that are very common in pregnancy. They're swollen rectal veins that may bleed or protrude through your anus. Hemorrhoids are caused by the increased pressure of your uterus, which interferes with blood flow to the rectal area, causing blood to pool in these veins. Symptoms include bleeding, itching and pain in and around your anus. The best approach is prevention, by avoiding constipation. The straining associated with constipation puts extra pressure on the veins and aggravates your symptoms. Once hemorrhoids develop, you can minimize the symptoms by keeping your rectal area clean and washing after each bowel movement, soaking in a warm bath, applying cold compresses and avoiding sitting for long periods. Hemorrhoids usually subside after pregnancy.

Try these strategies to help prevent constipation and hemorrhoids.

1. **Gradually increase your intake of dietary fibre** to 28 grams per day, the recommended intake during pregnancy. Foods like wheat bran, whole grains and fruit and vegetables contain insoluble fibre, which promotes bowel regularity. Two of the best ways to boost your fibre intake are to

start your day with a bowl of high-fibre breakfast cereal and to include a serving of legumes such as chickpeas, kidney beans, black beans or lentils in your daily diet. High-fibre cereals have at least 6 grams of fibre per serving, as stated on the package nutrition box. If you're constipated, choose a 100% bran cereal that provides 10 to 12 grams of fibre per serving. Mix 1/4 to 1/2 cup (60 to 125 ml) into your usual breakfast cereal. You'll find a list of higher-fibre foods in Chapter 1, page 29. But start slowly—consuming too much fibre too soon can cause bloating and gas, and it may even worsen your constipation.

2. **Drink plenty of water.** Aim for about 10 cups (2.4 L) each day, and more if you exercise. For insoluble fibre to work in your intestinal tract, it needs to absorb water first. By retaining water, fibre acts to increase stool bulk and promote regularity.

3. **Get regular exercise**—for example, take a brisk walk—to help keep your bowel movements regular.

4. **Check the dosage of your iron supplement.** Constipation may occur if you take a supplement supplying 100 milligrams of iron. This side effect often disappears within a week of first taking your iron supplement. If it persists, speak to your doctor or dietitian about decreasing the dosage. Many women report they feel better when they take their iron supplement before bedtime.

IRON-DEFICIENCY ANEMIA

Iron is an essential mineral in the production of red blood cells. During pregnancy, your blood volume increases nearly 50 percent, putting excessive demands on your body's ability to produce vital red blood cells. Your fetus also has specific iron requirements, especially during the last months of pregnancy, when iron stores are building up. When you're not pregnant, you need 18 milligrams of iron a day. When you're pregnant, you need 27 milligrams a day to prevent a deficiency.

During pregnancy, if you're not meeting those increased iron needs, your fetus draws from your iron stores, leaving you anemic and exhausted. Anemia is caused by a decline in the amount of hemoglobin in the blood. Hemoglobin is a protein found in red blood cells and it plays a very important role in carrying oxygen throughout your body. To build up hemoglobin concentrations, you need more iron to help increase the production of red blood cells. As a result of the increased iron demands of pregnancy, it's not possible to maintain your iron stores through diet alone.

This is why many nutritionists and doctors recommend that women take a prenatal vitamin-mineral supplement throughout their pregnancy. These supplements provide extra iron as well as calcium and folic acid (more on these nutrients later).

If you have anemia, you'll feel tired, weak and light-headed. You may also experience shortness of breath and heart palpitations. Anemia develops most often after the 20th week of pregnancy and is identified through blood tests that measure your hemoglobin levels. Your doctor may recommend that you take iron supplements throughout the second half of your pregnancy to avoid developing iron-deficiency anemia.

If you're diagnosed with iron-deficiency anemia, be sure to read Chapter 3, Anemia, where I discuss your recommended daily intake of iron, the best food sources of iron and how to enhance your body's absorption of this mineral.

RHESUS FACTOR INCOMPATIBILITY

Fairly early in your pregnancy, your blood will be tested for Rhesus (Rh) factor, a type of protein, or antigen, that's present in red blood cells. If your blood has the Rh antigen, you're Rh positive; if you don't have the protein, you're Rh negative. Problems occur if your fetus's blood has the Rh factor and your blood doesn't. If a small amount of your blood mixes with your developing baby's blood, which can happen, your body may respond as if you were allergic to your baby. Your body makes antibodies that can cross the placenta and attack your baby's blood, causing anemia and potentially life-threatening effects in your baby. When detected through proper prenatal care, this serious condition is now very rare.

GESTATIONAL DIABETES

Your body normally produces a hormone called insulin that controls the levels of blood sugar or glucose in your blood. If you have diabetes, your body doesn't produce enough insulin or doesn't use insulin effectively. During pregnancy, a small number of women develop gestational diabetes, even though they didn't have diabetes before they became pregnant. It's thought that elevated hormone levels produce metabolic changes during pregnancy and cause this condition.

In most cases, gestational diabetes doesn't cause symptoms and isn't a health risk for you. It does, however, create health risks for your baby. If this condition isn't treated, your baby is at greater risk of being still-born or of dying as a newborn. Gestational diabetes also can cause your fetus to have an excessive birth weight. When your baby is very large, you have an increased likelihood of Caesarean birth or birth injuries. Babies born to mothers with diabetes are also quite prone to hypoglycemia, or low blood sugar.

The symptoms of gestational diabetes aren't very obvious, so the condition must be detected by a glucose tolerance test. It usually develops in the second half of your pregnancy. You may be predisposed to this condition if you are obese, are over 30 years old or have a family history of diabetes. However, nearly half of the women with gestational diabetes have no risk factors at all. To manage this type of diabetes during your pregnancy, you should follow a diet planned for you by a registered dietitian, exercise regularly and have your blood-glucose level tested often. If your condition is severe, you may need insulin injections to control your blood-sugar levels; pregnant women who take daily insulin are three to four times more likely to have a baby with major birth defects.

Gestational diabetes usually disappears immediately after pregnancy, but you're at increased risk of encountering it again in another pregnancy. You're also more prone to developing diabetes in later life. Fortunately, there's no increased risk that your baby will develop diabetes, despite the fact that you had diabetes during pregnancy.

PRE-ECLAMPSIA

Swelling of your ankles and toes is very common and quite normal in pregnancy. Called edema, this condition indicates that your body is retaining water. But other types of swelling during pregnancy are causes of real concern. Swelling of your face and hands may be a warning sign of pre-eclampsia.

Pre-eclampsia, sometimes referred to as toxemia, develops during the last three months of pregnancy. The main indications of pre-eclampsia are high blood pressure and one or more of the following symptoms: protein in the urine, headache, blurred vision and intense stomach pain. Other symptoms include swelling or fluid retention (edema). However, it's possible to develop pre-eclampsia and have no obvious symptoms at all. Often, pre-eclampsia is detected only through a routine prenatal examination.

It's estimated that the incidence of pre-eclampsia has increased by nearly one-third over the past decade. This may be because more women over 35 are giving birth and multiple pregnancies are becoming more common, two risk factors for pre-eclampsia.

The exact cause of pre-eclampsia isn't yet known and there's no cure for the condition. It seriously restricts blood flow to the placenta, which may reduce the oxygen and nutrient supply to your fetus. This retards your baby's growth and causes fetal distress. It can also cause problems for your health by damaging your liver or kidneys, or by causing seizures and bleeding problems.

The first sign of pre-eclampsia is usually a sudden weight gain of more than 2 pounds (1 kg) in a week. This is due to fluid retention, not fat accumulation. You may also develop swelling in your hands and face, headaches and vision problems. The routine blood pressure tests that your doctor performs every month are the best way of detecting this condition in the early stages.

In mild cases, your doctor may suggest bedrest. By lying on your side, you enable blood to flow more freely to the placenta, increasing the nourishment to your fetus. Regular blood pressure, urine and blood tests will be necessary to check on the health of your baby. In more severe cases, you'll be hospitalized. Because pre-eclampsia compromises your baby's supply of nutrients and oxygen, it may be necessary to consider an early delivery. Even though the baby may be at risk because of a premature delivery, the dangerous conditions inside your uterus may create an even greater health risk. A discussion with your doctor will help you make an informed decision regarding the risks and benefits of an early birth. Once the baby is born, your blood pressure usually returns to normal. The condition may recur in later pregnancies, especially if you had a fairly severe case of pre-eclampsia.

The following nutrition strategies may help reduce your risk of developing pre-eclampsia:

- **Take extra calcium.** Observational studies have revealed that women who have higher calcium intakes also have a lower risk of developing high blood pressure during their pregnancies. In addition, a number of studies have found that taking calcium pills after the 20th week of pregnancy significantly reduces the risk of pre-eclampsia. In fact, it's thought that calcium supplementation can lower the risk of hypertension by 54 percent.[11] Canadian researchers analyzed the results of 14 studies involving more than 2500 pregnant women and concluded that taking 1500 to 2000 milligrams of calcium lowered blood pressure and reduced the risk of pre-eclampsia by 62 percent.[12]

Based on the evidence, the Canadian Hypertension Society recommends a calcium intake of 2000 milligrams per day to help lower blood pressure in women with pregnancy-induced hypertension. If you have a history of kidney disease or kidney stones, speak to your doctor before taking more calcium.

To meet your needs for calcium, you should already be consuming 1000 milligrams each day from your diet and prenatal supplement combined (this requires 3 cups/750 ml of milk, yogurt or calcium-enriched beverage in addition to the 250 milligrams of calcium that most prenatal supplements provide). To boost your intake to 2000 milligrams, take a 500 milligram calcium supplement twice daily. Take your calcium supplement two hours apart from your prenatal vitamin, since calcium inhibits your ability to absorb iron.

- **Get plenty of vitamins C and E.** These two antioxidants might be helpful in managing blood pressure throughout the second half of pregnancy. Compared to pregnant women with normal blood pressure, it appears that women with pre-eclampsia produce more free radicals, harmful oxygen compounds that roam the body and damage cells. Free radicals are a normal by-product of metabolism and your body has a built-in system of antioxidant enzymes to deal with them. Certain disease states, cigarette smoking, exposure to pollution and even heavy exercise can increase free radical production. It's thought that free radicals impair the ability of blood vessels to relax and dilate, and this can lead to pregnancy-induced high blood pressure. As antioxidants, vitamins C and E act as scavengers and neutralize free radicals before they can do harm.

  Researchers from Harvard University observed that, compared to women who consumed the most vitamin C, those whose daily diets provided less than 85 milligrams doubled their risk of pre-eclampsia. What's more, those women who got less than 35 milligrams per day had almost a fourfold higher risk for the condition.[13] British researchers studied women at risk for pre-eclampsia and found that taking vitamin C (1000 mg) and E (400 IU) supplements from the 16th through the 22nd week of their pregnancies lowered the risk of getting pre-eclampsia by 75 percent.[14]

During pregnancy, you need 85 milligrams of vitamin C each day. Vitamin C–rich foods include citrus fruit, citrus juices, cantaloupe, kiwi, mango, strawberries, broccoli, Brussels sprouts, cauliflower, red pepper and tomato juice. To supplement, take 500 milligrams of vitamin C once or twice daily. The daily upper limit is 2000 milligrams.

Your vitamin E requirements don't change when you become pregnant. You should be getting 15 IU each day from foods like wheat germ, nuts, seeds, vegetable oils, whole grains and kale. To supplement, take 400 IU of natural source vitamin E. The daily upper limit is 1500 IU.

BIRTH DEFECTS

About 3 to 5 percent of all babies are born with birth defects. Statistics indicate that birth defects account for the largest percentage of all infant deaths in North America. Many birth defects aren't preventable, because their cause is unknown. Researchers do know, however, that most birth defects occur in the first three months of pregnancy, often before a woman even knows she's pregnant. It's becoming increasingly evident that your state of health at the time of conception is one of the most important factors in protecting your baby from preventable malformations.

Neural tube defects (NTDs)

Neural tube defects (NTDs) are congenital malformations that occur during fetal life. They're caused by failure of the neural tube—what eventually forms the body's central nervous system—to close. NTDs are one of the most common congenital malformations seen among live-born infants in Canada. The most common neural tube defects are spina bifida and anencephaly.

It's been estimated that approximately eight hundred children a year in Canada are born with NTDs, half of whom will have spina bifida, a neural tube defect that prevents the vertebrae of the baby's spine from closing completely. In severe cases, the spinal cord protrudes outside the baby's body, limiting mobility and causing other neurological dysfunctions. Spina bifida can be surgically corrected, but surgical repair of the lesion is not always associated with improvement in motor function. Children with spina bifida often have long-term problems that require management by a healthcare team.

Folic acid (folate)

One nutrient known to prevent NTDs is folic acid. This is the synthetic form of folate, a B vitamin necessary for cell division and growth. Folate is also used to make red blood cells and DNA, the genetic blueprint of all cells. And it's essential to the normal development of your baby's spine, brain and skull during the early weeks of pregnancy.

Neural tube defects occur within the first four weeks of pregnancy, usually before a woman even knows she's pregnant. It's well established that taking folic acid before and during the early weeks of pregnancy is vital to preventing NTDs in the developing fetus. Since one-half of all pregnancies in Canada are unplanned, all women of childbearing age are urged to take a multivitamin providing 0.4 milligram of folic acid.

To reduce the risk of NTDs, the Society of Obstetricians and Gynaecologists of Canada advises healthy women to take a multivitamin with 0.4 to 1 milligram of folic acid for at least two to three months before becoming pregnant and throughout pregnancy and breastfeeding.

Women at high risk for NTDs—including women with epilepsy, type 1 diabetes, a family history of NTDs and those who are obese—should take a supplement with 5 milligrams of folic acid a few months prior to pregnancy and continue through the 12th week of pregnancy. After twelve weeks, a multivitamin with 0.4 to 1 milligram of folic acid can be taken. (Mounting evidence also suggests that women who aren't overweight and who are regular users of multivitamins before and during pregnancy have a lower risk of pre-eclampsia. Folic acid is needed for the development and function of blood vessels, a process thought to be disrupted in women with pre-eclampsia.)

Although a multivitamin with folic acid helps women meet increased folate requirements, pregnant women should also include folate-rich foods in their diet. Good food sources include lentils, black beans, cooked spinach, asparagus, avocado and artichokes. You'll find the folate content of selected foods in Chapter 1, page 19.

Other causes of birth defects

One vitamin you don't want to get too much of during your pregnancy is vitamin A. In fact, if you take a vitamin supplement, make sure it contains no more than 5000 international units (IU) of vitamin A. Most prenatal formulas provide 2500 IU of the vitamin. High daily intakes of supplemental vitamin A (more than 10,000 IU) are associated with birth defects. You may have read that some of the nutrient beta carotene is converted to vitamin A in the body. This is true, but it's not transformed to vitamin A efficiently enough to cause toxicity. Beta carotene in a supplement is considered safe.

Infectious diseases, such as rubella (German measles) and syphilis can also cause birth defects. Syphilis should be treated with an antibiotic before you become pregnant because it can cause bone and tooth deformities. If you have not had rubella, you should be vaccinated against the disease before you become pregnant. Because the vaccine can also pose problems for a developing fetus, you should wait three months after vaccination before becoming pregnant. A rubella infection in early pregnancy causes abnormalities in the heart, eyes and ears of your fetus.

Medications

Few clinical drug trials involve pregnant women, so the effects of most medications and drugs are still unknown. The same goes for herbal supplements. For this reason, it's sensible for you to avoid all medications throughout your pregnancy, unless prescribed by your doctor. If medications are necessary to manage a health risk, you should always ask for the lowest possible dosage, in order to minimize the impact on your baby. If you have a pre-existing medical condition, such as high blood pressure, diabetes or lupus, you shouldn't discontinue your medication; however, there may be safer drugs that you can take during your pregnancy. Discuss your concerns with your doctor, so that you can weigh the risks and benefits of changing your medication and make an informed decision.

Most medications, even over-the-counter drugs, are particularly dangerous for your fetus during the first trimester. This is the time when vital organs and systems are developing and medications can interfere with normal growth patterns, causing serious health risks and birth defects.

Nutrition guidelines for a healthy pregnancy

Now it's time to look at the whole picture: what and how much you need to eat, and what foods and beverages you should avoid during your pregnancy. Let's start by reviewing your nutrient requirements during this exciting time.

Recommended Dietary Allowance (RDA) for Key Nutrients During Pregnancy (Adults and Teens)

Nutrient	RDA: not pregnant	RDA: pregnant
Calories	1900–2200 calories/day	1st trimester: no increase 2nd and 3rd trimesters: add 300 calories/day
Protein	46 grams/day	1st trimester: no increase 2nd and 3rd trimesters: add 25 grams/day
Calcium	1000 milligrams/day	Adults: 1000 milligrams/day Teens: 1300 milligrams/day
Vitamin D	1000 IU (25 mcg)/day	2000 IU (50 mcg)/day
Iron	18 milligrams/day	27 milligrams/day (for entire pregnancy)
Zinc	8 milligrams/day	Adults: 11 milligrams/day Teens: 13 milligrams/day
Folate	400 micrograms/day	600 micrograms/day

A FOOD PLAN FOR PREGNANCY

With a few exceptions—for example, folate, vitamin D and iron, for which supplements are needed—the following diet shows how your nutrient requirements translate into food choices. Both pregnant women and teens can use this guide.

Food group servings	Food choices	Recommended daily
Grain foods (carbohydrates, iron, fibre; choose whole-grain as often as possible)		*6 to 10*
	Whole-grain bread	1 slice
	Bagel, large	1/4
	Roll, large	1/2
	Pita pocket	1/2
	Tortilla	6 inch (15 cm)
	Cereal, cold	3/4 cup (175 ml)
	Cereal, 100% bran	1/2 cup (125 ml)

Food group servings	Food choices	Recommended daily
	Cereal, hot	1/2 cup (125 ml)
	Crackers, soda	6
	Corn	1/2 cup (125 ml)
	Popcorn, plain	3 cups (750 ml)
	Grains, cooked	1/2 cup (125 ml)
	Pasta, cooked	1/2 cup (125 ml)
	Rice, cooked	1/3 cup (75 ml)
Vegetables & Fruit (carbohydrates, fibre, vitamins, minerals)		*7 to 10*
	Vegetables, cooked/raw	1/2 cup (125 ml)
	Vegetables, leafy green	1 cup (250 ml)
	Fruit, whole	1 piece
	Fruit, small (plums, apricots)	4
	Fruit, cut up	1 cup (250 ml)
	Berries	1 cup (250 ml)
	Juice, unsweetened	1/2 to 3/4 cup (125 to 175 ml)
Milk & Alternatives (8 grams protein per serving; protein, carbohydrates, calcium, vitamin D, vitamin A, zinc)		*3*
	Milk	1 cup (250 ml)
	Yogurt	3/4 cup (175 ml)
	Cheese	1-1/2 oz (45 g)
	Soy beverage, fortified	1 cup (250 ml)
Meat & Alternatives (7 grams protein per serving; protein, iron, zinc)		*6 to 9*
	Fish, lean meat, poultry	1 oz (30 g)
	Egg, whole	1
	Egg, whites only	2
	Legumes (beans, chickpeas, lentils)	1/3 cup (75 ml)
	Soy nuts	2 tbsp (30 ml)
	Tempeh	1/4 cup (60 ml)

Food group servings	Food choices	Recommended daily
	Tofu, firm	1/3 cup (75 ml)
	Texturized vegetable protein (TVP)	1/3 cup (75 ml)
	Veggie dog, small	1
Fats & Oils* *(essential fatty acids, vitamin E)*		*4 to 6*
	Butter, margarine, mayonnaise	1 tsp (5 ml)
	Nuts/seeds	1 tbsp (15 ml)
	Peanut and nut butters	1-1/2 tsp (7 ml)
	Salad dressing	2 tsp (10 ml)
	Vegetable oil	1 tsp (5 ml)
Water/Fluid		*10*
	Water	1 cup (250 ml)
	Herbal tea**	1 cup (250 ml)

All serving sizes are based on measures after cooking.

*To include sources of essential fatty acids in your diet, choose canola oil, walnut oil, flaxseed oil and nuts and seeds more often as your fat servings.

**Avoid herbal teas listed on page 301.

FOODS TO EAT MORE OF
Fish: Omega-3 fatty acids

There are two omega-3 fats in fish: docosahexaenoic acid (DHA) and eicosapentaenoic acid (EPA). When it comes to fetal health, DHA appears to be the most important omega-3 fatty acid. That's because it's very important for your baby's brain and eye development, especially during the third trimester. DHA accumulates in a developing baby's brain, and this increases three to five times during the final trimester.

How much DHA reaches your baby's brain depends on your diet during pregnancy. Animal studies suggest that offspring born to mothers who had DHA-deficient diets have behavioural problems and abnormal vision. Some research suggests that a lack of omega-3 fatty acids during your pregnancy can result in learning and behavioural disorders later in a child's life.

Mothers and their developing babies can get DHA in two ways: by eating 5 to 12 ounces (150 to 360 g) of oily fish each week or by taking a daily fish oil supplement. Good choices of fish that are high in omega-3 fatty acids but low in mercury include salmon, trout, sardines, herring, and Atlantic mackerel. If you don't eat fish, choose a fish oil supplement that supplies 500 milligrams of DHA and EPA combined per day. Avoid fish liver oil supplements, which are often high in vitamin A. Vegetarian DHA supplements are available; they're made from algae and supply 200 milligrams of DHA per tablet.

FISH AND MERCURY. Some species of fish contain high levels of mercury, which can accumulate in the body and affect the developing nervous system, especially the brain, of infants and young children. If a woman consumes too much mercury before and during her pregnancy, it may increase the risk of birth defects and learning disabilities in her child. Some, but not all, studies have found associations between a women's mercury exposure during pregnancy and her offspring's neurologic test scores during childhood.

Fortunately, the types of fish that provide the most omega-3 fatty acids are also low in mercury and can be safely enjoyed by pregnant women. Women who are pregnant or breastfeeding, and women who could become pregnant, should limit—or avoid, in my opinion—swordfish, shark, marlin, orange roughy, escolar, fresh and frozen tuna, king mackerel and canned albacore (white) tuna. Canned light tuna (e.g., skipjack, yellowfin, tongol) is low in mercury and safe to eat regularly. Health Canada advises that women (and children) limit their intake of high-mercury fish to a small portion once per month.

Folate-rich foods

I've already emphasized the importance of meeting your folate requirements to prevent neural tube defects. But this issue is so important that I want to mention it again. In addition to getting supplemental folic acid from your prenatal multivitamin or a separate folic acid supplement, aim to include at least two good sources of folate in your daily diet. Eat fruit, dark-green leafy vegetables, dried peas, beans and lentils, avocado, asparagus and orange juice. See the list in Chapter 1, page 19, for the best ways to get this important B vitamin in your diet.

FOODS, BEVERAGES AND HERBS TO LIMIT OR AVOID

Foods

Some foods have a greater potential for causing food poisoning, and some types of food poisoning are of particular concern during pregnancy. The hormonal changes of pregnancy affect a woman's immune system, making her more susceptible to food poisoning, especially listeriosis. To minimize your risk of food-borne illness, be extra careful to practice safe food handling during your pregnancy.

Foods to Avoid

Type of food poisoning	Risky foods
Listeriosis can cause miscarriage during the first three months of pregnancy and illness or stillbirth later in pregnancy.	Hot dogs Non-dried deli meats (e.g., mortadella, ham) Soft and semi-soft cheeses (e.g., feta, brie, Camembert and, if made from unpasteurized milk, blue-veined cheese) Refrigerated meat pâtés and meat spreads Refrigerated smoked seafood and smoked fish Raw or undercooked meat, poultry, fish
E. coli infection can cross the placenta and infect your growing baby.	Undercooked beef products Unpasteurized milk Contaminated water and mayonnaise Improperly processed cider

Beverages

Coffee (caffeine)

Caffeine is a stimulant and can cause irritability, nervousness and insomnia. Not only does it cross the placenta and reach the fetus, it also acts as a diuretic, dehydrating your body of valuable fluid. The evidence for coffee's ill effect on pregnancy remains unclear at this time. Researchers have found that high levels of caffeine, equivalent to more than 6 cups (1500 ml) of coffee per day, are associated with miscarriage.[15] And according to Canadian researchers, even less might be harmful. An analysis of studies conducted from 1966 to 1996 concluded that consuming as little as 150 milligrams of caffeine each day (1 to 2 cups/250 to 500 ml of coffee) slightly increased the risk of miscarriage and of low-birthweight babies.[16] However, the researchers did note that they were unable to determine whether this finding was related to the woman's age at pregnancy, cigarette smoking or alcohol use.

Based on the evidence at hand, Health Canada advises that you limit your caffeine intake to a daily maximum of 200 milligrams. See Chapter 1, page 11, for the caffeine content of selected beverages and foods.

Alcoholic beverages

There's no question about this advice: Avoid consuming alcohol during pregnancy. Alcohol can cross the placenta and, in the case of heavy drinking (at least four drinks per day), it can cause fetal alcohol syndrome in newborns. Babies born with fetal alcohol syndrome have lower birth weights, smaller heads, abnormal facial features, heart defects and mental retardation. Even occasional, moderate drinking might harm your baby. Fetal alcohol syndrome is seen in 30 percent to 40 percent of infants whose mothers drank at least 2 ounces (60 ml) of absolute alcohol per day during the first trimester. Mild forms of this disorder have also occurred when women drank 1 ounce (30 ml) of alcohol per day or indulged in binge drinking.

Herbs and herbal supplements

Although herbs are considered "natural," very few herbs are considered safe for pregnant women. Herbs may be milder than prescription medications, but many contain natural ingredients that can cause miscarriage or premature birth, harm your developing baby and even jeopardize your health. The truth is, very few studies have tested the safety of herbal supplements in pregnancy. If you use herbal products, do so very cautiously.

Herbal Supplements to Avoid During Pregnancy

Alder buckthorn	Essential oils	Pokeroot
Aloe vera	Feverfew	Rhubarb (safe to use as a
Angelica	Ginger root* (safe in cooking)	food)
Barberry	Ginseng	Rue
Birthroot	Goldenseal	Sage (safe to use in cooking)
Black cohosh, blue cohosh	Gotu kola	Sarsaparilla
Blessed thistle	Juniper berries	Scotch broom
Bloodroot	Kava kava	Senna
Cascara sagrada	Licorice root	Shepherd's purse
Coltsfoot	Mistletoe	Southernwood
Comfrey	Mugwort	Squill
Cotton root	Nutmeg (safe to use in	St. John's wort
Damiana	cooking)	Tansy
Devil's claw	Osha	Uva ursi
Dong quai	Parsley (safe to use in cooking)	Wild yam
Echinacea	Pennyroyal	Wormwood
Ephedra (Ma huang)	Pleurisy root	Yarrow

*Ginger may be safe when taken appropriately, for a short period of time, to treat severe morning sickness. See page 271 for more about ginger and morning sickness.

Herbal Supplements Considered Safe During Pregnancy

Bilberry	Ginkgo biloba	Raspberry leaf
Cranberry	Grape seed extract	Valerian root
Evening primrose oil	Green tea extract	

Although these supplements are considered safe to use during pregnancy, keep in mind that very little research has been conducted in pregnant women. Be sure to inform your doctor if you take an herbal product.

Safe Herbal Teas

Chamomile	Linden flower*
Citrus peel	Orange peel
Ginger	Rosehip
Lemon balm	

*Not recommended if you have a pre-existing heart condition.

Because herbal teas often possess drug-like properties, it's wise to brew them weakly and *consume no more than 2 to 3 cups (500 to 750 ml) per day during your pregnancy*. If you have a plant or pollen allergy, be careful not to use teas that may contain herbs related to plants to which you have known allergies. For instance, if you're allergic to plants in the Asteracease/Compositae family (ragweed, daisy, marigold and chrysanthemums), you should avoid chamomile and echinacea.

17
Breastfeeding

Once again, this chapter isn't formatted quite like the others. Because breastfeeding isn't a medical condition that requires prevention or management, there's no Bottom Line summary at the end.

Nature has designed breast milk as the perfect first food for your baby. It is nutritionally superior to all other forms of infant food and is ideally suited to the developmental needs of a newborn human. A growing body of research indicates that breast milk protects babies from illness, provides the basis for good brain growth and promotes early bonding between mother and child. The Canadian Paediatric Society recommends exclusive breastfeeding (that means no supplementing with formula) for at least the first six months of your baby's life. In combination with complementary foods, breastfeeding can be successfully continued until your child is over 2 years old.

Essentially, your breasts are a network of milk-producing glands, called alveoli, supported within an envelope of fibrous and fatty tissue. Each breast contains fifteen to twenty glands, connected by milk ducts to your nipple. The alveoli don't mature until they're stimulated by the hormonal surge of estrogen and progesterone that occurs during pregnancy. As these hormone levels increase, small reservoirs of milk develop behind the nipples.

The actual process of breastfeeding or lactation is stimulated by the sucking action of your baby. Nerve endings in the pigmented tissue (areola) that surrounds the nipple are triggered by the pressure of your baby's tongue. They instantly send a signal to the hypothalamus and pituitary glands in your brain to initiate the flow of milk. These glands release the hormone prolactin to stimulate milk production, and the hormone oxytocin to contract the muscle fibres around the milk glands, which forces the milk into the duct network. The combined action of these two hormones results in the letdown sensation that most women recognize as essential to successful breastfeeding.

Although the composition of breast milk may change as your baby develops, there are only three main types of breast milk:

1. **Colostrum** is produced in the first few days after birth and is released before normal lactation begins. It's the perfect food for newborns and especially rich in nutrients and antibodies. Appearing as a thin, yellow fluid, colostrum has a very high calorie and protein content and it protects your baby against infection. Because colostrum is so beneficial for your baby, you should consider breastfeeding for the first few days after birth, even if you have decided to bottle-feed your baby later.
2. **Foremilk** is a thinner type of milk that's released from your breast at the beginning of a feeding. It is normally lower in fat content and is intended to satisfy your baby's thirst and fluid needs.
3. **Hindmilk** follows foremilk during a feeding. It has a higher fat and calorie content and is important to your baby's growth and overall good health. To ensure that your newborn receives the nutritional benefits of both foremilk and hindmilk, encourage your baby to drain one breast completely before moving on to the other.

Almost every woman can breastfeed. The size and shape of your breasts and nipples don't affect your ability to produce an adequate milk supply for your baby. There are very few medical or environmental reasons why you shouldn't breastfeed. Only if you are taking specific medications or have a serious illness, such as HIV infection, AIDS, tuberculosis, hepatitis or kidney or heart problems, or if your baby has certain medical conditions, would you be advised not to breastfeed.

Breast versus bottle

INFANT BENEFITS OF BREASTFEEDING

At one time, breastfeeding was not a popular choice among women. In 1963, only 38 percent of Canadian women breastfed their babies.[1] As research began to document the many benefits of breast milk, those numbers have risen dramatically. Recent studies indicate that nearly 75 percent of all Canadian babies are breastfed, at least initially.[2]

- **Protection from infection.** Many studies have revealed that babies fed only breast milk for the first four to six months are less likely to get respiratory tract infections, ear infections, urinary tract infections, stomach infections and diarrhea. Some studies even suggest that breastfeeding can protect infants from infections for years after nursing.[3]

- **Prevention of allergies and asthma.** Hay fever, asthma, eczema and food allergies are often referred to as atopic diseases or atopy. Atopic diseases have one thing in common—they're allergic disorders caused by the body eliciting an immune response. This immune reaction triggers the release of massive quantities of chemicals that cause symptoms in the skin, the cardiovascular system, the gastrointestinal tract or respiratory system.

  Plenty of evidence shows that exclusive breastfeeding for the first four months can lower your baby's risk of developing an atopic disease, especially if you or your partner is affected by one.[4-7] In fact, infants with a parent or sibling with an allergic disease are at greater risk of developing atopy during infancy or childhood. A review of twelve studies found that exclusive breastfeeding reduced the risk of asthma by 30 percent in children without a family history of atopy, and by 48 percent in children with a family history.[8]

- **Promotion of intelligence.** Several studies have reported that nutrients in breast milk have a positive effect on intellectual development in childhood. Compared to babies who are not breastfed, those who are breastfed for at least four months score higher on verbal IQ and performance tests. And it seems that the longer a woman breastfeeds her child, the greater the effect.[9-13] Researchers for the University of Chicago recently reviewed forty studies on the subject and concluded that breastfeeding does indeed promote intelligence.[14] Many studies measure infant IQ scores at 12 or 18 months of age, but not all. Other studies suggest that the positive effects of breastfeeding on intelligence persist into childhood and possibly even adulthood. Danish researchers studied 3250 young adults and found that the longer they were breastfed as babies, the better they scored on IQ tests at 18 years of age.[15]

- **Prevention of SIDS.** Sudden infant death syndrome (SIDS) refers to the sudden and unexpected death of an apparently healthy baby. Typically, a peacefully sleeping baby simply never wakes up, for reasons that remain elusive. SIDS affects one out of every 750 babies born in Canada. It normally occurs between 2 and 4 months of age; it rarely occurs before 2 weeks or after 6 months of age. Over the past twenty years, the incidence of SIDS has fallen in Canada, mainly because researchers have identified strategies that can help reduce an infant's risk. Although one of the most important preventive measures a parent can take is to place the baby on his or her back to sleep, breastfeeding may also offer some protection.

A handful of studies have linked breastfeeding to a lower risk of SIDS. American researchers analyzed twenty-three studies on the risk of SIDS in bottle-fed infants compared to breastfed infants and found that bottle-feeding was associated with double the risk. Nineteen of the twenty-three studies favoured breastfeeding as a protective measure against SIDS.[16] It's not entirely clear why breastfeeding may cut the risk of SIDS; however, some researchers believe that the immune-enhancing properties of breast milk play a role.

Other studies suggest that, compared to formula-fed infants, breastfed babies have lower blood pressure during childhood and adolescence, are less likely to be obese and have a lower risk of leukemia.[17-26]

- **Protection again many common illnesses.** Approximately 80 percent of the cells in breast milk are macrophages, cells that kill bacteria, fungi and viruses. Breast milk provides antibodies that give your baby varying degrees of protection against illnesses such as ear infections, pneumonia, bronchitis, diabetes mellitus, German measles and staphylococcal infections. Breastfeeding may also offer a protective effect against chronic digestive diseases.

- **Allergy free and sterile.** Although breast milk contains more than one hundred ingredients that aren't found in infant formula, your baby will never develop an allergy to your milk. Occasionally, you may eat something that affects your milk and your baby may react to that particular food; however, if you eliminate that food from your diet, the problem should disappear. Milk that comes directly from your breast is sterile, eliminating the dangers of bacteria in bottles or in water that hasn't been properly sterilized. As an additional benefit, the exercise of sucking at the breast strengthens your baby's jaws, promoting good jaw development and straight, healthy teeth.

MATERNAL BENEFITS OF BREASTFEEDING

The benefits of breastfeeding are not limited to your baby. As a mother, you'll find that breastfeeding has many practical advantages:

- **Bonding with your baby.** Breastfeeding helps build a special bond between you and your baby. When you nurse, that skin-to-skin contact, cuddling and holding can help your newborn feel more secure and comforted. Breastfeeding moms may also have increased self-confidence and feelings of closeness with their babies. However, there's no question that the act of feeding your baby—whether breast milk or formula—elicits very warm, protective and powerful emotions in mothers.

- **Convenience.** Breastfeeding saves time and money. There's no buying, measuring or mixing of formula. And there are no bottles to sterilize and warm. It takes just a second to provide breast milk to your hungry baby.

- **Getting back into shape.** Immediately after birth, your baby's sucking causes your body to release oxytocin, a hormone that causes your uterus to contract. This helps shrink your uterus more quickly to its original size and lessens any bleeding a woman may have after giving birth. (Oxytocin also helps initiate the letdown of your milk by causing the tiny muscles around your milk glands to contract and squeeze.)

    Breastfeeding also burns up extra calories (as many as 500 per day), so it can make it easier to lose those pregnancy pounds. Nursing for at least five to six months mobilizes fat from your lower body, which can promote weight loss. After the first month, most breast-feeding women gradually lose 1 to 2 pounds (0.5 to 1 kg) per month, though some lose as much as 4 pounds (1.8 kg) each month. Not all women lose weight and some may even gain a little weight during breastfeeding.

    But be forewarned: Breastfeeding alone won't necessarily help you get your pre-pregnancy figure back. Other factors seem to have a greater effect on your total weight loss—your age, your pre-pregnancy weight and how you gained weight when you were pregnant. And let's not forget that exercise and healthy eating count too.

Many of my clients report that breastfeeding makes them feel hungry all the time. It's sometimes difficult to lose that last 10 pounds (4.5 kg) when your appetite kicks into high gear. Breastfeeding isn't the time to diet. Eating too few calories will slow down your milk production and cause you to lose protein, not fat.

- **Protection from cancer.** Breastfeeding for the first six months may protect your future health too. Exclusive breastfeeding delays the return of ovulation and the menstrual cycle. This prolonged suppression of the menstrual cycle seems to be linked to a lower risk of breast, ovarian and possibly uterine cancers.

There's good evidence that breastfeeding reduces the risk of premenopausal breast cancer, so women with a family history of the disease might especially benefit from nursing. *The Lancet*, a medical journal, reported a 2002 analysis of forty-seven studies in thirty countries that included more than 50,000 women with breast cancer and 96,973 women without the disease. The researchers concluded that the longer women breastfeed, the greater the protection from breast cancer. They went on to say that the lack of or short duration of breastfeeding in developed countries is a major contributor to the high incidence of breast cancer in these countries.[27]

DRAWBACKS OF BREASTFEEDING

Despite its many advantages, breastfeeding can be inconvenient and often requires a complete change in lifestyle, affecting everything from the clothing you wear to the places you go. You're very closely tied to your baby while breastfeeding and, in some cases, your partner may not always be supportive of your decision.

You can overcome the inconvenience of breastfeeding by occasionally expressing and storing your breast milk. This gives you the freedom to leave your infant with a babysitter and allows your partner to share in the feeding routines. Bottles and nipples for storing breast milk should be sterilized and the expressed milk should be refrigerated immediately. It can be stored for up to forty-eight hours in the fridge or frozen for up to three months. Don't thaw or warm breast milk on the stove or in the microwave, as excessive heat can destroy vital nutrients.

In the early weeks, breastfeeding can be painful. Until your body adjusts to the new demands, your nipples may become cracked and sore and your breasts may become swollen and hard. A warm shower and manual expression of a small amount of excess milk may help to relieve the discomfort of this engorgement. There's also a possibility that you may develop clogged milk ducts, which can lead to a painful infection called mastitis. Most breastfeeding problems can be solved quite easily, although some do require medical attention.

When you decide to stop breastfeeding, or if you choose not to breast-feed at all, your breasts will eventually stop producing milk. Until this happens, though, your breasts may become swollen and painful. A well-fitted bra and ice packs or pain relievers may help to ease your discomfort until your milk dries up completely.

PROS AND CONS OF BOTTLE-FEEDING

If you're considering an alternative to breastfeeding, or would like to combine breast- and bottle-feeding, the Canadian Paediatric Society recommends that you use commercial, iron-fortified formulas until your baby is at least 9 to 12 months old. Whole cow's milk may be introduced at 1 year, but skim milk and partly skimmed milk—1% and 2% milk fat—are not recommended for the first two years. Soy, rice or other vegetarian beverages are incomplete sources of nutrition and are also not recom-mended for the first two years. However, you may use soy-based formulas if your child can't have dairy-based products for reasons of health, culture or religion.

Most women choose bottle-feeding over breastfeeding because it is convenient and allows for more personal freedom. Your partner can easily share in the feeding responsibilities, and you may feel more comfortable feeding your baby in public with a bottle. When bottle-feeding, you should always take care that all bottles and nipples are carefully cleaned and that infant formulas are stored properly.

One of the biggest disadvantages of bottle-feeding is the potential for overfeeding. Because there's a predetermined amount of formula in each bottle, you may be tempted to feed your baby more than he or she needs. To avoid this, you shouldn't encourage your child to finish every bottle. Instead, allow your baby to take only as much formula as he or she needs to satisfy hunger. You can offer your baby water between feedings, but try to limit other fluids, such as fruit juice, so that you don't interfere with your baby's intake of nutrient-rich formula.

Tips for breastfeeding success

A recent national survey indicated that over 40 percent of women stop breastfeeding before the recommended four-month minimum time period. The most common reasons given for stopping are inconvenience or a perceived lack of milk supply. Although breastfeeding usually comes naturally to both mother and child, these tips may help you prevent some of the common problems that often contribute to an early decision to stop breastfeeding:

- **Start early.** Begin within an hour of delivery, if possible, when your baby's sucking instinct is quite strong.
- **Nurse on demand.** Frequent nursing stimulates your breasts to produce a good milk supply. Crying is considered a late indicator of hunger.
- **No supplements.** The more often your baby feeds at your breast, the more milk you'll produce. Breast milk satisfies both hunger and thirst, so extra fluids are usually not needed. Don't offer water or formula supplements that might interfere with your baby's appetite.
- **No artificial nipples.** The sucking action needed for pacifiers is different from the sucking action of breastfeeding. Don't confuse your baby while he or she is learning to feed. Delay giving a nipple substitute for several weeks.
- **Eat well and rest often.** To produce enough milk you need to eat a balanced diet, including at least 500 extra calories and 8 to 12 cups (2 to 3 L) of fluid a day. Rest frequently to prevent infections, which are aggravated by fatigue.
- **Proper position.** To avoid sore nipples, your baby should be encouraged to open wide and to take your nipple far back into his or her mouth.
- **Air-dry nipples.** Until your nipples become accustomed to the sucking action, air-dry them or gently blow them dry with a hair dryer after feedings.
- **Natural healing.** If your nipples dry out and crack, coat them with breast milk or natural moisturizers to help healing. Vitamin E or lanolin may also be used to protect your nipples, although your baby may react to these substances.

- **Watch for infection.** The signs of infection include fever, breast redness and painful lumps. Make sure you get appropriate medical attention.

Nourishing your newborn

At one time or another, most breastfeeding mothers worry whether breast milk is really providing their babies with enough nourishment. It's reassuring to know that infants lose as much as 7 percent of their birth weight during the first week of life. Normally, your baby will start to gain weight within a few days and should regain all of his or her birth weight within ten days. During the first three months of life, your infant will gain approximately 2 pounds (1 kg) per month, or an ounce a day. In the third to sixth month, he or she will gain about 18 to 26 ounces. Ideally, your baby should have doubled his or her birth weight by the age of 4 months.

Healthy newborns should be fed approximately eight to twelve times every twenty-four hours, usually spending 10 to 15 minutes on each breast. In the first few weeks after birth, it's not recommended for your baby to go longer than four hours without a feeding.

One of the easiest ways to determine whether your baby is feeding well is to check the number of wet diapers he or she is producing. A normal newborn wets six to eight diapers a day and has two to three bowel movements. A healthy baby should be content after most feedings, and have a vigorous cry, firm skin and a good sucking reflex. Although all of these signs indicate successful breastfeeding, it's highly recommended that you and your baby visit a doctor within two to four days of birth for a thorough evaluation. Your doctor will check your baby's growth, monitor his or her fluid intake and ensure that his or her digestive system is working properly. Breastfeeding malnutrition or dehydration is a potentially serious condition that can be easily identified through a routine medical examination.

STRATEGIES FOR BREASTFEEDING

The quality and quantity of breast milk that you produce is primarily dependent on your calorie and fluid intake. Even if your diet is not perfect, you should still be able to produce good-quality milk for your baby. Your body adapts to the nutritional demands of your child by drawing on nutrients already in your system. For example, you may actually lose bone mass during breastfeeding because your body acquires calcium by pulling it out of your bones into your bloodstream. Fortunately, this is a temporary condition; once you stop breastfeeding or begin to menstruate, your bone mass gradually returns to normal.

In order to stay healthy while caring for your baby, you should always eat a balanced diet. To replace the calories lost through breastfeeding, it's necessary to add an extra 500 calories to your daily intake. This should include an extra 25 grams of protein. The chart below outlines your extra nutrient requirements for breastfeeding and how to meet these needs from your diet.

Recommended Dietary Allowance (RDA) for Key Nutrients During Breastfeeding (Adults and Teens)

Nutrient	Not breastfeeding	Breastfeeding
Calories	2200 calories/day	2700 calories/day Do not eat less than 1800 calories/day You may need extra calories if you are: • a breastfeeding teenager • a woman breastfeeding more than one infant • a woman who is underweight or did not gain adequate weight during the pregnancy • a woman breastfeeding while pregnant
Protein	46 grams/day	71 grams/day If you're breastfeeding more than one baby, you may need extra protein.
Calcium	1000 milligrams/day	Adults: 1000 milligrams/day Teens: 1300 milligrams/day
Vitamin D	1000 IU (25 mcg)/day	2000 IU (50 mcg)/day
Iron	18 milligrams/day	Adults: 9 milligrams/day Teens: 10 milligrams/day
Zinc	8 milligrams/day	Adults: 12 milligrams/day Teens: 14 milligrams/day
Folate	400 micrograms/day	500 micrograms/day

A FOOD PLAN FOR BREASTFEEDING

Here's how your nutrient requirements translate into food choices. Both breastfeeding women and breastfeeding teens can use this guide.

Food group	Food choices	Recommended daily servings
Grain foods (carbohydrates, iron, fibre; choose whole grain as often as possible)		8 to 12
	Whole-grain bread	1 slice
	Bagel, large	1/4
	Roll, large	1/2
	Pita pocket	1/2
	Tortilla	6 inch (15 cm)
	Cereal, cold	3/4 cup (175 ml)
	Cereal, 100% bran	1/2 cup (125 ml)
	Cereal, hot	1/2 cup (125 ml)
	Crackers, soda	6
	Corn	1/2 cup (125 ml)
	Popcorn, plain	3 cups (750 ml)
	Grains, cooked	1/2 cup (125 ml)
	Pasta, cooked	1/2 cup (125 ml)
	Rice, cooked	1/3 cup (75 ml)
Vegetables & Fruit (carbohydrates, fibre, vitamins, minerals)		7 to 10
	Vegetables, cooked/raw	1/2 cup (125 ml)
	Vegetables, leafy green	1 cup (250 ml)
	Fruit, whole	1 piece
	Fruit, small (plums, apricots)	4
	Fruit, cut up	1 cup (250 ml)
	Berries	1 cup (250 ml)
	Juice, unsweetened	1/2 to 3/4 cup (125 to 175 ml)

Food group	Food choices	Recommended daily servings
Milk & Alternatives (8 grams protein per serving; protein, carbohydrates, calcium, vitamin D, vitamin A, zinc)		3
	Milk	1 cup (250 ml)
	Yogurt	3/4 cup (175 ml)
	Cheese	1-1/2 oz (45 g)
	Soy beverage, fortified	1 cup (250 ml)
Meat & Alternatives (7 grams protein per serving; protein, iron, zinc)		6 to 9
	Fish, lean meat, poultry	1 oz (30 g)
	Egg, whole	1
	Egg, whites only	2
	Legumes (beans, chickpeas, lentils)	1/3 cup (75 ml)
	Soy nuts	2 tbsp (30 ml)
	Tempeh	1/4 cup (60 ml)
	Tofu, firm	1/3 cup (75 ml)
	Texturized vegetable protein (TVP)	1/3 cup (75 ml)
	Veggie dog, small	1
	Veggie burger	1/2
*Fats & Oils** (essential fatty acids, vitamin E)		4 to 6
	Butter, margarine, mayonnaise	1 tsp (5 ml)
	Nuts/seeds	1 tbsp (15 ml)
	Nut butter	1-1/2 tsp (7 ml)
	Salad dressing	2 tsp (10 ml)
	Vegetable oil	1 tsp (5 ml)
	Flaxseed, ground	2 tbsp (30 ml)
Water/Fluid		12
	Water	1 cup (250 ml)

All serving sizes are based on measures after cooking.

*To meet the increased requirements for ALA (an omega-3 fatty acid) during breastfeeding, include canola oil, walnut oil, flaxseed oil and ground flaxseed as your fat servings.

Foods to limit or avoid

Offending foods

Many women can eat anything they like without causing any problems in their infant. But occasionally, a sensitive baby might react to something you've eaten. Your baby experiencing gas and fussiness may be a sign that something in your diet is making its way into your breast milk.

If your baby is fussy two to eight hours after you ate the suspect food, remove it from your diet for at least three days. If this pleases your baby, you've probably found the culprit! Sometimes it's just a matter of eating less of the offending food. Try reintroducing a small amount of the food and monitor your infant's behaviour. Although no two babies are alike, here is a list of foods that could trigger fussiness:

- strongly spiced foods containing chili powder, curry powder, cumin, garlic and onion
- gas-producing vegetables such as cabbage, onion, garlic, broccoli, Brussels sprouts, cauliflower, peppers and turnip
- citrus fruit such as oranges, tangerines, grapefruit, lemons and limes
- chocolate
- milk, soy, eggs, fish, corn, peanuts and nuts

Caffeine

I recommend that you avoid consuming large amounts of caffeine while breastfeeding. Most women can have 1 or 2 cups (250 to 500 ml) of coffee (up to 300 milligrams of caffeine) without affecting their babies. Amounts greater than this can stimulate your baby, causing irritability and wakefulness. Large doses of caffeine may also interfere with the availability of iron from breast milk and impair your infant's iron stores. Take a moment to review all sources of caffeine in your diet—coffee, tea, iced tea, soft drinks, chocolate and some over-the-counter medications. You'll find a comprehensive list of foods and their caffeine content in Chapter 1, page 11. If you suspect that caffeine is bothering your baby, eliminate it from your diet for one week to see if it makes a difference.

Alcohol

You may have heard that drinking a beer helps promote the letdown of milk. The truth? There's not a stitch of scientific evidence to support this notion. Even if beer does increase milk production, research suggests that the presence of alcohol in breast milk can alter its flavour and decrease the amount of breast milk an infant drinks by 23 percent.[28]

Once you consume alcohol, it passes into your breast milk at a concentration similar to that found in your bloodstream. Although a nursing infant is actually exposed to only a fraction of the alcohol a mother drinks, newborns detoxify alcohol much more slowly than adults do. Even a small amount of alcohol, consumed regularly, can affect your baby. Drinking alcohol, even in moderate amounts, can impair a baby's motor development and disrupt his or her sleep patterns. Drinking large amounts of alcohol can impair the flow of breast milk, not to mention the growth and development of your baby.

Occasional drinking while breastfeeding hasn't been linked with overt harm to infants, but the possibility of adverse effects hasn't been ruled out either. Until a safe level of alcohol in breast milk is established, it's safest to feed your baby breast milk that doesn't have any alcohol in it. If you plan to enjoy the occasional drink or two, you'll need to alter your breastfeeding schedule to allow the alcohol to clear from your bloodstream before you nurse. For each alcoholic drink, wait one hour before feeding your baby. So if you consume two drinks, you need to wait two hours after the last drink. If you're out for an evening that entails a few drinks, make sure you store enough breast milk in advance.

OTHER NUTRITIONAL CONSIDERATIONS WHILE BREASTFEEDING
Multivitamin and mineral supplement
A varied, well-balanced healthy diet will meet your daily requirements for most nutrients during breastfeeding. However, there are circumstances when taking a multivitamin and mineral supplement—or continuing to take your prenatal vitamin—is a wise idea:

- You find it difficult to eat regularly during the day or make healthy food choices.
- You're a complete vegetarian (vegan) and you don't use vitamin B12–fortified foods such as soy beverages.
- You're concerned about meeting your iron needs because you eat very little red meat.
- You avoid dairy products and don't choose calcium-fortified products such as soy milk or orange juice.

A good-quality multivitamin and mineral supplement will help you meet your nutrient needs, with the exception of vitamin D, during and after breastfeeding. If you're lacking calcium in your diet, I recommend that you take calcium supplements. For every serving of milk or milk alternative you don't get—aim for three a day—take a 300 milligram calcium citrate supplement. Make an effort to choose nutritious, wholesome foods every day.

Vitamin D supplements

According to the Canadian Paediatric Society (CPS), Canadian mothers and babies, especially those in northern communities, aren't getting enough vitamin D. Vitamin D deficiency—prevalent among pregnant women, exclusively breastfed infants and northern Aboriginal populations—can pose serious dangers to the development of a fetus and infant, yet is easily preventable through supplements. Vitamin D can also help protect babies against certain illnesses in childhood and later life.

The CPS recommends that all babies who are exclusively breastfed receive a supplement of 400 IU per day, and that babies in the North (above 55 degrees latitude) get 800 IU per day during the winter months (from October to April).

Breastfeeding (and pregnant) women should supplement with 2000 IU of vitamin D per day. You'll learn more about vitamin D supplements in Chapter 1, page 13.

Prevention of allergies

If you, your partner or one of your children suffers with allergies, your baby has a higher risk for developing an allergic disease such as eczema, hay fever, asthma or food allergies. To lessen your child's risk for developing an allergic disease (atopy), it's a wise idea to eliminate highly allergenic foods from your diet while you're breastfeeding. In fact, a recent analysis of three studies, involving 210 allergic mothers, found that following an "antigen avoidance" diet during breastfeeding protected their children from atopic eczema for the first twelve to eighteen months.[29]

Common foods that cause an allergic reaction include cow's milk, egg whites, shellfish, fish, wheat, soybeans, peanuts and nuts. An allergic reaction can occur when some of the food protein is absorbed from the intestine intact, instead of being digested into smaller particles as most proteins are. Once the intact protein is in the bloodstream, your body recognizes it as a foreign invader (an antigen). Your body's immune system then produces antibodies to halt the "invasion." As your immune system attempts to fight off the antigen, symptoms appear throughout the body such as swelling of the lips, stomach cramps, vomiting, diarrhea, hives, rashes or eczema, and wheezing or breathing problems.

If stray proteins enter your bloodstream, they can make their way into your breast milk. The earlier and more often an infant ingests a food, the greater the chance it will become an allergen. That's because a baby's immune system isn't functional until 6 months of age, when the digestive system can produce its own immunoglobins to defend against foreign substances. An immature intestinal tract is also more permeable to food allergens, so they enter the bloodstream more readily.

In infants, reactions to food most commonly involve the gastrointestinal system and include spitting up, diarrhea (watery loose stools in a greater number and volume than usual), cramping, constipation, gas and poor weight gain. But often skin reactions such as eczema, hives, rash and itching occur too.

If your baby is at greater risk for developing an allergic disease, you might decide to eliminate potential allergens from your diet while you breastfeed. If you go this route, you must ensure that your nutrient needs are met by including other foods in your diet that provide similar nutrients. I recommend that you consult with a registered dietitian to help you map out a healthy meal plan for breastfeeding. To find a dietitian in your area, visit www.dietitians.ca.

If there's no history of food allergy in your immediate family, there's no need to avoid allergenic foods while you're breastfeeding.

Weaning to solids

Nutritionally, your baby won't need solid foods before the age of 4 to 6 months. By then, your infant will have established the tongue and mouth movements necessary for swallowing solid foods and will be developmentally ready to try new tastes, textures and methods of feeding. A gradual weaning over weeks or months is the easiest way to introduce solid food. You can begin by replacing one breastfeeding a day with unsweetened fruit juice or formula, offering it in a cup or a bottle. By the time your baby is 1 year old, he or she should be eating a variety of foods from Canada's Food Guide.

IRON-FORTIFIED FOODS

You should be aware that infants are quite susceptible to developing iron-deficiency anemia. For the first four to six months of life, your healthy baby is protected against iron deficiency by elevated levels of hemoglobin in red blood cells, which store up to 75 percent of his or her total iron requirements. Those resources are depleted as your baby grows and you'll need to add more iron to his or her diet.

As I mentioned earlier, an iron-fortified infant formula is recommended for bottle-fed babies because cow's milk doesn't supply enough iron for your baby's needs. Unfortunately, breast milk doesn't supply enough iron either—it contains only 0.3 to 0.5 milligram of iron per litre. To prevent an iron deficiency, the Canadian Paediatric Society recommends a single grain, iron-fortified cereal such as rice as your baby's first solid food. This should be introduced at 4 to 6 months of age.

When you decide to introduce solid food to your infant, you should offer only one new food at a time. That way, if your baby has an allergic reaction or digestive difficulties, you'll know which food caused the problem. To prevent food sensitivities, you should avoid giving your baby cow's milk, wheat, shellfish, egg whites and chocolate until he or she is at least 1 year old.

DIETARY FAT

An infant's calorie and nutrient requirements are higher than those for any other age group. If you restrict the fat in your infant's diet, it may lead to an inadequate energy intake, a deficiency of essential fatty acids and failure to thrive. For this reason, dietary fat shouldn't be restricted in children under the age of 2 years.

HONEY

Don't feed your baby honey or foods that contain honey until he or she is at least 1 year of age. This sweetener may contain microbial spores that cause botulism. In infants, but not older children and adults, these spores can germinate in the intestine and produce a toxin that's then absorbed. Symptoms of infant botulism include poor feeding, constipation, loss of tension in the muscles, weakness and difficulty breathing. Spores that cause botulism have also been found in corn syrup; however, no case of infant botulism has ever been linked to corn syrup.

FLUORIDE SUPPLEMENTS

Dental cavities aren't a big issue in Canada, due mainly to the addition of fluoride to our drinking water. However, the increased availability of fluoride not only in drinking water but also in foods prepared with fluoridated water, toothpaste, mouthwashes, multivitamin and mineral supplements and so on seems to be giving rise to a different problem, something called dental fluorosis. This cosmetic condition shows up on the teeth as white specks, brown-grey stains or pitting.

For this reason fluoride supplements aren't recommended from birth as they once were. If you live in an area that has little or no fluoride in the water, a supplemental dose of 250 micrograms is recommended from 6 months to 3 years of age.

HERBAL SUPPLEMENTS AND HERBAL TEAS

As is the case during your pregnancy, you need to use caution with herbs. Very little research has been conducted about the use of herbs during breastfeeding. We do know that some herbs may have side effects such as nausea and vomiting, others have drug-like effects and some can cause reactions in your baby. Here's a list of herbs that are unsafe to use during breastfeeding.

Herbs and Herbal Supplements to Avoid During Breastfeeding

Aloe vera	Cornsilk	Hawthorn
Alder buckthorn	Dong quai	Horseradish (safe as a food)
Burdock	Ephedra	Licorice root
Cascara sagrada	Eucalyptus	Pennyroyal
Chamomile*	Fenugreek	Sassafras
Black cohosh, blue cohosh	Feverfew	Senna
Coltsfoot	Ginseng	St. John's wort
Comfrey	Goldenseal	Yarrow

*Taken as a tea, chamomile probably poses no danger to your baby.

Major brands of herbal teas, those that contain an herb only for essence and those that don't contain large amounts of an unusual herb are generally safe to drink when breastfeeding. Brew your herbal tea weakly and don't consume more than two cups (500 ml) per day.

PART 6

HORMONAL HEALTH

18

Premenstrual syndrome (PMS)

Does your life feel out of control for one week out of every month? Does your mood swing from depression to anger at the drop of a hat? Do you feel emotional, tearful and anxious? Do your insatiable cravings for junk food only aggravate the suddenly too-tight fit of your clothes? If you answered yes to one or more of these questions, then you're only too aware that these are symptoms of premenstrual syndrome (PMS). If you suffer from PMS, you're not alone. Countless women all over the world struggle to cope with symptoms like these each day.

For some women, the physical and emotional changes caused by PMS are so severe that they interfere with the ability to function at work or interact with family and friends. When PMS symptoms seriously undermine quality of life, the condition is called *premenstrual dysphoric disorder* (PMDD)—a complex medical disorder that affects only a small percentage of women. It's thought to be an excessive reaction to the normal hormonal changes associated with the menstrual cycle.

Your monthly cycle

The symptoms of PMS appear during the last two weeks of the menstrual cycle, referred to as the luteal phase of your cycle. There are three distinct phases in each menstrual cycle: the follicular phase, ovulation and the luteal phase. Two areas of the brain, the hypothalamus and the pituitary gland, control all the hormonal changes that regulate each of these distinct stages.

The menstrual cycle begins when the hypothalamus produces gonadotropin-releasing hormones (GnRH). These hormones pass into the pituitary gland and trigger the release of luteinizing hormone (LH) and follicle-stimulating hormone (FSH). Working in combination, these two hormones promote the growth of follicles, tiny sac-like structures located in the ovaries. Each follicle surrounds an ovum, or egg. Between ten to twenty follicles will enlarge, but normally only one egg is released during each menstrual cycle. Throughout this time of growth, the follicles produce most of the female sex hormone estrogen that circulates in your body. This is the follicular phase of your cycle, and it lasts from the first day of your period until you ovulate.

Ovulation occurs in the middle of the menstrual cycle, near day 14, when hormone surges trigger one follicle to burst and release its egg. Over the next thirty-six hours, the egg travels through one of your Fallopian tubes to reach the uterus.

After ovulation, your body enters the luteal phase: The outer wall of the burst follicle remains in the ovary, transforming into a mass of tissue called the corpus luteum. This tissue begins to secrete another female sex hormone, progesterone, which prepares the uterus for pregnancy. If the egg isn't fertilized and pregnancy doesn't occur, the levels of estrogen and progesterone immediately begin to drop. The lining of the uterus and the unfertilized egg are no longer needed and are eliminated from the body through menstruation. This completes the menstrual cycle and the entire process starts all over again.

What causes PMS?

Researchers don't know exactly what triggers PMS. One of the most popular theories suggests that PMS is caused by an imbalance in the levels of estrogen and progesterone. Symptoms may develop because you have too much estrogen and not enough progesterone in your system during the last two weeks of the menstrual cycle. Estrogen affects the kidneys and causes sodium and water retention. Alterations in estrogen and progesterone can also affect the levels of natural brain chemicals called neurotransmitters. It's thought that deficiencies in serotonin and dopamine, two neurotransmitters that affect mood and emotion, may be responsible for the mood swings typical of PMS.

Excessive levels of a hormone called prolactin may be responsible for breast tenderness and swelling. Prolactin is responsible for stimulating the breast changes and milk production necessary for breastfeeding.

Nutrient deficiencies may account for certain symptoms of PMS. For instance, breast tenderness may also be caused by a lack of essential fats in the diet, which play an important role in regulating pain and inflammation. A deficiency of calcium may cause agitation, irritability and depression. In addition, low calcium levels may stimulate an overproduction of parathyroid hormones, which are believed to influence mood and mental function by interacting with the brain chemical serotonin. Dietary deficiencies of vitamin B6, magnesium and zinc or excessive consumption of caffeine, salt, alcohol and red meat may also trigger PMS.

Finally, it's possible that PMS is associated with medical conditions that have a nutritional component, such as hypoglycemia (low blood sugar) or hypothyroidism (low thyroid-hormone level).

Symptoms

PMS is a collection of emotional, psychological and physical symptoms that develop during the seven to fourteen days before the start of your menstrual period. There are more than 150 documented symptoms, with the most common being depression. PMS symptoms tend to fall into two main categories:

1. **Physical symptoms** include breast tenderness and swelling, bloating, fluid retention, weight gain, headaches, food cravings (especially for sweet or salty foods), acne, muscle pain, backaches, fatigue, dizziness, sleep disturbances, constipation or diarrhea. Many of these physical symptoms are caused by fluid retention, especially weight gain. In my private practice, women gain an average of 2 to 4 pounds (1 to 1.8 kg) during the premenstrual week. Heavier women may gain as much as 7 or 8 pounds (3 to 3.5 kg). Fluid retention can also cause abdominal bloating. And if you experience constipation, it only adds to the misery of bloating and weight gain.
2. **Emotional or psychological symptoms** include mood swings, depression, irritability, aggressiveness or hostility, anxiety, crying spells,

changes in sex drive, difficulty concentrating and feelings of low self-esteem.

PMS symptoms vary from woman to woman and they can also be different from one menstrual cycle to the next. In PMS, symptoms get worse as your menstrual cycle progresses and are relieved when your period begins. When you reach menopause, PMS normally disappears, although the symptoms may recur if you take hormone replacement therapy during your post-menopausal years.

Who's at risk?

Most women suffer from some type of premenstrual discomfort. In fact, as many as 80 percent of all women experience one or more of the symptoms associated with PMS. But research indicates that 20 percent to 30 percent of women have moderate to severe PMS that interferes with daily functioning. It's estimated that 2 percent to 6 percent of women have PMDD.[1]

PMS can begin any time after puberty. Research suggests that you're more susceptible if you're under a lot of stress, you're younger than 34 years or you drink alcohol.[2] Although heredity may also play a role, PMS symptoms aren't consistent in families and vary considerably among female relatives.

Diagnosis

It can be difficult to diagnose PMS because the symptoms mimic those of many other disorders. Before your doctor can diagnose PMS, he or she must first eliminate the presence of another medical condition such as clinical depression, hypothyroidism, chronic fatigue syndrome, diabetes or irritable bowel syndrome.

The classic indicator of PMS is the timing of your symptoms. Your doctor will try to determine if your symptoms occur consistently around ovulation and continue until the beginning of your period. For the diagnosis of PMS to be correct, there must be a symptom-free interval between menstruation and the next ovulation near day 14 of your cycle. If your symptoms persist during all phases of your menstrual cycle, then you may be suffering from some other medical disorder. To help your doctor with the diagnosis, you may be asked to keep a menstrual diary, where you record your physical and emotional symptoms every day for several months. Because there are no laboratory tests that identify PMS, this diary is one of the most important tools used to assess your condition. To make the diagnosis of PMS, your doctor will look for a pattern of symptoms that occur regularly and have a negative impact on your ability to manage personal relationships and function normally at home and at work.

Your doctor will also review your medical and psychiatric history and conduct a thorough physical examination, including a pelvic exam. In some cases, laboratory tests may be needed to rule out other medical conditions.

Conventional treatment

Treating PMS can be just as difficult as diagnosing it. That's because the condition affects different women in so many different ways. Most conventional treatment approaches are directed at relieving symptoms and improving the quality of life. Before you embark on a medication to treat a symptom, try implementing the nutritional approaches in the Managing PMS section below for three menstrual cycles. If dietary and/or other lifestyle changes don't improve your PMS within three months, your doctor may suggest medications to reduce your symptoms. Although the following drugs can help alleviate symptoms, keep in mind that some of them have side effects that may cause problems of their own:

1. **Diuretics.** These drugs eliminate excess fluid from your body by increasing urine production; they're often used to treat premenstrual swelling of hands, feet and face.
2. **Analgesics (pain killers).** The most effective of these for headaches, menstrual cramps and pelvic pain are non-steroidal anti-inflammatory medications (NSAIDs) such as ibuprofen (Advil, Motrin) and naproxen (Anaprox).
3. **Antidepressants.** Widely used to treat the depression and mood disorders associated with PMS, these medications increase the level of natural brain chemicals that are affected by the female sex hormones. Selective serotonin reuptake inhibitors (SSRIs) such as fluoxetine

(Prozac) and paroxetine (Paxil) are the most effective in reducing the psychological symptoms of PMS.

4. **Oral contraceptives.** These are often prescribed to women to even out hormonal fluctuations. Although some women benefit from these pills, others experience no change in their symptoms. Some women find that their symptoms are worsened by birth control pills.

5. **Ovarian suppressors.** Drugs such as Danocrine (a synthetic hormone related to the male sex hormone testosterone) are sometimes used to halt the menstrual cycle. Studies show that when menstruation stops, PMS stops too. Although the results of this type of treatment are usually very good, women often don't want to go to such extreme measures to manage their condition. Side effects of ovarian suppressors include the development of menopausal symptoms, such as vaginal dryness and hot flashes.

Managing PMS

Fortunately, there are some fairly simple modifications to your diet and lifestyle that can help you manage and prevent the physical and emotional symptoms of PMS. During the worst phases of PMS, drug therapy may be necessary to improve your quality of life.

DIETARY STRATEGIES
Meal timing
Plan to eat three meals *and* one or two midday snacks. Levels of neurotransmitters in the brain are susceptible to fluctuations in the levels of nutrients in your bloodstream, so any drastic change in normal eating patterns—such as crash dieting, bingeing, or meal or snack skipping—can alter neurotransmitter levels and mood. The hormonal fluctuations of PMS also make you more susceptible to having a low blood-sugar level, which can cause low energy, increased appetite and hunger, irritability and headache.

Carbohydrates
Studies have found that high-carbohydrate meals produce a calming, relaxing effect by influencing the level of serotonin in the brain. Researchers have linked high serotonin levels with happier moods and low levels with mild depression and irritability in women with PMS. One study

found that meals high in carbohydrates improved mood in young women within 30 minutes of consumption.[3] Another study found that when women with PMS drank a high-carbohydrate beverage, their mood improved within 90 minutes.[4]

Carbohydrate-rich foods like whole-grain bread, cereal, rice and pasta contain an amino acid called tryptophan, which normally competes for entry into the brain with other amino acids found in protein-rich foods like chicken, meat or fish. If your mood is affected by PMS, eat high-carbohydrate meals that contain very little protein. This allows tryptophan to get into the brain, where it's used to make the neurotransmitter serotonin. Try pasta with tomato sauce, a toasted whole-grain bagel with jam or a bowl of cereal with low-fat milk.

A liquid dietary supplement called PMS Escape (Enzymatic Therapy), available in the United States, has been clinically proven to reduce mood swings, irritability and carbohydrate cravings and to increase energy levels. It's thought that it reduces PMS symptoms by increasing the concentration of serotonin in the brain. PMS Escape is a flavoured, powdered drink mix made from a blend of carbohydrates, vitamins and minerals.

You might also consider trying sports carbohydrate-replacement drinks. These are sold at health food stores and sporting good stores as powder mixes or ready to drink and come in a variety of flavours.

Carbohydrates: Low glycemic index

There was a time when nutritionists encouraged people to get the majority of their carbohydrates from starchy foods like bread, pasta and rice, rather than simple sugars in desserts, candy and juice. This was because starchy foods have more nutrients than sugar and we thought that they were digested and absorbed in the bloodstream more slowly, leading to more stable blood-sugar or blood-glucose levels and better energy levels. Today, however, we know that all starchy foods are not created equal. For example, the carbohydrates in a white bagel are absorbed into your bloodstream at a faster rate than carbohydrates in a bowl of bran cereal. It turns out that starchy foods vary widely in how quickly they're converted to blood glucose.

Nutritionists now classify carbohydrate foods according to their glycemic index (GI), or how quickly they cause a rise in blood sugar. Foods with a low GI raise your blood sugar more slowly than foods with a high GI. When you eat a food that quickly raises your blood sugar you get a burst of energy. But this spike in sugar also causes your pancreas to release a large amount of insulin into your bloodstream. Since insulin's job is to lower your blood sugar, your quick energy boost is followed by a crash. That can lead to increased hunger and carbohydrate cravings.

Foods with a low GI, on the other hand, take longer to digest and lead to a gradual, slow rise in blood glucose. You don't get the insulin surge, and the energy from low GI food lasts longer. The glycemic index of a food depends on cooking time, fibre content, fat content and ripeness.

To help reduce hunger and food cravings, emphasize low glycemic-index carbohydrates in your meals and snacks. Here are some examples:

Foods with Low Glycemic Index

Bread, Cereals, Grain foods & Potatoes

Sourdough bread

Whole-grain pumpernickel bread

100% bran cereal

All-Bran Buds cereal with Psyllium, Kellogg's

Red River Hot Cereal

Barley

Brown rice

Bulgur

Pasta

New potatoes

Red- or white-skinned potatoes

Sweet potatoes

Legumes

Baked beans

Chickpeas

Kidney beans

Lentils

Soybeans

Fruit

Apple

Apricots, dried
Cherries
Grapes
Orange
Peach
Plum
Dairy products
Milk
Yogurt

Dietary fat

A few studies have found that when women with PMS are put on a low-fat diet, they suffer fewer and less-intense PMS symptoms.[5-7] Diets consisting of 15 percent to 20 percent calories from fat are associated with less water retention, less weight gain and fewer menstrual cramps. A low-fat diet may affect PMS symptoms by influencing the levels of hormones in the body, especially estrogen.

To reduce your intake of dietary fat, in particular saturated fat, choose lower-fat animal foods such as lean meat and poultry breast, and milk and yogurt with 1% or less milk fat. Avoid or limit your intake of processed meats such as bacon, sausage, hot dogs and salami. Use added fats and oils sparingly. Include oily fish such as salmon, trout and sardines in your diet twice per week to increase your intake of omega-3 fat, a type of fat that may help ease feelings of depression.

Use the following chart to help you trim excess animal fat in your diet.

Lower-Fat Food Choices

Dairy products	
Milk	Skim, 1% milk fat (MF)
Cheese	Products with less than 20% MF
Cottage cheese	Products with 1% MF or less
Sour cream	Products with 7% MF or less
Yogurt	Products with less than 1.5% MF

Meat, Poultry & Eggs

Red meat	Flank steak, inside round, sirloin, eye of round, extra-lean ground beef, venison
Pork	Centre-cut pork chops, pork tenderloin, pork leg (inside round, roast), baked ham, deli ham, back bacon
Poultry	Skinless chicken breast, turkey breast, ground turkey
Eggs	Egg whites (2 whites replace 1 whole egg). You'll find egg whites beside the fresh eggs in your grocery store.

Alcohol and caffeine

You read earlier that women who drink alcohol are at greater risk for PMS. Alcoholic beverages can trigger or worsen many PMS symptoms, including fatigue, irritability, depression, bloating, increased appetite and fluid retention. Alcohol has a dehydrating effect on the body, which can leave you feeling sluggish. It can also cause fatigue by interfering with the body's ability to sleep soundly. If you suffer with PMS, avoid alcohol completely during the seven to fourteen days before your menstrual period. During the rest of the month, you should consume no more than seven drinks per week (maximum one a day).

Caffeine can also worsen irritability, anxiety, headaches, diarrhea, fatigue and breast tenderness. As little as two small cups of coffee in the morning can affect your sleep that same night by blocking the brain's production of a natural sleep-inducing chemical called adenosine.

If your PMS symptoms include irritability, anxiousness or general fatigue, consume no more than 200 milligrams of caffeine daily, and preferably none. Switch to low-caffeine beverages like tea or hot chocolate or caffeine-free alternatives such as decaf coffee, herbal tea, cereal coffee, juice, milk or water. The caffeine content of selected beverages and foods is outlined in Chapter 1, page 11.

VITAMINS AND MINERALS

Vitamin B6

In 1999, British researchers analyzed the results from nine clinical trials involving 940 women with PMS.[8] They concluded that B6 supplementation was significantly better than the placebo treatment in relieving PMS symptoms, especially depression. A study from the University of Reading in Great Britain, published after the 1999 review, found that 50 milligrams of B6 combined with 200 milligrams of magnesium had a significant but modest effect on reducing anxiety-related PMS symptoms, including nervous tension, mood swings, irritability and anxiety.[9] More recently, a study of 60 females suffering from PMS found that 100 milligrams of B6 taken daily for three months led to a significant reduction in overall PMS symptoms, including breast tenderness and depression.[10]

The body needs B6 for the production of two brain chemicals that have a potent effect on mood, serotonin and dopamine. Dopamine also regulates the secretion of prolactin, a hormone that may be linked to PMS.

To use B6 for PMS, take 50 to 100 milligrams per day. Daily doses over 100 milligrams don't appear to have additional benefit and may increase the risk of adverse effects. Supplementing with too much B6 for a period of time has toxic effects, including irreversible nerve damage. The safe daily upper limit is 100 milligrams.

Vitamin E

Three randomized clinical trials revealed that vitamin E supplements improved PMS-related depression, anxiety, headache, food cravings and insomnia.[11–13] In one study, women with PMS were given 150 international units (IU), 300 IU or 600 IU of vitamin E. All doses were more effective at relieving symptoms than the placebo pill. How vitamin E works to help ease PMS isn't understood.

The richest sources of vitamin E are vegetable oils, nuts, seeds and wheat germ. Leafy green vegetables (especially kale) are also good sources. But when you consider that 2 tablespoons (30 ml) of grapeseed oil—a cooking oil rich in vitamin E—provides only 11.5 IU, you can see why you must rely on a supplement to increase intake to an effective dose. To supplement, take 200 to 400 IU of vitamin E per day. The daily upper limit is 1500 IU. If you have diabetes or heart disease, don't take high-dose vitamin E supplements.

Calcium and Vitamin D

Research has determined that blood-calcium and blood–vitamin D levels are lower in women with PMS and that calcium supplementation can reduce the severity of PMS symptoms. A well-designed study of 466 women found that those who took 1200 milligrams of supplemental calcium daily for three months had a significant reduction in PMS symptoms, especially mood swings, low back pain, food cravings and fluid retention. The majority of women experienced a 50 percent reduction in overall symptoms (compared with a 36 percent improvement among women who took the placebo pill). The strongest improvement was observed during the third menstrual cycle, which implies that the effect of calcium supplements increases with continued use.[14]

Meeting your daily calcium and vitamin D requirements might also reduce the risk of developing PMS in the first place. In a large study of women aged 27 to 44 who were followed for ten years, compared to those who consumed the least calcium each day (529 milligrams), women with the highest intake from foods (1283 milligrams) were 30 percent less likely to develop PMS. A high vitamin D intake lowered the risk of PMS by 40 percent.[15]

It's thought that increasing estrogen levels that occur during the week before the menstrual period cause a decline in circulating levels of calcium and vitamin D, which triggers PMS symptoms. (Interestingly, the symptoms of PMS and hypocalcemia—low calcium in the blood—are strikingly similar).

CALCIUM. The recommended dietary allowance (RDA) for calcium is 1000 to 1500 milligrams, depending on your age. The best food sources include milk, yogurt, cheese, fortified soy and rice beverages, fortified orange juice, tofu, salmon (with bones), kale, bok choy, broccoli and Swiss chard. If your diet lacks calcium, as is the case for many Canadians, take a calcium supplement to ensure that you're meeting your daily requirement. See Chapter 1, page 14, for more information on calcium requirements, calcium-rich foods and calcium supplements.

VITAMIN D. The recommended daily intake is 1000 international units (IU) for adults. Best food sources are fluid milk, fortified soy and rice beverages, oily fish, egg yolks, butter and margarine. However, it's not possible for adults to consume 1000 IU each day from foods alone. For this reason, it's necessary to take a vitamin D supplement in the fall and winter, and year-round if you are over the age of 50, have dark-coloured skin, don't expose your skin to sunshine in the summer months or go outdoors often, or wear clothing that covers most of your skin. See Chapter 1, page 13, to learn more about vitamin D supplements.

Magnesium

Several studies have reported lower levels of magnesium in women with PMS.[16,17] Research has also determined that increasing your intake of this mineral can improve symptoms of depression, anxiety, fluid retention and breast tenderness. In one study, women who took 250 milligrams of magnesium each day reduced overall PMS symptoms by 35 percent after three months.[18-20]

Magnesium is found in all body cells and fluids, where it's needed to maintain fluid balance by pumping sodium and potassium in and out of cells. It's also used by over three hundred enzymes, including those that produce energy and reduce pain. Vitamin D is needed for magnesium absorption, so it's possible that women deficient in vitamin D will also have low levels of magnesium.

The best sources of magnesium are whole foods, including unrefined grains, nuts, seeds, legumes, dried fruit and green vegetables. Studies have determined a daily dose of 200 to 360 milligrams of supplemental magnesium to be effective in easing PMS symptoms. If you take calcium supplements, buy one with magnesium added. A 2:1 calcium citrate supplement generally gives you 300 milligrams of calcium and 150 milligrams of magnesium. Depending on your diet, you might need to take one of these supplements two or three times a day.

If you don't need supplemental calcium, buy a supplement made from magnesium citrate; the body absorbs this form of the mineral more efficiently. The safe upper limit for magnesium is 350 milligrams per day from a supplement—more than this can cause diarrhea, nausea and stomach cramps.

Sodium

Without a doubt, fluid retention, bloating and weight gain are the most common PMS complaints among my clients. High levels of estrogen associated with PMS can cause the kidneys to retain water and sodium. Eliminating table salt and foods high in sodium the week before your period can help prevent swollen hands and feet. Although this is especially important after ovulation, it's prudent to reduce your sodium intake every day of the month. Most women in Canada consume excessive amounts of sodium—which can increase the risk of high blood pressure and osteoporosis.

To help cut back on sodium, read nutrition labels and choose commercial food products that have lower sodium contents. Eating fewer processed foods and restaurant meals is one of the key strategies to desalting your diet. Most of the salt we consume every day comes from processed and prepared foods—only one-fourth comes from the saltshaker. To further reduce your sodium intake, avoid the saltshaker at the table and minimize the use of salt when you cook. Women need only 1500 milligrams of sodium each day for health. Aim for less than 2300 milligrams of sodium each day (that's 1 teaspoon/5 ml of table salt). Season your foods with herbs, spices, flavoured vinegars and fruit juices. You'll find strategies to reduce your sodium intake in Chapter 1, page 9.

HERBAL REMEDIES
Chasteberry *(Vitex agnus-castus)*
For more than forty years European physicians have been prescribing this herbal remedy to regulate the menstrual cycle and ease PMS symptoms. In some women, taking chasteberry seems to decrease symptoms of PMS, especially breast pain or tenderness (mastalgia), edema, constipation, irritability, depressed mood or mood alterations, anger and headache.[21–25]

Chasteberry also appears to be effective in treating premenstrual dysphoric disorder (PMDD). In an eight-week study, the herb was comparable to the drug fluoxetine at relieving overall symptoms. However, chasteberry seemed somewhat more effective for physical symptoms such as breast tenderness, swelling, cramps and food cravings, while the medication seemed somewhat more effective for psychological symptoms such as depression, irritability, insomnia, nervous tension and feeling out of control.[26]

Choose a product standardized to contain 6 percent agnuside since this is what has been used in most of the clinical trials. The recommended dose varies and will depend on the formulation of chasteberry. Extracts are typically used in doses of 20 to 240 milligrams per day. Keep in mind that it takes at least four weeks for the herb to start working and several months for it to reach its full effect. Mild side effects may include nausea, headache and skin rash.

Evening primrose *(Oenothera biennis)* oil
Supplements of evening primrose oil are a rich source of gamma-linolenic acid (GLA), a fatty acid. The body uses GLA to make special compounds

called prostaglandins that decrease inflammation and pain. Researchers studying women with PMS have focused on a beneficial prostaglandin called PGE1.

GLA is formed in the body from linoleic acid, an essential fatty acid found in vegetable oils, nuts and seeds. Some experts believe that women with PMS have a reduced ability to make PGE1 from linoleic acid in the diet and that this can cause symptoms such as breast pain and tenderness, irritability, depression and headache. Many dietary factors, such as animal fat, alcohol and hydrogenated vegetable oils, can also interfere with the conversion of linoleic acid to GLA. The enzyme responsible for this conversion requires zinc, magnesium and vitamins B6 and C to function properly, so a high-fat diet that's missing important vitamins and minerals can hamper GLA production and contribute to low levels of PGE1.

A number of studies have investigated the effectiveness of evening primrose oil in alleviating PMS symptoms. A handful of studies in the 1980s found that daily supplements of evening primrose oil outperformed the placebo treatment in improving PMS symptoms of breast tenderness, irritability and depression. However, recent studies haven't found evening primrose oil to be an effective treatment for PMS as a whole, possibly because the doses used were too low or the supplement wasn't taken for long enough.

Evening primrose oil does appear to offer promise for treating breast pain and tenderness. Research has shown the supplement to be as effective as certain drugs used to treat cyclic breast pain. Investigators from the University of Wales in Great Britain concluded that evening primrose oil was the best first-line therapy for cyclic breast pain, providing relief with essentially no side effects.[27–29]

Buy a supplement standardized to contain 9 percent GLA. For cyclic breast pain, take 3 to 4 grams per day, split in two equal doses. Start by taking three 500 milligram capsules at breakfast, and repeat at dinner. For PMS, take 2 to 4 grams per day, in divided doses. It can take three menstrual cycles to feel the effects of evening primrose oil and up to eight months for full effectiveness.

Ginkgo biloba

The finding that ginkgo helped women with PMS occurred by accident. Women who were taking ginkgo for brain health noticed that fluid retention associated with their menstrual cycle lessened while they were on the herb. Then, in 1993, researchers from France conducted a formal study of

143 women with PMS.[30] They found ginkgo to be significantly more effective than the placebo in treating PMS-related breast tenderness, abdominal bloating and swollen hands, legs and feet. The women in the study took ginkgo on day 16 of their cycle and continued until day 5 of their next cycle, at which time they stopped. They resumed taking the herbal remedy on day 16.

The recommended dose of ginkgo is 80 milligrams twice daily. Start on day 16 (ovulation) and continue until the fifth day of your next period (day 5). Buy a product standardized to contain 24 percent ginkgo flavone glycosides.

A small number of women have reported that the herb caused mild stomach upset. Ginkgo shouldn't be taken with blood-thinning drugs such as warfarin (Coumadin) or heparin unless your doctor is monitoring you.

St. John's wort *(Hypericum perforatum)*

This yellow-flowered plant has long been heralded for its ability to balance emotions. It's widely used in Europe to treat both mild depression and seasonal affective disorder. A 2008 review of studies conducted in 1200 patients suffering from mild depression concluded that St. John's wort provided a beneficial effect and led to a substantial increase in rates of remission.[31] A small pilot study found that St. John's wort taken daily for two months improved symptoms of PMS by roughly 50 percent in some women.[32] However, because the herbal remedy interacts with so many different medications—including oral contraceptives—this might not be a viable option for some women.

Experts believe the herb eases depression by keeping brain serotonin levels high for a longer period of time, the same way that antidepressant drugs Paxil, Zoloft and Prozac do.

Buy a St. John's wort supplement that's standardized to 0.3 percent hyperforin content, the extract used in most clinical studies of mild and moderate depression. The recommended dose is 300 milligrams taken three times daily.

St. John's wort has been reported to cause sensitivity to sunlight in very light-skinned individuals. The herb also has the potential to interact with a number of medications. If you're currently taking a prescription antidepressant drug, don't take it concurrently with St. John's wort. Be sure to consult your physician before stopping any medication.

OTHER NATURAL HEALTH PRODUCTS
Omega-3 fatty acid supplement

The omega-3 fatty acids DHA (docosahexaenoic acid) and EPA (eicosapen-taenoic acid) in fish oil are essential to healthy brain cell function. EPA, in particular, seems more influential on mood. Studies have found that people who are depressed have lower levels of omega-3 fatty acids in their bloodstream. Omega-3 fatty acids also promote the production of anti-inflammatory compounds in the body, which could possibly help reduce menstrual cramping and pain. A preliminary three-month study conducted in 70 women with PMS found that a daily supplement of krill oil (2 grams) resulted in a significant reduction in both emotional symptoms and the use of painkillers. Although these findings are positive, their validity is limited due to flaws in the study's design.[33] (Krill are very small, shrimp-like crustaceans; they serve as a primary food for whales and sharks. Krill oil supplements have a lower DHA and EPA content than supplements made from fish oil.)

If you want to try krill oil, take 2000 milligrams (2 grams) per day. The brand used in the clinical trial was Neptune Krill Oil (Neptune Technologies & Bioresources Inc.).

To improve PMS-related mood swings, you may also consider taking an omega-3 fatty acid supplement that contains a high amount of EPA.

LIFESTYLE FACTORS
Exercise

Regular exercise is an excellent way to manage your PMS symptoms. Start with a program of regular aerobic exercise for 30 minutes, at least four times each week. Activities such as brisk walking, jogging, stair climbing, biking or swimming offer many other health benefits, in addition to reducing your PMS discomfort.

Reduce stress

There's no question that PMS is closely related to stress. Reducing the stress in your life and promoting more time for relaxation will go a long way towards improving your quality of life and minimizing the effects of PMS. Deep-breathing exercises, biofeedback and progressive muscle relaxation techniques can be very effective in helping you control your response to PMS symptoms.

THE BOTTOM LINE...
Leslie's recommendations for managing premenstrual syndrome (PMS)

1. Eat once every three hours to keep your blood-sugar levels stable. Plan for between-meal snacks.
2. Eat a high-carbohydrate diet. Carbohydrate-rich foods like whole grains, pasta, cereal, rice and fruit trigger the production of serotonin, a brain neurotransmitter associated with relaxed, happier moods.
3. Choose low-glycemic carbohydrate foods that get digested and converted to blood sugar more slowly than other carbohydrate-containing foods to stabilize your energy levels and keep hunger and food cravings at bay.
4. Eat a low-fat diet, as this may help to reduce the level of circulating estrogen.
5. Avoid alcohol for seven to fourteen days before your period since it causes fatigue and may affect your mood.
6. To help reduce irritability, anxiety and general fatigue, aim for no more than 200 milligrams of caffeine per day (and preferably none).
7. If your PMS symptoms include depression, boost your intake of vitamin B6. Take 50 to 100 milligrams of B6 per day. Don't exceed 100 milligrams daily.
8. To help improve mood swings, anxiety, headache, food cravings and insomnia, increase your intake of vitamin E–rich foods. Consider supplementing your diet with 200 to 400 IU of vitamin E each day.
9. To help with mood swings, low back pain, food cravings and fluid retention, get 1200 milligrams of calcium every day from foods and supplements.
10. Supplement your daily diet with 1000 IU of vitamin D. Choose a supplement made from vitamin D3 rather than vitamin D2, since D3 is the more active form in the body.
11. Add magnesium-rich foods to your diet. Getting more magnesium may help improve mood swings, anxiety, fluid retention and headache. To supplement, take 250 milligrams of magnesium citrate once daily. Alternatively, choose a calcium supplement with magnesium added. Don't take more than 350 milligrams per day.

12. To reduce or prevent fluid retention, swelling, bloating and weight gain, reduce your daily sodium intake to no more than 2300 milligrams of sodium each day.

13. Once your diet and nutritional intake is up to speed, try taking chasteberry (*Vitex agnus-castus*) for overall PMS relief. The dosage will depend on the formulation.

14. If you suffer from breast tenderness and breast pain each month, consider trying evening primrose oil. Take 3 to 4 grams daily, in divided doses. For relief from overall PMS symptoms, take 2 to 4 grams per day, in divided doses. Buy a product that's standardized to 9 percent GLA.

15. If fluid retention is your only PMS symptom, try 80 milligrams of ginkgo biloba twice daily. Start on day 16 (ovulation) and continue until the fifth day of your next period (day 5). Buy a product standardized to contain 24 percent ginkgo flavone glycosides.

16. If vitamin B6 has not helped your monthly depression, try St. John's wort. Take 300 milligrams three times daily. Buy a product standardized to contain 0.3 percent hyperforin. This herb may interact with a number of prescription medications.

17. To improve PMS-related mood swings, consider taking an omega-3 fatty acid supplement that contains a high amount of EPA.

19
Perimenopause

If you're a woman in your mid- to late 40s or early 50s, chances are you're experiencing changes in your monthly menstrual cycle, not to mention myriad uncomfortable physical symptoms.

The signs and symptoms associated with menopause occur over a period of time called *perimenopause*, which literally means "around menopause." For many women, the first sign of perimenopause is an erratic menstrual cycle—skipped, lighter or shorter periods. The hallmark of this countdown to menopause is a fluctuating level of the female sex hormones, estrogen and progesterone. Estrogen highs can bring on PMS-like symptoms, including mood swings, fluid retention and headache, whereas estrogen lows promise hot flashes, vaginal dryness and forgetfulness.

You're considered to have reached *menopause* when a year has passed since your last period. Although it can vary, the average age at which a Canadian woman hits menopause is 51. It's at this time that women enter *post-menopause*, the phase of life in which the risk for heart disease, osteoporosis and breast cancer increases. I have devoted a separate chapter to each of the health concerns associated with the post-menopausal years.

Your menstrual cycle

In order to understand what happens to your body during menopause, it helps to know how your hormones normally act during the childbearing years. The menstrual cycle is governed by the interaction of four hormones: luteinizing hormone, follicle-stimulating hormone (FSH), estrogen and progesterone. By definition, the first day of the menstrual cycle—day 1—is the first day bleeding commences. A woman's menstrual cycle lasts 25 to 36 days; most women don't have cycles that last exactly 28 days. The cycle ends just before the next menstrual period.

Bleeding, or menstruation, occurs after estrogen and progesterone levels decrease at the end of the previous cycle. During the early part of your monthly cycle, the ovaries produce estrogen. The brain responds to this increasing estrogen level by telling the pituitary gland to release follicle-stimulating hormone (FSH) and luteinizing hormone (LH). These two hormones, in turn, act on your ovaries. FSH causes egg follicles to develop and release estrogen. When the circulating estrogen rises to a critical level, the pituitary gland releases a surge of LH. This influx of LH causes ovulation by telling the follicle to release a mature egg.

The ruptured egg follicle then turns into a gland called the corpus luteum, which produces progesterone after ovulation. During the last 14 days of the menstrual cycle, progesterone prepares your body for pregnancy by thickening the lining of your uterus. If conception doesn't occur, the corpus luteum becomes smaller, estrogen and progesterone levels fall and the uterine lining sheds, resulting in the next menstrual period.

What causes perimenopause?

For the menstrual cycle to occur regularly, the ovaries must produce enough estrogen and progesterone. As a woman gets older, her supply of eggs and follicles dwindles, resulting in lower levels of estrogen and progesterone. During the years before menopause, declining levels of estrogen and progesterone cause irregular periods—periods may be skipped and they may be lighter. With lower levels of hormones, periods become shorter and eventually cease.

Symptoms

MENSTRUAL IRREGULARITY

As ovulation becomes more erratic, the intervals between periods can become longer or shorter and menstrual flow may become lighter or heavier. Many women also skip periods for a number of months.

VAGINAL CHANGES

The tissues of the vagina and urethra (opening to the bladder) become thinner, less elastic and drier with declining estrogen levels. This can result in decreased lubrication, burning, itching, urinary tract infections and uncomfortable sexual intercourse.

HOT FLASHES AND NIGHT SWEATS

Hot flashes, without a doubt, are the most commonly reported symptom of menopause, occurring in up to 85 percent of North American women.[1,2] It's estimated that for 10 percent to 15 percent of women they're severe enough to interfere with daily life. On average, hot flashes persist for three to five years, but in 50 percent of women, they last up to five years.

A warning signal or aura often precedes a hot flash. A hot flash may begin as a pressure in the head, a headache or a wave of nausea. A sensation of heat then starts in the head and neck and spreads to the torso, arms and entire body. Sweating follows and is most intense in the upper body. Clothing may become soaked, particularly if hot flashes occur during sleep (night sweats is the term for hot flashes that occur during sleep). Chills or shakes may follow as a result of a drop in body temperature. The entire event can last from a few seconds to several minutes, and it may take an hour for chills to subside.

Scientists believe that when estrogen levels drop, your body's temperature control system malfunctions. It senses that you're too hot, even though your body temperature is normal, and attempts to cool you down by increasing your heartbeat and sending more blood to your skin, especially in your head and neck. Blood vessels in your skin then dilate, which causes heat to escape from your body. As a result, your skin flushes and you sweat. Hot flashes are actually your body's way of cooling you down.

INSOMNIA

Night sweats often cause disrupted sleep. Although many women have no difficulty going back to sleep, some simply cannot. Night after night of little sleep leaves you exhausted, and that's when other perimenopausal symptoms can take over your life. Fatigue caused by lack of sleep can lead to irritability, depression and forgetfulness. Many experts believe that there's something else going on to interrupt sleep, something that's not related to hot flashes during sleep.

MOOD SWINGS

Most women describe the mood swings of perimenopause like those of premenstrual syndrome (PMS). They talk about crying at the drop of a hat, or blowing up at a spouse for no good reason. These feelings can be disruptive to both your personal life and work life. Not all women experience mood swings during the transition years. Studies show that if a woman has had a hysterectomy she's more likely to feel depressed. Women who are irritable and cranky during PMS tend to experience those same mood swings during perimenopause.

Mood swings are partly due to a loss of estrogen. Although we don't fully understand what's going on in the body, we do know that natural chemicals in the brain, called neurotransmitters, respond to hormonal fluctuations of the menstrual cycle. Some of these chemicals stimulate nerves that make us more alert. Others interact with nerves to calm us down. The hormonal ups and downs of perimenopause may also make us more sensitive to feelings and emotions. You'll find nutritional strategies that may help you manage mild to moderate depression presented in Chapter 13, Depression.

MEMORY PROBLEMS

During perimenopause there are a few things happening to your body that may cause forgetfulness. For one, there's an aging process going on. The older we get, the more short-term memory we lose. Menopausal symptoms such as insomnia and fatigue can also cause memory problems. Evidence suggests that estrogen affects the brain chemistry and structure that's involved in memory, and that the loss of estrogen associated with menopause may be largely responsible for memory decline.

HEAVY BLEEDING

Most women experience some change to their monthly cycle. The first sign of perimenopause is irregular menstruation. Your periods may stop suddenly or may become lighter and closer together, and then stop. On the other hand, some women experience heavy bleeding during their periods—usually caused by an imbalance of estrogen and progesterone. When ovulation doesn't occur, progesterone isn't produced. This means that estrogen continues to build up the uterine lining, which becomes very thick and releases a lot of blood when it sheds in response to a drop in estrogen levels. As estrogen levels decline with approaching menopause, heavy bleeding becomes less of an issue.

In some cases, heavy bleeding can be the sign of another health disorder: polyps, a fibroid or, less commonly, cancer. Alert your gynecologist if your periods last more than seven days, if you bleed between your periods or if your menstrual flow becomes much heavier than usual.

If heavy flow has plagued you for some time and your energy level is dragging, ask your family doctor to measure your iron level. Your *hemoglobin* level measures circulating iron in red blood cells, and your *ferritin* level measures the amount of iron stored in your liver, spleen and bone marrow. A blood test will determine if you have an iron deficiency and may indicate the need for single iron supplements.

Who's at risk?

Perimenopausal symptoms can affect women ten years before menopause, when hormonal changes kick in. Today in Canada 3.9 million women are between the ages of 40 and 54, the phase of life when levels of certain hormones are changing and dwindling. Although perimenopause can start in a woman's late 30s, most women begin noticing symptoms in their 40s.

Not all women experience the uncomfortable symptoms associated with perimenopause. Although research is lacking in this area, there are a few factors that might increase your risk for suffering one or more of the side effects of midlife hormonal fluctuations. Ask yourself the following questions:

- Are you in your mid- to late 40s?
- Did your mother experience any perimenopausal symptoms?
- Do you suffer from nasty premenstrual symptoms, especially mood swings?
- Have you never delivered a baby? (Some research suggests that never having a baby may increase the risk of early menopause.)
- Do you eat a diet that's high in animal fat and lacking fruit, vegetables and fibre?
- Do you drink too much alcohol and coffee?
- Do you smoke cigarettes?

- Is your life full of stress and tension?
- Do you lack adequate sleep on a regular basis?
- Do you lack regular exercise?

Answering yes to one or two of these questions doesn't mean you're at greater risk of experiencing perimenopausal symtoms. However, a greater number of affirmative answers does increase the likelihood.

Conventional treatment

Perimenopause itself requires no medical treatment. Instead, treatments focus on relieving symptoms and reducing the risk of osteoporosis and heart disease that may occur during the post-menopausal years. Possible treatments include:

- **short-term hormone replacement therapy** (estrogen plus progestin) to reduce hot flashes
- **oral contraceptives** to regulate periods and reduce hot flashes and vaginal dryness
- **progestin therapy** to regulate periods in women who can't take oral contraceptives
- **endometrial ablation** to provide relief from heavy bleeding by destroying the lining of the endometrium using a laser, electrical energy or heat

Managing perimenopause

Maintaining a healthy weight, getting regular exercise and managing stress helps many women ease perimenopausal symptoms. As well, a number of specific nutrition strategies may benefit some women. Although the list of alternative therapies below isn't all encompassing, it highlights a few important strategies. If you're looking for a more comprehensive guide to managing perimenopausal symptoms, pick up a copy of my book *Leslie Beck's Nutrition Guide to Menopause* (Penguin Canada).

DIETARY STRATEGIES
Trigger beverages and foods

Eliminate foods in the diet that can worsen hot flashes, insomnia or mood swings. Caffeine-containing beverages and foods like coffee, tea, colas and dark chocolate trigger hot flashes and can affect the quality of your sleep. Start by avoiding caffeine in the afternoon. Replace these beverages with caffeine-free or decaffeinated beverages like herbal tea, mineral water, fruit and vegetable juice, and decaf coffee. Medications such as Midol, Excedrin and Anacin also provide a fair amount of caffeine. The caffeine content of various beverages and foods can be found in Chapter 1, page 11.

Reduce alcohol intake to no more than one drink a day, and preferably none if you're experiencing hot flashes or you're under stress. Drinking alcoholic beverages can bring on a hot flash, interrupt sleep and affect mood. To lessen its effect, drink alcohol only with a meal. When alcohol is consumed on an empty stomach, 20 percent is absorbed directly across the walls of your stomach, reaching your brain within a minute. When the stomach is full of food, alcohol is less able to reach the stomach wall and pass through, so its effect on the brain is delayed. When you're socializing, have no more than one drink per hour. Since the liver can't metabolize alcohol any faster than this, drinking slowly ensures that your blood-alcohol concentration doesn't rise. To slow your pace, alternate one alcoholic drink with a non-alcoholic drink. One drink is equivalent to 5 ounces (145 ml) of wine, 12 ounces (340 ml) of beer, 10 ounces (300 ml) of wine cooler or 1-1/2 ounces (45 ml) of 80-proof (40 percent) distilled spirits.

If you're experiencing hot flashes, avoid spicy foods. Many women complain that certain spices can trigger a hot flash.

Soy foods and isoflavones

Diets rich in soy may explain why women living in China and Japan have a 20 percent incidence of hot flashes compared with women in Western countries who have an 85 percent incidence.[3] Well-controlled studies have found that soy foods can modestly ease hot flashes.[4-6] A twelve-week Italian study looked at the effects of soy protein and hot flashes in 104 women aged 48 to 61. The study found that, compared with the placebo group, the women who consumed 60 grams of soy protein powder reported a 26 percent reduction in the average number of hot flashes by week 3 and a 33 percent reduction by week 4.

Although soy tends to decrease both the frequency and severity of hot flashes, its effects are generally modest or mild. And all the studies found that participating women who received the placebo also experienced some improvement. It's thought that soy isoflavones might be more effective in women who have a higher number of hot flashes.

Soybeans contain naturally occurring compounds called isoflavones, a type of phyto(plant)estrogen. Genistein and daidzein are the most active soy isoflavones and have been the focus of much research. Isoflavones have a similar structure to the hormone estrogen and, as a result, have a weak estrogenic effect in the body. Even though isoflavones in soy are about fifty times less potent than estrogen, they still offer a source of estrogen. When a woman's estrogen levels are low during perimenopause, a regular intake of foods like roasted soy nuts, soy beverages and tofu can help reduce hot flashes.

Experts believe that a daily intake of 40 to 80 milligrams of phytoestrogens is required to help alleviate hot flashes and reduce other health risks.[7] Soy foods vary in the amount of isoflavones they contain, with even the same type of food made by different manufacturers differing in isoflavone content.

Isoflavone Content of Selected Soy Foods

Soy food	Serving size	Isoflavone content (milligrams)
Roasted soy nuts	1/4 cup (60 ml)	40–60 mg
Soy beverage, So Nice	1 cup (250 ml)	60 mg
Soy beverage, most brands	1 cup (250 ml)	20–25 mg
Soy flour	1/4 cup (60 ml)	28 mg
Soy hot dog	1	15 mg
Soy protein isolate powder	1 oz (30 g)	30 mg
Soybeans, cooked or canned	1/2 cup (125 ml)	14 mg
Tempeh, cooked	3 oz (90 g)	48 mg
Texturized vegetable protein, dry	1/2 cup (125 ml)	30–120 mg
Tofu, firm	3 oz (90 g)	22 mg
Tofu, soft	3 oz (90 g)	28 mg

Source: USDA Database for the Isoflavone Content of Selected Foods, Release 2.0, September 2008. Available at: www.ars.usda.gov/SP2UserFiles/Place/12354500/Data/isoflav/Isoflav_R2.pdf.

Wondering how to use soy foods? To get you started, try some of my suggestions below:

- Use a calcium-fortified soy beverage on cereal or in a breakfast smoothie.
- Add canned soybeans to chili or soup.
- Cube firm tofu and add to homemade or store-bought soups.
- Grill firm tofu on the barbecue: Marinate tofu in balsamic vinegar or brush with hoisin sauce and then make tofu kebabs with vegetables.
- Substitute firm tofu for ricotta cheese in lasagna and cheesecake recipes.
- Use silken tofu in creamy salad dressing, smoothie or dip recipes.
- In recipes for baked goods, replace one-quarter of the all-purpose flour with soy flour.
- Add roasted soy nuts to a green salad or enjoy them on their own as a snack.
- Replace ground meat with soy ground round in chili, pasta sauce and tacos.
- Try veggie burgers (made with soy protein) and veggie dogs on the grill.

Carbohydrates

If you're experiencing sleep problems, try eating a small serving of a carbohydrate-rich food—like milk, cereal or a slice of toast—before bedtime. Such foods provide the brain with an amino acid called trypto-phan, a building block in the manufacture of serotonin, a brain chemical that has been shown to facilitate sleep, improve mood, diminish pain and even reduce appetite.

This recommendation isn't intended to make you gain weight, so eat a small portion or drink a glass of low-fat milk or soy beverage. If your insomnia hasn't improved after one week, look at other factors that may be disrupting sleep.

If you're feeling depressed or irritable, eat high-carbohydrate meals that contain very little protein. Protein foods such as chicken, meat or fish provide the body with many different amino acids that compete with tryptophan for entry into the brain. Try pasta with tomato sauce, a toasted whole-grain bagel with jam or a bowl of cereal with low-fat milk.

If you're suffering from fuzzy thinking, include carbohydrates in your breakfast. Studies in children and adults have shown that, compared with breakfast-skippers, individuals who eat a morning meal score higher on tests of mental performance that same morning.[8-10] The speed of information retrieval (a component of memory) seems to be affected the most by skipping breakfast. Breakfast foods such as whole-grain cereal, fruit, yogurt and whole-grain toast supply brain cells with glucose, their primary energy source. After a night of fasting, a low blood-glucose level needs to be replenished in the morning.

VITAMINS AND MINERALS
Vitamin B12

Many studies have found that vitamin B12 promotes sleep, especially in people with sleep disorders.[11-14] Researchers in Japan have used 1.5 to 3 milligrams of the vitamin each day to restore normal sleep patterns in patients. B12 is thought to restore sleep by working with melatonin, a hormone that's involved in maintaining the body's internal clock. A deficiency of vitamin B12 may cause disturbances in melatonin release.

The recommended dietary intake for vitamin B12 for healthy women is 2.4 micrograms. Vitamin B12 is found in all animal foods: meat, poultry, fish, eggs and dairy products. If you're eating these foods every day, chances are you're meeting your B12 needs. Foods fortified with the vitamin include soy beverages, rice beverages and breakfast cereals (but check labels to be sure).

Strict vegetarians, women who take acid-blocking medication and women over the age of 50 must get B12 from foods fortified with the vitamin or by taking a multivitamin. As we age, we produce less stomach acid, which results in an inability to properly absorb the B12 in foods. Single supplements of vitamin B12 come in 500 or 1000 microgram strengths.

Choline

Although not an official vitamin, choline is a member of the B vitamin family. It's found in egg yolks, organ meats and legumes, and it's used as a building block for a memory neurotransmitter called acetylcholine. Supplements of choline have been shown to enhance memory and reaction time in animals, particularly aging animals. Researchers believe that choline supplements will improve brain tasks only if you're deficient in the nutrient. Stress and aging can deplete choline levels.

It's not known if supplemental choline can improve memory in people who have normal levels of choline, but it's important to meet your daily requirements. Healthy women need 425 milligrams of choline each day. The best food sources are egg yolks, liver and other organ meats, brewer's yeast, wheat germ, soybeans, peanuts and green peas.

Supplemental choline is available as lecithin supplements. The maximum safe limit is 3500 milligrams (3.5 grams) of choline a day. High doses of choline can cause low blood pressure and a fishy body odour in some people.

Iron

If you're experiencing heavy menstrual flow, it's extremely important to eat an iron-rich diet. Iron is used by red blood cells to form hemoglobin, the molecule that transports oxygen from your lungs to your cells. If your diet falls short of iron, or if your body loses iron faster than your diet can replace it, red blood cell levels drop and less oxygen is delivered to your tissues. Symptoms of iron deficiency include weakness, lethargy and fatigue on exertion. Iron deficiency is a progressive condition. Even if your iron stores aren't low enough to diagnose anemia, symptoms of iron deficiency can still be felt.

Women who are menstruating require 18 milligrams of iron per day. Post-menopausal women need 8 milligrams. The best iron sources are lean beef, tofu, legumes, enriched breakfast cereals, whole-grain breads, raisins, dried apricots, prune juice, spinach and peas. Iron in food comes in two forms: heme iron in animal foods and nonheme iron in plant foods. Heme iron is the most efficiently absorbed and is found in red meat, chicken, eggs and fish. Nonheme iron is less efficiently absorbed. See Chapter 3, page 62, for tips on how to enhance iron absorption.

A multivitamin and mineral supplement is recommended for women with higher iron requirements. Most formulas provide 10 milligrams, but you can find some that provide up to 18 milligrams. If you're experiencing persistent heavy bleeding, the recommended daily intake might not be enough to meet your needs. Sometimes 100 milligram tablets of supplemental iron are recommended to replenish depleted iron stores. Single iron supplements should be taken only under the supervision of your dietitian or doctor. Take single iron supplements for three months and then have your blood retested. Once iron stores are replenished, iron supplements should be discontinued. To prevent constipation associated with high doses of iron, increase your fibre and fluid intake. See Chapter 3, Anemia, for more information about iron supplementation.

HERBAL REMEDIES
Black cohosh *(Cimicifuga racemosa)* for hot flashes
Based on clinical experience and findings from controlled scientific studies, black cohosh is the most promising herbal remedy for treating hot flashes. In studies lasting six months to one year, black cohosh extracts seem to modestly reduce symptoms of menopause, such as hot flashes. The most consistent evidence is for a specific commercial extract called Remifemin (Enzymatic Therapy/PhytoPharmica). This extract is standardized to contain 1 milligram triterpene glycosides, calculated as 27-deoxyactein per 20 milligram tablet. Studies have found that it significantly reduces menopausal symptoms and hot flash frequency compared to a placebo. Preliminary evidence suggests that the herbal remedy is comparable to low-dose transdermal estradiol (Estraderm) for relieving menopausal symptoms. Research using other formulations of black cohosh is less consistent.[15-17]

Exactly how the herb works is still under scientific debate. It exerts estrogen-like effects, but its active ingredients don't bind to estrogen receptors or influence estrogen levels in the blood. Experiments in animals have demonstrated that black cohosh doesn't stimulate the growth of estrogen-dependent tumours. Instead, the herb—through the naturally occurring triterpene glycosides compounds it contains—may exert its effect by interacting with certain brain receptors.

Buy a product standardized to contain 2.5 percent triterpene glycosides. The typical dose is 40 milligrams taken twice daily. The type of black cohosh used in virtually all the scientific research is sold under the name Remifemin. This product is sold in 20 milligram strength, since a recent study has shown that the herb is equally effective at this lower dose.

Once you start using black cohosh, it may take up to four weeks to notice an effect. Mild stomach upset and headache may occur.

Valerian *(Valeriana officinalis)* for insomnia
Scientists have learned that valerian promotes sleep by weakly binding to two brain receptors, GABA receptors and benzodiazepine receptors.

Several small studies conducted among patients with sleep disorders have found valerian reduces the time it takes to fall asleep and improves the quality of sleep. In one double-blind study conducted in Germany, 44 percent of patients taking valerian reported perfect sleep and 89 percent reported improved sleep compared with those taking the placebo pill. Another small study found that individuals with mild insomnia who took 450 milligrams of valerian before bedtime experienced a significant decrease in sleep problems. The same researchers studied 128 individuals and found that compared with the placebo, 400 milligrams of valerian produced a significant improvement in sleep quality in people who considered themselves poor sleepers.[18-22]

Unlike commonly prescribed sleeping pills, valerian doesn't lead to dependency or addiction. Nor does it produce a morning drug hangover.

The recommended dose is 400 to 900 milligrams in capsule or tablet form, two hours before bedtime, for up to twenty-eight days. For tinctures (1:5), take 1 to 3 millilitres (15 to 20 drops) in water several times per day, or try 5 millilitres before bedtime. The herb works best when used over a period of time. Don't take valerian with alcohol or sedative medications.

THE BOTTOM LINE....
Leslie's recommendations for managing perimenopause

1. Eliminate beverages and foods from your diet that can trigger or worsen perimenopausal symptoms. Caffeinated beverages, alcoholic beverages and spicy foods are good places to start.
2. Add 1 serving of soy food to your diet each day. Once you've found a few soy foods you like, ensure you're getting 40 to 80 milligrams of isoflavones each day.
3. If you can't fall asleep at night, try a light carbohydrate-rich snack 30 minutes before bedtime to increase the level of serotonin in your brain.
4. Make sure you get enough B12 in your diet to help promote deep sleep. If you can't get enough B12 through food, or if you don't produce enough stomach acid for its absorption, take a B12 supplement of 500 or 1000 micrograms once daily.
5. To help your brain make more of the memory neurotransmitter acetylcholine, increase your intake of foods rich in choline, a fat-like B vitamin. Good sources are eggs, legumes and organ meats. If these

foods aren't on your A-list, consider taking a choline or lecithin supplement.

6. If you experience heavy flow during your periods, increase your intake of iron-rich foods. Make sure your multivitamin and mineral supplement has 10 to 18 milligrams of iron. At menopause, when you're no longer menstruating, switch to a regular formula that supplies 5 to 10 milligrams of iron. If heavy flow has plagued you for some time and your energy level is dragging, ask your family doctor to measure your iron level to determine if you have an iron deficiency. If you're diagnosed with iron-deficiency anemia, take a 100 milligram iron supplement two or three times a day after meals. Once iron supplements are discontinued, return to your multivitamin and mineral supplement.

7. To help ease hot flashes, try a standardized extract of black cohosh. Take 40 milligrams of the herb twice daily, morning and evening.

8. To help treat insomnia, consider taking 400 to 900 milligrams of standardized extract of valerian. Take the herb two hours before going to bed.

20

Polycystic ovary syndrome (PCOS)

Sometimes referred to as Stein-Leventhal syndrome, polycystic ovary syndrome (PCOS) is the most common cause of menstrual problems in women. The disorder affects as many as 10 percent of all premenopausal women, and many don't even know they have it. Furthermore, up to 10 percent of women with PCOS are infertile. PCOS also affects other body systems and is linked with a number of serious long-term health problems, including diabetes and heart disease.

For reasons not yet fully understood, women with PCOS produce unusually high levels of estrogen, luteinizing hormone and male hormones called androgens. This disrupts the normal menstrual cycle and encourages the formation of cysts in the ovaries, making PCOS one of the leading causes of infertility. The hormone imbalances observed in PCOS produce symptoms such as severe acne, excessive hair growth and obesity. There's no cure for PCOS and its treatment varies according to the symptoms.

What causes PCOS?

Hormones control many of your body's internal processes. They're produced and regulated by an interrelated series of glands called the endocrine system. Two tiny glands located in the brain, the hypothalamus and the pituitary gland, monitor and balance the normal activity of the endocrine system. The pituitary gland helps control the cycles of the female reproductive system: It secretes luteinizing hormone (LH), which stimulates the ovaries to release mature eggs and to produce the female sex hormones, estrogen and progesterone. LH is also necessary for the production of androgens, male sex hormones that are present in small quantities in every woman.

PCOS is thought to develop when the pituitary gland malfunctions and secretes an overabundance of LH, triggering an increase in the production of androgens, which results in a corresponding increase in estrogen levels. PCOS causes the production of these three hormones to remain at high levels, disrupting the natural hormonal balance of the menstrual cycle. Excess production of male hormones may interfere with insulin production.

PCOS usually develops during puberty at the time when menstruation would normally begin. The elevated level of LH in the bloodstream interferes with the normal functioning of the ovaries. The excess hormones prevent eggs from maturing properly, which often results in the failure to ovulate, called anovulation. Failure to release an egg prevents or delays the onset of menstruation in young girls and may cause mature women to experience irregular or skipped periods. PCOS can also cause heavy vaginal bleeding that can lead to iron-deficiency anemia.

The hormonal imbalance seen in women with PCOS also causes cysts (fluid-filled sacs) to accumulate in the ovaries. These cysts are eggs that matured but were never released because of abnormal hormone levels. Polycystic (meaning "many cysts") ovaries are covered with a tough, thick outer layer and may grow as much as two to five times larger than normal. These cysts interfere with the activity of the ovaries and contribute to the infertility problems associated with PCOS.

Symptoms and associated medical conditions

The symptoms of PCOS are physically debilitating and often psychologically damaging. Although the syndrome affects each woman a little differently, the primary symptoms include:

- abnormal, irregular or absent periods
- infertility
- mood swings
- weight gain or obesity
- elevated blood glucose—30 to 40 percent of women with PCOS have high blood-sugar levels[1]

- high blood pressure
- high blood cholesterol
- increased hair growth (hirsutism)
- male-pattern baldness
- acne
- oily skin
- heavy, persistent vaginal bleeding
- iron-deficiency anemia

In addition to infertility, women with PCOS face other reproductive concerns. Approximately one-third of all pregnancies in women with the condition end in miscarriage.[2] There's also an increased risk of pregnancy disorders such as pre-eclampsia, gestational diabetes, premature labour and stillbirth. The reproductive problems that plague women suffering from PCOS make it one of the most heartbreaking and frustrating medical disorders.

PCOS disrupts normal physical development by stimulating the production of higher levels of androgens, or male hormones. This causes some women to acquire secondary male characteristics such as frontal balding, deepening of the voice and increased muscle mass. One of the most common symptoms in women with PCOS is hirsutism, a condition that causes body and facial hair to follow a male growth pattern. Women with hirsutism grow excessive amounts of coarse hair on their face, legs, chest and groin. Studies have shown that hirsutism causes high levels of stress and frequent bouts of depression in women.

Obesity is another serious complication that affects nearly 50 percent of all women with PCOS. Obesity contributes to the already high levels of estrogen associated with this disorder. Androgens are converted to estrogen in body fat, and the greater the amount of body fat a woman has, the higher the level of estrogen. Excess estrogen in the bloodstream can trigger severe acne and has been associated with increased risk of endometrial, ovarian and breast cancer.

PCOS is a disorder that progresses fairly slowly, but unfortunately the symptoms tend to worsen over time. Research indicates that women with PCOS have a higher risk of developing insulin resistance, a condition that's further aggravated by obesity. Insulin is a hormone secreted by your pancreas. By attaching to special receptors on your cells, insulin promotes your cells to take in and store glucose and protein, the nutrients your body needs to function and produce energy. Unfortunately, insulin activity can break down as a result of insulin resistance, which is caused by defective insulin receptors that insulin cannot attach to correctly. As a result, insulin is unable to do its job properly and glucose is unable to enter the cells, where it's needed for energy.

Insulin resistance causes a high level of insulin to remain in the bloodstream, causing hyperinsulinemia. These high insulin levels can lead to type 2 diabetes and heart disease. In fact, studies indicate that women with PCOS have at least seven times the risk of heart attack compared to other women. Many women with PCOS and insulin resistance have high blood pressure, low levels of HDL (good) cholesterol and high levels of blood triglycerides, a type of blood fat implicated in the development of heart disease. High blood insulin can also cause weight gain, since the body tries to protect itself by turning excess insulin into fat.

Most women with PCOS have some degree of insulin resistance and many go on to develop full-blown diabetes. It's been estimated that by the age of 40, as many as 40 percent of women with PCOS will have type 2 diabetes or impaired glucose tolerance. It's becoming more evident that insulin resistance plays a very important role in both the cause and symptoms of PCOS. Treatment directed at reducing insulin resistance can restore ovulation, decrease the levels of male hormones, lower triglycerides and elevated blood pressure and promote weight loss.

Who's at risk?

Women can develop PCOS as early as their preteens, or the condition may appear at any time throughout the childbearing years. Most women, however, begin to experience symptoms at menarche, the onset of menstruation. PCOS becomes less common as women get older and rarely develops after menopause. But the health consequences of the disorder, such as type 2 diabetes resulting from insulin resistance, persist into the menopausal years.

Although there isn't enough evidence to prove a genetic link to the disease, many women with PCOS have a mother or a sister with similar symptoms.

Diagnosis

There's no single test for PCOS. A preliminary diagnosis is usually made on the basis of symptoms. Identifying PCOS is often very difficult since the symptoms can vary significantly from woman to woman. To diagnose the condition, your physician will normally begin with a full physical exam and a medical history. He or she will be looking for signs such as menstrual irregularities and the presence of male characteristics such as hirsutism, balding and acne.

Blood tests will be performed to check for excessive levels of androgens, estrogen and luteinizing hormone. An ultrasound may be suggested to look for polycystic ovaries. However, it's important to keep in mind that close to one-quarter of women who don't have PCOS show evidence of cysts in their ovaries. Enlarged ovaries may be a symptom of another medical disorder, so ultrasound results aren't considered true indicators of PCOS. Blood-screening tests for cholesterol, glucose and insulin may also be required to determine the full extent of PCOS-related health risks.

Conventional treatment

Since PCOS has no cure, treatment is usually directed at managing the primary symptoms, especially hirsutism, menstrual irregularities and infertility. The choice of treatment depends on the type and severity of symptoms, a woman's stage of life and her plans regarding pregnancy.

For women not planning to become pregnant, oral contraceptives can control menstrual irregularities. Birth control pills inhibit the production and activity of androgens and therefore help reduce acne, lower the risk of ovarian and endometrial cancer, and slow hair growth for women with hirsutism. Oral contraceptives aren't recommended for menopausal women or for women with risk factors for certain heart or blood diseases.

Antiandrogen drugs (e.g., spironolactone, Diane 35) are also effective in reducing growth of unwanted hair. To further minimize the effects of hirsutism, many women remove excessive hair by shaving, waxing or using depilatories or electrolysis.

For women planning to have children, the treatment of choice is usually the fertility drug clomiphene citrate (Clomid). Clomiphene stimulates the ovaries to release eggs. Studies indicate that 80 percent of women with PCOS ovulate in response to clomiphene, but only 50 percent of these women become pregnant.[3] If clomiphene doesn't work well for you, your physician may try to induce ovulation with a variety of hormone supplements, including follicle-stimulating hormone (FSH) and gonadotropin-releasing hormone (GnRH) drugs such as leuprolide (Lupron) and nafarelin (Synarel).

To lower health risks such as type 2 diabetes and heart disease, your doctor may prescribe an insulin-sensitizing drug—such as metformin (Glucophage)—to decrease insulin resistance and delay or prevent the development of type 2 diabetes. These medications also reduce androgen production and restore normal menstrual cycles.

Although medications such as the ones discussed above do have proven benefits, don't overlook one of the simplest and most effective methods of treating PCOS: weight loss. Losing excess weight reduces your insulin resistance, lowers the secretion of androgens and lowers your estrogen levels. This may help eliminate excessive hair growth, restore regular menstrual periods and improve your chances of becoming pregnant, as well as enhance your overall health and well-being.

At present, PCOS is treated on a symptom-by-symptom basis with medication, dietary changes and exercise. Researchers continue to investigate both the causes of this syndrome and improved treatment options. If you have PCOS, the changes I list below may help you manage your condition so that you can lead a healthier and more satisfying life.

Managing PCOS

DIETARY STRATEGIES
Weight control

Obesity and overweight, especially abdominal obesity, is present in over half of women with PCOS and has a marked impact on the progression of the syndrome. Excess abdominal fat worsens the symptoms of PCOS by increasing insulin resistance and further elevating levels of male hormones. As a result, weight loss is central to the treatment strategies for PCOS. Research has demonstrated that losing weight if you're obese enhances the body's sensitivity to insulin, normalizes hormone levels and restores menstrual regularity.[4-10] Studies have shown that losing more than

5 percent of body weight can restore fertility in obese women with PCOS.[11,12]

To determine if you're at a healthy weight, see Chapter 2, page 37, to calculate your body mass index (BMI) and waist circumference. Having a BMI of between 25 and 29.9 indicates overweight and a BMI of 30 or greater is defined as obese. Having a waist circumference greater than 31.5 inches (80 cm) is associated with health risks. Use the strategies outlined in Chapter 2 to promote safe, gradual weight loss. In addition, pay special attention to the following:

1. **Reduce your portions of carbohydrate-containing foods.** Lower-carbohydrate diets are recommended with PCOS. Eating smaller portions of carbohydrates not only reduces your calorie intake but also helps to reduce high levels of blood insulin. That's because, once digested into glucose units, carbohydrate foods trigger the release of insulin in the bloodstream. But don't give up all carbohydrate-containing foods. I don't recommend high-protein diets that eliminate all starchy foods, fruit and milk products. Over the long run this isn't healthy, nor is it sustainable.

2. **Get rid of excess sugar—natural and refined.** Too much sugar in the diet contributes to high blood-triglyceride levels, something that shows up on blood tests of a number of women with PCOS.

Carbohydrates: Low glycemic index

Unfortunately, insulin resistance makes weight loss more difficult to achieve. To help improve insulin resistance and lower blood-insulin levels, it's important to eat smaller portions of carbohydrate-rich foods and to choose the right types of carbohydrate foods. When you eat a carbohydrate-rich food, whether it's bread, pasta, yogurt, an apple or fruit juice, the carbohydrate is broken down into glucose and absorbed into your bloodstream. Blood sugar (glucose) rises, signalling the pancreas to release insulin into the bloodstream. Insulin then clears sugar from your blood, taking it into your cells, where it's used for energy. If you have insulin resistance, insulin can't perform this task properly and some sugar remains in the blood, causing more insulin to be released. This results in a chronically high insulin level that, over time, increases the risk of type 2 diabetes and heart disease.

Carbohydrate foods are digested and absorbed at different rates. Some foods are digested slowly and result in a steady, slow rise in blood sugar, which means that less insulin is secreted into the blood. Slow carbohydrates have what's called a low glycemic-index (GI) value. Foods with a high glycemic-index value are digested and absorbed more quickly, causing much higher insulin levels.

To prevent an excessive surge of insulin after eating, meals and snacks should emphasize foods with a low GI value. Foods such as whole-grain pumpernickel bread, steel-cut oatmeal, 100% bran cereal, legumes, yogurt and soy milk all have a low GI value. For a list of selected foods ranked by their glycemic-index value, see Chapter 5, Hypoglycemia, page 85. Use the chart below to help you replace higher-glycemic carbohydrates with lower-glycemic ones.

High-glycemic food	Low-glycemic food
Bread, white or whole wheat	Whole-grain pumpernickel, whole-grain rye, sourdough
Most processed breakfast cereals (Corn Flakes, Puffed Rice, Special K)	100% bran (All-Bran Original, All-Bran Buds), Mueslix, oatmeal
Instant rice	Basmati rice, brown rice, wild rice
Mashed potato	Beans or pasta
Bananas	Apples, nectarines, oranges, peaches
Snack foods: chips, cookies, crackers	Dried apricots, fruit (as above), latte, low-fat smoothie, milk, popcorn, yogurt

Studies have also demonstrated that a calorie-reduced diet that's moderate, not high, in carbohydrates is effective in promoting weight loss in women with PCOS. Studies have assigned participants to weight-loss diets with 40 percent of calories derived from low GI carbohydrates.[13-15] A registered dietitian (visit www.dietitians.ca) can help design a lower-carbohydrate weight-loss plan for you.

VITAMINS AND MINERALS
Calcium and Vitamin D

Gonadotropin-releasing hormone (GnRH) drugs such as leuprolide (Lupron) and nafarelin (Synarel) improve PCOS symptoms by causing a deficiency of estrogen, a hormone that also prevents bones from losing calcium. As a result, GnRH drugs cause accelerated bone loss, which may be partially irreversible.

A six-month Italian study of 44 women with PCOS showed that those women receiving a GnRH medication experienced a significant decrease in bone density.[16] Women given the drug in combination with the antiandrogen drug spironolactone didn't show any change in bone density. Spironolactone offers a bone-sparing effect in this situation. Your doctor may prescribe another medication along with a GnRH drug to offset the bone loss. The jury is still out on whether some of these drug combinations (called add-back regimens) actually prevent bone loss.

To help minimize bone loss if you're taking a GnRH drug, it's very important to meet your recommended daily intakes for calcium and vitamin D, two nutrients critical for bone health.

CALCIUM. The recommended dietary allowance (RDA) is 1000 to 1300 milligrams, depending on your age. The best food sources are milk, yogurt, cheese, fortified soy and rice beverages, fortified orange juice, tofu, salmon (with bones), kale, bok choy, broccoli and Swiss chard. If your diet falls short of calcium, make up the difference by taking a calcium supplement once or twice daily. See Chapter 1, page 16, for more information about calcium supplements.

VITAMIN D. The recommended daily intake is 1000 international units (IU) for adults and 400 IU for children and teenagers. Best food sources are fluid milk, fortified soy and rice beverages, oily fish, egg yolks, butter and margarine. However, it's not possible for adults to consume 1000 IU each day from foods alone. For this reason, it's necessary to take a vitamin D supplement in the fall and winter, and year-round if you are over the age of 50, have dark-coloured skin, don't expose your skin to sunshine in the summer months or go outdoors often, or wear clothing that covers most of your skin. See Chapter 1, page 13, to learn about vitamin D supplements.

Chromium

The body uses this mineral to make glucose tolerance factor (GTF), a compound thought to help maintain normal blood-sugar levels by increasing insulin receptor sensitivity. A deficiency of chromium causes impaired glucose tolerance, increased cholesterol and triglyceride levels, and decreased HDL (good) cholesterol levels. Research suggests that when taken as a supplement, chromium can help reduce high blood cholesterol and triglycerides and stabilize blood-sugar levels. A handful of studies have demonstrated that chromium supplementation reduces blood glucose and improves glucose tolerance in women with PCOS. However, taking chromium didn't improve hormone levels or the frequency of ovulation.[17,18]

The recommended dietary intake for women is 25 micrograms of chromium per day. Good food sources include apples with the skin, green peas, chicken breast, refried beans, mushrooms, oysters, wheat germ and brewer's yeast. Processed foods, refined foods with a high glycemic-index value such as white bread, white rice, white potatoes, refined breakfast cereals and cereal bars, sugar and sweets contain very little chromium.

If you're concerned that you're not getting enough chromium in your diet, check your multivitamin and mineral supplement to see how much it contains. Most brands supply 25 to 50 micrograms. If you choose to take a separate chromium supplement, take 200 micrograms per day. Supplements made from chromium picolinate and chromium nicotinate are thought to be absorbed more efficiently than those made from chromium chloride. Don't exceed 400 micrograms per day.

OTHER NATURAL HEALTH PRODUCTS
Inositol

Although not an official vitamin, this natural compound is closely related to the B vitamin family. Inositol is found in foods mainly as phytic acid, a fibrous compound. Good sources include citrus fruit, whole grains, legumes, nuts and seeds. When you eat these foods, intestinal bacteria liberate inositol from phytic acid.

Once in the body, inositol is an essential component of cell membranes. It promotes the export of fat from cells in the liver and intestine. Supplements of inositol are thought to improve insulin sensitivity and have been used to treat symptoms of PCOS. In one study of 44 obese women, 1200 milligrams of inositol taken once daily for six to eight weeks decreased blood triglycerides and testosterone levels, reduced blood pressure and caused ovulation.[19] Previous studies suggest that people with insulin resistance and type 2 diabetes might be deficient in inositol.

The recommended dose for PCOS is 1200 milligrams per day. When choosing a supplement, look for D-chiro-inositol. No adverse effects of inositol have been reported. Inositol supplements may be difficult to find, since few companies manufacture them.

THE BOTTOM LINE...
Leslie's recommendations for managing polycystic ovary syndrome (PCOS)

1. If you're overweight, embark on a weight-loss program. Losing weight is a cornerstone in the management of PCOS. Enlist the help of a professional. Contact the Dietitians of Canada (www.dietitians.ca) for a referral to a nutritionist in your community.
   * To get you started losing weight, practice my tips in Chapter 2.
   * Follow a diet that's lower in carbohydrates, but don't eliminate all carbohydrate foods. This will help women with insulin resistance lose weight more effectively.
2. Choose low glycemic-index carbohydrate foods.
3. Increase your intake of calcium and vitamin D, especially if you're taking a gonadotropin-releasing hormone drug such as Lupron or Synarel. These medications promote an estrogen deficiency that can cause bone loss.
4. Increase your intake of foods rich in chromium, a mineral that helps insulin work properly. Consider taking a 200 microgram chromium supplement if you have insulin resistance.
5. Consider supplementing your daily diet with 1200 milligrams of inositol, a relative of the B vitamins.

21
Thyroid Disease

Disorders of the thyroid gland are more common among Canadians than diabetes or heart disease. Your tiny, butterfly-shaped thyroid gland is located in front of your windpipe. Although it weighs only an ounce, this gland is the command centre for many organs in your body, including your heart, brain and liver, as it regulates metabolism and cell growth. The symptoms of thyroid disorders are often difficult to read, for both the woman affected and her physician. In fact, many women don't even know they have a thyroid problem. If left untreated, thyroid disease can cause serious health problems.

Thyroid disease affects the production of thyroid hormones. Hypothyroidism results from an underactive gland that produces insufficient thyroid hormones. In hyperthyroidism, the opposite is true. As you'll read below, each disorder has unique causes, symptoms and treatments.

Graves' disease
(Graves' hyperthyroidism)

Graves' disease is an autoimmune condition caused by an overactive thyroid gland. It occurs approximately five times more often in women than in men and is considered to be the most common cause of hyperthyroidism. Women who suffer from Graves' disease experience symptoms such as rapid weight loss, increased pulse rate, sweating, nervousness, insomnia and a thickening of the skin on the shins. In 50 percent of all cases, Graves' disease causes the eyes to protrude, due to swelling and inflammation of the tissues around the eyes. Fortunately, Graves' disease can be controlled fairly easily. It's treated with anti-thyroid drugs, radioactive iodine or surgical removal of the thyroid gland.

WHAT CAUSES GRAVES' DISEASE?

Your thyroid gland produces a steady supply of two major thyroid hormones, T4 (thyroxine) and T3 (triiodothyronine). When you're healthy, the pituitary gland located in your brain releases thyroid-stimulating hormone (TSH), which then triggers the release of T3 and T4. These thyroid hormones travel in your bloodstream to various organs in your body and control your body temperature, influence your heart rate and determine the speed of all your internal chemical processes. In a nutshell, thyroid hormones act to control your body's metabolic rate, the speed at which you burn calories. When T3 and T4 are at normal levels, the amount of TSH in your blood levels off.

When your thyroid gland becomes overactive, it secretes too many thyroid hormones, causing your cells to work harder and your metabolism to speed up by 60 percent to 100 percent. This condition is known as hyperthyroidism and is characterized by a high metabolic rate. Hyperthyroidism causes a range of symptoms, including pounding heartbeats, profuse sweating, increased blood pressure, fatigue, weakness and general feelings of anxiousness, irritability and nervousness. When your levels of T3 and T4 are too high, TSH is suppressed. Measuring the level of TSH in your blood allows your doctor to check your thyroid function and thyroid hormone levels.

Several factors may trigger hyperthyroidism, but Graves' disease—in North America at least—causes 90 percent of all cases. This disorder is named after the Irish physician Robert Graves who first described it in 1835. The condition is also referred to as diffuse toxic goiter, thyrotoxicosis or Basedow's disease.

Graves' disease is an autoimmune condition. Under normal circumstances, the immune system produces antibodies that protect the body from foreign invaders, such as bacteria and viruses. In Graves' disease, the immune system malfunctions and produces a protein called thyroid-stimulating antibody that causes the thyroid gland to overproduce thyroid hormones.

At this point, little is known about the exact causes of Graves' disease. Scientists have determined that it tends to run in families, but they don't understand the circumstances that trigger the condition in certain individuals. It's thought that severe emotional stress may be a factor. Stress can increase the blood levels of cortisone and adrenaline, two hormones that help prepare the body for a stressful event. Cortisone and adrenaline may affect the production of antibodies in the immune system. Yet many women with Graves' disease have very little stress in their lives, which suggests that there must be other factors at work. It's possible that environmental conditions may cause immune system malfunctions, triggering the problems of an overactive thyroid.

Graves' disease has a strong association with eye disease. The antibodies that stimulate the overproduction of thyroid hormones also react with the proteins in the eye muscle, as well as the connective tissue and fat around the eyeball. This causes swelling and inflammation of the tissues, resulting in protruding eyes. Again, very little is known about the connection between Graves' hyperthyroidism and eye disease.

Thyroid hormones also have an effect on the reproductive system. Women with Graves' disease may find that their menstrual periods decrease, and younger girls may experience a delay in the onset of menstruation. For many women, an overactive thyroid gland is connected with infertility. Fortunately, once the condition has been treated successfully, fertility is usually quickly restored.

If left untreated, Graves' disease increases the risk of miscarriage or birth defects and may, in rare cases, lead to death. However, if properly diagnosed, the condition can be safely and effectively controlled.

SYMPTOMS

Women with Graves' hyperthyroidism experience many of the following symptoms:

- nervousness and irritability
- fast heartbeat
- sleeplessness
- heat intolerance
- high blood pressure
- increased perspiration
- shakiness and tremors
- muscle weakness, especially in upper arms and thighs
- confusion
- increased appetite
- weight loss

- frequent bowel movements
- eye changes, including puffiness and a constant stare
- sensitivity to light, increased tear formation
- fine, brittle hair and thinning skin
- lighter or less frequent menstrual periods

In addition to the symptoms of hyperthyroidism listed above, Graves' disease is characterized by three other distinctive symptoms:

1. The thyroid gland may become quite enlarged, causing a bulge in the neck. This is called a goiter and develops because the immune antibodies overstimulate the entire gland.
2. Sometimes people with Graves' disease develop a lumpy, reddish thickening of the skin in front of the shins, known as pretibial myxedema. If you develop this symptom, you'll find that the thickened skin may be itchy and red and may feel quite hard.
3. Fifty percent of people with Graves' disease have eyes that protrude out of their sockets, due to a buildup of deposits and fluid in the orbit of the eye. As a result, the muscles that move the eye aren't able to function properly, causing double or blurred vision. Eyelids may not close properly because they're swollen with fluid, exposing the eye to injury from foreign particles. Eyes will hurt and will be red and watery.

WHO'S AT RISK?

About 75 percent of all autoimmune diseases occur in women, hitting them most often between the ages of 30 and 40.[1] In North America, hyperthyroidism (from all causes) affects more women than men. In Canada, Graves' disease affects approximately one in every one hundred people, and it looks like it's becoming more common.[2] You may be at risk of developing Graves' disease if you:

- are a woman between the ages of 20 and 40
- are a woman who has given birth within the last six months
- have experienced thyroid disease before
- have been overtreated for hypothyroidism
- have other autoimmune conditions (e.g., Hashimoto's thyroiditis, diabetes mellitus, rheumatoid arthritis, lupus, pernicious anemia or vitiligo)

Diseases of the immune system tend to run in families. Graves' disease has been identified as an inherited condition, although not every member of an afflicted family will develop the disorder. Cigarette smoking and stress may also increase the risk for Graves' disease.[3]

DIAGNOSIS

Usually, your doctor will be able to make an initial diagnosis of hyperthyroidism based on a history and investigation of your symptoms. The appearance of a goiter and protruding eyes are strong indicators of Graves' disease.

To confirm the diagnosis, your physician may suggest a simple blood test to measure the level of thyroid hormone in your bloodstream. If the laboratory results are unclear, a test to measure your blood levels of thyroid-stimulating hormone (TSH) may be necessary. The TSH test is a very sensitive diagnostic tool and is often used to identify cases of hyperthyroidism, even before symptoms appear. Once hyperthyroidism has been diagnosed, your doctor may also send you for a CAT scan, an ultrasound or an MRI. These tests are used to obtain a clear picture of your thyroid gland, which will help determine the exact cause of your overactive thyroid problems.

CONVENTIONAL TREATMENT

The treatment for hyperthyroidism varies according to the needs and symptoms of each woman. In developing a treatment plan, your physician considers your age, the severity of your illness, the symptoms you're experiencing and other medical conditions that you may have.

There are three main approaches to treating the problems associated with hyperthyroidism and Graves' disease:

1. **Medication.** Antithyroid drugs such as Tapazole (methimazole) and Propyl-Thyracil (propylthiouracil) are most commonly used to treat hyperthyroidism. They slow down the activity of the thyroid gland by suppressing the release of thyroid hormones. The doses of these medications are adjusted according to the level of thyroid hormone in your blood. Antithyroid drugs are usually prescribed in mild cases of hyperthyroidism and for children, young adults or the elderly with the disease.
2. **Radioactive iodine.** Since antithyroid drugs don't cure hyperthyroidism, you may be treated with radioactive iodine to achieve a

long-term solution. A small dose of radioactive iodine is taken by mouth and travels from your stomach to your thyroid gland, where it destroys some of the cells. Treatment is usually designed to destroy only enough thyroid cells to bring thyroid hormone production back to a normal level. Treatment with radioactive iodine usually causes your thyroid gland to slow down to the point where it underproduces thyroid hormones, creating a condition known as hypothyroidism. This is easily treated by taking a daily thyroid hormone pill called Synthroid (levothyroxine) to restore normal blood levels.

3. **Surgery.** Hyperthyroidism can be permanently cured by surgically removing the thyroid gland in a procedure called a thyroidectomy. This may be considered if you have a large goiter, if you have a negative reaction to antithyroid medication or if you're in a younger age group. Once the thyroid gland is removed, the cause of hyperthyroidism is eliminated. However, you'll probably become hypothyroid and thus require thyroid replacement medication for the rest of your life.

In addition to one or more of these treatments, your doctor will usually prescribe beta-blocking drugs such as Inderal (propranolol), Tenormin (atenolol) and Lopressor (metoprolol). Beta-blockers don't control abnormal thyroid function but are useful in managing symptoms such as increased heart rate, elevated blood pressure and nervousness until other forms of treatment can be started. These drugs block the action of the thyroid hormone circulating in your bloodstream, slowing your heart rate and reducing feelings of nervousness and irritability. They're not suitable for people who have asthma or heart failure, as they may cause these conditions to worsen.

Eye symptoms

Any eye changes you experience because of Graves' disease usually improve once the hyperthyroidism is under control. In some cases, however, the condition progresses despite all thyroid gland treatments. In these situations, strong drugs such as oral steroids (prednisone) or immunosuppressants (cyclosporin) may be used to minimize swelling and reduce pressure on the optic nerve.

Your specialist may consider radioactive treatments and surgery to remove some bone from the eye orbit to reduce swelling and prevent nerve damage. Simple ways to help you cope with your eye changes include using eye drops and eye lubricants, sleeping with the head of your bed elevated and wearing eyeglasses with prisms to improve double vision. If you're a cigarette smoker, bear in mind that smoking makes eye symptoms worse and reduces your response to treatment.

Fertility

Women who have been treated for Graves' hyperthyroid usually have no difficulty becoming pregnant, since normal fertility is restored once the condition is under control. If you've been given radioactive iodine, you should wait six months after treatment before becoming pregnant.

If you're pregnant and require treatment for Graves' disease, you should be aware that radioactive iodine treatment isn't recommended during pregnancy and surgery, and should be avoided for fear of causing a miscarriage. Because pregnancy has a suppressive effect on the immune system, you can consider treatment with a low-dose antithyroid drug. However, be careful to avoid higher doses, as these medications can cross the placenta and affect your baby's thyroid gland. Radioactive treatments should also be avoided while breastfeeding, but antithyroid drugs in lower doses appear to be safe for both nursing mothers and babies.

Hypothyroidism

Hypothyroidism develops when your thyroid gland doesn't produce enough thyroid hormones to meet your body's needs. An underactive thyroid gland causes your metabolic rate to slow down, making you feel slow, sluggish and constantly tired. Thyroid deficiencies have also been known to cause infertility or miscarriages in early pregnancy.

Hypothyroidism affects ten times more women than men. It usually strikes after age 40 and is common in elderly women. Hypothyroidism usually develops when your body's immune system malfunctions, causing damage to the thyroid gland. It can also occur after treatment for hyperthyroidism, or an overactive thyroid. In most cases, hypothyroidism is a permanent condition that requires lifelong treatment with thyroid hormone drugs.

WHAT CAUSES HYPOTHYROIDISM?

The thyroid gland is a small organ with a big job. Located in your neck, just below your Adam's apple, the thyroid controls and coordinates your main body functions, or metabolism. It produces two thyroid hormones, thyroxine (T4) and triiodothyronine (T3), which circulate through your bloodstream and act on almost every organ in your body. These hormones maintain a healthy metabolic rate by controlling the speed at which your body burns calories to use energy.

A well-functioning thyroid gland is essential to normal growth and development. If your thyroid doesn't produce enough thyroid hormones, all your bodily functions slow down. You begin to feel sluggish and tired and may develop a variety of other uncomfortable symptoms. As the condition becomes more advanced, you could experience serious health problems.

The most common type of hypothyroidism is known as Hashimoto's thyroiditis or chronic thyroiditis. It's an autoimmune disease caused by a malfunction of your immune system. In this case, the immune system begins to produce antithyroid antibodies that attack your thyroid gland. The damage caused by these antibodies prevents the thyroid from producing adequate levels of thyroid hormones. People with Hashimoto's thyroiditis often develop a painless thyroid lump or goiter that can be seen at the lower front of their throat.

Hypothyroidism can also be caused by:

- surgery to remove the thyroid gland (usually a treatment for thyroid cancer, and in some cases for overactive thyroid)
- radioactive iodine therapy (usually used to treat overactive thyroid conditions)
- X-rays, especially of the head and neck
- treatment with certain medications, such as lithium
- obesity
- pregnancy and postpartum conditions
- iodine deficiencies
- absence of a thyroid gland at birth (all babies in Canada are screened for hypothyroidism to detect this condition)
- genetic predisposition

Another version of the disorder, known as secondary hypothyroidism, may develop if you have an abnormality in an area of your brain called the hypothalamic-pituitary axis. The pituitary gland helps the thyroid gland regulate the production of T3 and T4 by releasing thyroid-stimulating hormone (TSH). The hypothalamus gland performs a similar function by producing thyrotropin-releasing hormone (TRH). If these two glands don't secrete enough hormones to trigger your thyroid gland to function, you may experience the hormonal deficiencies that lead to hypothyroidism.

SYMPTOMS

The symptoms of hypothyroidism vary in severity, depending on the decrease in thyroid hormone levels and the length of time that a deficiency has been present. Most of the time, the symptoms are fairly mild. In the early stages of the disorder, symptoms may not be noticeable at all and you may still feel quite well. However, research indicates that people with mild hypothyroidism go on to develop more severe thyroid problems in later years.

When you have more severe hypothyroidism, you may begin to feel slow, sluggish, tired and run down. You may also feel depressed and lose interest in your normal activities. Additional hypothyroid symptoms include:

- increased sensitivity to cold
- muscle swelling or cramps, especially in your arms and legs
- weight gain
- dry, itchy skin
- constipation
- increased menstrual flow
- tingling or numbness in your hands and feet
- coarseness or loss of hair
- memory loss and mental impairment
- infertility or miscarriages
- a slow heart rate
- dull facial expression, droopy eyelids and hoarse voice
- high blood pressure

Naturally, you won't develop all of these symptoms, but you can certainly expect to experience some of them. Because hypothyroidism progresses gradually, worsening over a period of months or years, you may not even realize how unwell you feel until your thyroid condition is corrected with hormone medication.

WHO'S AT RISK?

Two out of every one hundred Canadians have an underactive thyroid gland.[4] Thyroid disease can affect anyone, but hypothyroidism is ten times more common in women than in men. The risk of hypothyroidism increases considerably as you age. It usually strikes after age 40 and is common in elderly women. In fact, up to 10 percent of women over the age of 65 show evidence of hypothyroidism.[5] Although the condition most often affects middle-aged and older adults, it can develop in infants and teenagers.

Hashimoto's thyroiditis has been associated with a genetic component, so your risk may be greater if you have a close relative, such as a parent or grandparent, with a related autoimmune disease.

Some women also develop thyroid conditions during or immediately after pregnancy. Thyroiditis is especially common during the period following the birth of the baby, when it can often be confused with postpartum depression.

If you've had surgery or received radioactive iodine therapy to treat thyroid conditions such as hyperthyroidism, Graves' disease or thyroid cancer, you may be predisposed to hypothyroidism. Irradiation of the head and neck through X-rays or cancer treatment may also predispose you to thyroid problems.

In countries outside North America, one of the most common causes of hypothyroidism is iodine deficiency. This mineral is an essential component of thyroid hormones. People who don't have natural sources of iodine in their diet, such as fish and other seafood, are at high risk of developing hypothyroidism. In Canada and the United States, the problem has been virtually eliminated because iodine has been added to table salt.

DIAGNOSIS

Current tests for thyroid disorders are quite sensitive and precise, making it possible to get a very accurate diagnosis of hypothyroidism. If your doctor suspects that your symptoms are caused by an underactive thyroid gland, he or she will order blood tests to confirm the diagnosis. One test will measure the level of T4 in your blood; if you have hypothyroidism, the T4 levels will be low. When your condition is mild, however, it's possible that your blood levels of both T4 and T3 could measure in the normal range. In that case, you may be tested for the level of TSH in your blood—a high TSH level will confirm the diagnosis of thyroid failure.

Sometimes, an additional test may be necessary to detect the presence of antithyroid antibodies in your blood. This will help your doctor determine if your hypothyroidism is caused by the immune condition Hashimoto's thyroiditis. Elderly people may also undergo further laboratory testing to find out if the thyroid condition is putting extra stress on the heart or raising blood pressure or cholesterol levels.

CONVENTIONAL TREATMENT

In most cases, hypothyroidism is a permanent condition that requires a lifetime of treatment. The goal of treatment is to provide your body with enough thyroid hormones to maintain an efficient metabolic rate. At present, the prescription of a thyroid supplement is the only effective treatment for this disorder. The supplement is usually a form of synthetic T4, a small pill taken daily. Although the supplement contains only T4, the various organs in your body can convert the hormone into the more powerful T3 as needed.

There are also some thyroid supplements that are made from hormones extracted from animal thyroids. These aren't often prescribed today because their potency levels are inconsistent. They also contain T3, which can cause heart problems, especially in older people or those with heart conditions.

Your doctor determines your daily dosage of thyroid replacement hormones based on your age, sex, weight, thyroid function and other medications. Usually, you'll start with a low dose and increase it gradually until your blood levels of T4 and TSH are within normal range. Hypothyroidism is an ongoing process and your dosage may change as your thyroid function deteriorates. Regular blood tests help your doctor adjust your thyroid hormone medication to suit your needs. If you become pregnant, the dose may need to be increased. Older people need less thyroxine, so your dosage may be lowered as you age. Once your medication levels have been properly adjusted, you should feel energetic, healthy and symptom-free—and able to resume a completely normal life.

Managing thyroid disease

DIETARY STRATEGIES
Weight control

Weight gain is a concern for women with both types of thyroid disease—hyperthyroidism and hypothyroidism. Some research suggests that up to 50 percent of women with hyperthyroidism report weight problems after therapy. Weight gain can occur for two reasons. First, when your thyroid hormones return to lower, normal levels your metabolic rate slows down. This means your body burns fewer calories each day. Second, if you don't reduce your food intake to match your lower metabolism, the pounds can creep on. To prevent weight loss when they're experiencing the disease, many women increase their food intake; having gotten used to eating more, it can be easy to continue doing that even after treatment has ended.

In the case of an underactive thyroid gland, you're also at risk of gaining weight. A deficiency of thyroid hormones leads to a general decline in the rate at which your body burns carbohydrates, protein and fat for energy. As a result, weight gain is common. And it's more difficult (but not impossible) to lose weight if your thyroid hormone levels aren't in a correct balance.

If you have Graves' disease and now weigh more than you did before you were afflicted with the condition or if you're suffering from hypothyroidism and have difficulty controlling your weight, examine your eating habits to determine where you're going wrong. Keep a food diary for two weeks. Just writing down what you eat often highlights your dietary discrepancies. I always have my clients keep a food diary before they come to see me. They're often surprised to learn how much and what they eat. There's nothing like seeing it in black and white! For some women, keeping a daily journal is all the motivation they need to make healthy food choices and lose weight.

For some other strategies that will help you lose your excess weight, read the section on weight control in Chapter 2.

Managing Graves' hyperthyroidism

The nutritional approaches I discuss below are intended to help offset side effects associated with various types of treatment for Graves' disease. In addition to keeping you well during and after your course of therapy for this disease, my strategies will also improve your overall health and feeling of well-being.

DIETARY STRATEGIES

Vitamins and minerals

Antioxidants

Research suggests that hyperthyroidism is associated with a decrease in antioxidants and an increase in oxidative stress brought on by free radical molecules. It's also thought that oxidative stress caused by free radicals can contribute to the tissue damage caused by hyperthyroidism.[6-9] Free radicals are highly reactive oxygen molecules that are produced by normal body processes. Dietary antioxidants such as vitamins C and E, beta carotene and selenium quench harmful free radicals and prevent them from causing damage to body cells.

Studies that measured levels of antioxidant nutrients in the blood and thyroid tissue of women with Graves' disease have observed decreased levels of beta carotene and vitamin E.[10,11] Another study looked at the effect of a daily vitamin C supplement in 24 women undergoing antithyroid drug therapy for Graves' disease.[12] At the beginning of the study, the researchers found that, compared with healthy women who served as controls, those with hyperthyroidism had higher levels of oxidized compounds and lower levels of antioxidant enzymes in their blood. After taking 1000 milligrams of vitamin C for one month, these women had significant increases in antioxidant enzymes.

Research conducted in women taking Tapazole (methimazole) for Graves' disease found that a mixed antioxidant supplement (vitamins C and E, beta carotene and selenium) increased antioxidant enzymes in the body and was associated with achieving normal thyroid hormone levels at a faster rate than medication alone.[13,14]

If you're undergoing antithyroid drug treatment for Graves' disease, increase your intake of antioxidants from diet and supplements. As an alternative to supplementing antioxidants singly (see below), mixed antioxidant supplements are available (e.g., SISU Supreme Antioxidant 6, SISU Ester ACES Plus and Jamieson Formula NT-OX).

VITAMIN C. The recommended dietary allowance (RDA) is 75 and 90 milli-grams for women and men, respectively (smokers need an additional 35 milligrams). Best food sources include citrus fruit, citrus juices, cantaloupe, kiwi, mango, strawberries, broccoli, Brussels sprouts, cauli-flower, red pepper and tomato juice. To supplement, take 500 milligrams of vitamin C once daily. The daily upper limit is 2000 milligrams.

VITAMIN E. The RDA is 22 international units (IU). Best food sources include wheat germ, nuts, seeds, vegetable oils, whole grains and kale. To supplement take 400 IU of natural source vitamin E. Buy a "mixed" vitamin E supplement if possible. The daily upper limit is 1500 IU.

BETA CAROTENE. No RDA has been established for beta carotene. Best food sources are orange and dark-green produce, including carrots, sweet potato, winter squash, broccoli, collard greens, kale, spinach, apricots, cantaloupe, peaches, nectarines, mango and papaya. Most beta carotene supplements supply 10,000 to 25,000 IU of beta carotene. If you're a smoker, don't take high-dose beta carotene supplements.

SELENIUM. The RDA is 55 micrograms. Best food sources include Brazil nuts, shrimp, salmon, halibut, crab, fish, pork, organ meats, wheat bran, whole-wheat bread, brown rice, onion, garlic and mushrooms. To supplement take 100 to 200 micrograms per day. The daily upper limit is 400 micrograms.

Calcium and Vitamin D

It's well documented that hyperthyroidism causes a higher rate of bone breakdown. Some studies, but not all, have found that antithyroid medication has a harmful effect on bone density. To further explore the effect of antithyroid medication on bone loss, French researchers summarized the results from 41 studies in 1250 patients.[15] Their results showed that medications like Tapazole (methimazole) and Propyl-Thyracil (propylthiouracil), which suppress thyroid hormone secretion, cause significant bone loss in the lower spine and hip in post-menopausal women.

There's also evidence that women with Graves' disease are more susceptible to calcium and vitamin D deficiency during the winter months.[16] Deficiencies of these two nutrients are linked with a higher risk of tetany following surgery for Graves' disease. Tetany—usually caused by very low calcium levels in the blood—is characterized by pain, twitching, cramps and spasms of the muscles. Mild tetany is characterized by tingling in the fingers, toes, lips and tongue. Low calcium levels can be caused by a lack of vitamin D. Fortunately, tetany can be successfully treated with adequate calcium and vitamin D.

To protect your bones and lower the risk of post-operative tetany, make sure you meet your daily requirements for each nutrient (see Chapter 1 for more information on food sources and supplements).

CALCIUM. Consume 1500 milligrams of calcium per day to help offset increased bone loss. Best food sources are milk, yogurt, cheese, fortified soy and rice beverages, fortified orange juice, tofu, salmon (with bones), kale, bok choy, broccoli and Swiss chard. Take a calcium supplement once or twice daily to ensure that you reach an intake of 1500 milligrams.

VITAMIN D. Consume 1000 IU of vitamin D daily from a supplement. Best food sources are fluid milk, fortified soy and rice beverages, oily fish, egg yolks, butter and margarine; however, diet won't provide enough vitamin D to meet your needs. To determine how much extra vitamin D you need to take, calculate how much you're already consuming from your multivitamin and calcium supplements, subtract that from your RDA and make up the difference. Vitamin D is available in 400 and 1000 IU doses.

Iodine

This trace mineral is an integral part of T3 and T4, the two thyroid hormones released by the thyroid gland. Our major source of iodine is the ocean—seafood and seawater are excellent sources of the mineral. As you move further inland, the amount of iodine in foods varies and generally reflects the amount in the soil that plants grow in or animals graze on. Land that was once under the ocean contains plenty of iodine. In Canada and the United States, the soil around the Great Lakes is iodine-poor. However, the fortification of table salt with iodine in Canada has eliminated health problems caused by iodine deficiency.

If your body is deficient in iodine on an ongoing basis, the production of thyroid hormones will slow down. This will eventually lead to hypothyroidism. But if you eat salty processed foods and fast foods, or if you add table salt to your meals, you're certainly not at risk for consuming too little iodine.

It may seem odd, but too much iodine in the diet can also cause hypothyroidism. Excess iodine can result in low thyroid hormone levels by halting the activity of enzymes needed for their production. There have been cases of people who develop hypothyroidism by taking in too much iodine in the form of iodine-rich seaweed and kelp on a daily basis.

Obviously a lack of iodine won't lead to Graves' hyperthyroidism. But if you do have Graves' disease, shortchanging your diet of this indispensable mineral might influence your remission rate after treatment with antithyroid drugs. An American study of 69 patients who took antithyroid medication for Graves' disease suggests that the more iodine in the diet, the longer the rate of remission, or how long the disease remained dormant.[17]

The recommended daily intake for iodine is 160 micrograms per day. Women need to consume an additional 25 and 50 micrograms each day during pregnancy and breastfeeding respectively. It's estimated that North Americans consume 200 to 600 micrograms of iodine per day, well above our requirements. Some of this iodine excess may come from our growing dependence on fast and processed foods, since these foods contribute a generous amount of salt to our daily diet. Besides iodized salt, other food sources of iodine include seafood, bread, dairy products, plants grown in iodine-rich soil, and meat and poultry from animals raised on iodine-rich soil.

If you have Graves' disease and antithyroid drugs are a part of your treatment regime, make sure you include iodine-rich foods in your diet. This is particularly true if you live in an area with iodine-poor soil, if you avoid fast food and salty foods, and if you don't add table salt to your meals. Consider bringing back the salt shaker—but a little is all you need. Don't exceed 600 micrograms per day.

Managing hypothyroidism

DIETARY STRATEGIES
Lowering high LDL blood cholesterol
Hypothyroidism is linked with a greater risk of early heart disease, as thyroid hormones influence the level of blood cholesterol. Indeed, many studies find that patients suffering from a deficiency of thyroid hormones, whether they have overt symptoms or not, have higher levels of total cholesterol, LDL (bad) cholesterol and triglycerides.[18-24] And the more severe the hypothyroidism, the higher the cholesterol level.

Researchers have also learned that people with a sluggish thyroid gland have LDL cholesterol particles that are more readily oxidized by harmful free radical molecules. Free radicals are reactive oxygen molecules that roam the body and damage cells. When free radicals oxidize your LDL cholesterol, this cholesterol has a greater tendency to stick to artery walls. Although having a high level of LDL cholesterol is not good, having oxidized LDL cholesterol is worse. Your body does have ways of protecting itself from free radicals though. Special enzymes in the body and certain nutrients in foods act as antioxidants and help to keep free radical activity in check.

If you have high blood cholesterol, there are many dietary changes you can make to help lower your levels to the normal range. I strongly recommend that you read the cholesterol-lowering strategies in Chapter 12, Heart Disease and High LDL Cholesterol. You'll learn what foods and nutrients to add to your diet and what foods to limit.

Soy foods

You may have heard that eating large amounts of soy can block the production of thyroid hormones and result in an underactive thyroid and goiter (an enlarged thyroid gland). It's true that raw soybeans contain compounds that prevent the body's ability to use iodine. But heating soybeans eliminates these effects, and all soy foods, from tofu to soy nuts, are manufactured using heat. Goiter appears to only occur in people who are iodine deficient (the mineral is needed for normal thyroid function). In developed countries, salt is fortified with iodine to prevent deficiency. It's possible, however, that people who eat soy foods and who don't get enough iodine from their diet could be at risk for goiter.

Over the past fifteen years, a handful of studies have found no effect of soy foods on thyroid function or thyroid hormone levels in healthy adults and people with hypothyroidism who aren't iodine deficient.[25-27]

VITAMINS AND MINERALS
B Vitamins

Some, but not all, studies have found that people with hypothyroidism may have higher blood levels of homocysteine, a known risk factor for early heart disease.[28-30] Homocysteine is an amino acid that everyone produces. Under normal circumstances it's converted to other harmless amino acids with the help of three B vitamins: folate, B6 and B12. When this conversion doesn't occur rapidly enough because of a deficiency of B vitamins or a genetic defect, homocysteine can accumulate in the blood.

High levels of homocysteine can damage blood vessel walls and promote the buildup of cholesterol deposits. Research suggests that elevated homocysteine levels seen in patients with hypothyroidism are accompanied by low blood-folate levels.

Getting adequate amounts of B vitamins is an important way to keep your blood homocysteine at a healthy level. The best food sources for each B vitamin are as follows:

B Vitamin	Good Food Sources
Folate	Whole grains, wheat germ, lentils, artichokes, asparagus, broccoli, leafy greens, spinach (cooked) and orange juice
Vitamin B6	Whole grains, meat, poultry, fish, legumes, potatoes and bananas
Vitamin B12	All animal foods, including meat, poultry, fish, dairy products and eggs, as well as fortified soy and rice beverages

Including good food sources of B vitamins in your diet and taking a daily multivitamin and mineral pill will ensure that you meet your requirements for all B vitamins. A standard multivitamin provides 100 percent to 300 percent of the recommended dietary allowance for each nutrient.

If your blood-homocysteine level is elevated, your doctor may advise you to take a single supplement of folic acid. A daily dose of 0.8 to 1 milligrams of folic acid is sufficient to lower elevated blood homocysteine. Choose a folic acid supplement with vitamin B12 added. I don't recommend taking single folic acid supplements indefinitely; discontinue them once your homocysteine level is lowered to the acceptable range. A multivitamin that supplies 0.4 milligrams of folic acid is sufficient.

Many B complex supplements also supply a higher dose of folic acid than standard multivitamins. One word of warning if you opt for a high-potency B vitamin supplement: Vitamin B3, or niacin, can cause flushing when taken in amounts greater than 35 milligrams. This is a harmless reaction that causes your face, chest and arms to feel hot and tingly. The reaction usually passes within 20 to 30 minutes. To avoid this niacin flush (1) take your supplement right after eating a meal, (2) buy a supplement with less than 35 milligrams of niacin or (3) buy a multivitamin or B complex supplement that contains niacinamide rather than niacin (niacinamide is non-flushing).

Iodine

If the body is shortchanged of iodine on an ongoing basis, the production of thyroid hormones slows down and eventually hypothyroidism develops. However, the fortification of table salt with iodine in Canada and the United States has eliminated health problems caused by iodine deficiency. If you eat processed foods, restaurant meals and/or fast foods, or you add table salt to your meals, you're not at risk for consuming too little iodine.

Excess iodine in the diet can also cause hypothyroidism by halting the activity of enzymes needed for production of thyroid hormones. There have been cases of people developing hypothyroidism by taking in too much iodine in the form of iodine-rich seaweed and kelp supplements on a daily basis.[31]

The recommended daily intake for iodine is 150 micrograms per day. It's estimated that North Americans consume 200 to 600 micrograms of iodine per day—well above requirements. Some of this iodine excess may come from our growing dependence on fast and processed foods, since these foods contribute a generous amount of salt to our daily diet. Besides iodized salt, other food sources of iodine include seafood, bread, dairy products, plants grown in iodine-rich soil and meat and poultry from animals raised on iodine-rich soil.

Selenium

This trace mineral is an important component of an enzyme that produces the thyroid hormone T3. Researchers have learned that a selenium deficiency in older adults is strongly associated with lower levels of the T3 hormone.[32] The relationship between impaired selenium status and reduced thyroid hormone levels may be partially responsible for the hypothyroidism that's often diagnosed in elderly women. Despite this, a recent study of 501 adults aged 60 to 74 living in the United Kingdom failed to show an effect of selenium supplements on thyroid function.[33] However, a study conducted in pregnant women with thyroid antibodies in their bloodstream found that taking 200 micrograms of selenium versus a placebo during and after pregnancy was associated with reduced inflammation of the thyroid and a lower risk of developing hypothyroidism. (Pregnant women who test positive for thyroid antibodies are more prone to develop hypothyroidism after pregnancy.)[34] Other research suggests that a daily selenium supplement can reduce thyroid antibodies in patients with autoimmune thyroidosis (e.g., Hashimoto's thyroiditis).[35]

The best food sources of selenium include seafood and meat. Whole-wheat bread, wheat bran, wheat germ, oats, brown rice, Brazil nuts, Swiss chard and garlic are other good sources. Dietary intake from plant foods varies according to the selenium content of the soil in which the foods were grown.

People at greatest risk for a selenium deficiency are those who eat a vegetarian diet based on plant foods grown in low-selenium areas. But because most of us eat supermarket foods that have been transported from areas throughout Canada, the United States, Mexico or South America, selenium deficiency is uncommon.

If you're considering a supplement, check your multivitamin first. Some high-potency brands contain up to 100 micrograms of selenium. If you're using single selenium supplements, a 200 microgram dose is plenty. You might want to choose one that contains selenomethionine or selenium-rich yeast, since these organic forms of the mineral appear to be more available to the body.

The daily upper limit for selenium from foods and supplements is 400 micrograms per day. Over time, consuming too much selenium has toxic effects, including hair and nail loss, gastrointestinal upset, skin rash, garlic-breath odour, fatigue, irritability and nervous-system abnormalities.

Iron and calcium supplements

If you're taking levothyroxine (Synthroid) and also being treated for an iron deficiency, take your medication and your iron pill two to three hours apart rather than at the same time. Studies have found that iron supplements can reduce the body's absorption of levothyroxine.[36,37] It's possible that impaired absorption of your medication could make you hypothyroid and increase your medication requirements.

If you're taking iron supplements to correct an iron deficiency, your doctor will monitor your thyroid hormone levels closely. Iron pills should be taken only if your doctor has diagnosed you with iron deficiency. If you're taking them of your own accord, be sure to let your physician know.

Calcium supplements can also interfere with the absorption of levothyroxine, primarily when the two are taken at or near the same time. To avoid an interaction, take your calcium supplements four hours before or after taking levothyroxine.

THE BOTTOM LINE...
Leslie's recommendations for managing thyroid disease

1. If you've gained excess weight after treatment for Graves' disease or if you have hypothyroidism and are concerned about your body weight, embark on a healthy eating and exercise program. Start by keeping a food diary for two weeks to pinpoint areas that need improvement.
2. Don't skimp on iodine. The best sources of iodine are iodized table salt (all salt in Canada is fortified with iodine), seafood, plants grown on iodine-rich soil and foods from animals that graze on iodine-rich soil. But don't get too much iodine, as intakes greater than 600 micrograms per day may lead to hypothyroidism. To keep your iodine intake within reason, avoid eating large quantities of kelp, dulse or other sea vegetables on a daily basis.

Graves' Disease
1. Boost your intake of dietary antioxidants, including vitamins C and E and beta carotene.
2. Get more calcium and vitamin D in your daily diet. You need 1000 or 1500 milligrams of calcium and 1000 IU of vitamin D each day.

Hypothyroidism
1. If your doctor has determined that you have high blood-cholesterol levels, read Chapter 12, Heart Disease and High LDL Cholesterol, to get all my nutrition strategies to bring the levels down.
2. Boost your intake of B vitamins, in particular folate, B6 and B12.
3. Be sure you're getting enough selenium. The best food sources include seafood, meat, whole-wheat products, wheat bran, wheat germ, Brazil nuts, Swiss chard and garlic. If you take a supplement, don't exceed 200 micrograms per day.
4. If you're taking calcium supplements or single iron supplements, don't take either with your thyroid medication, since iron can reduce your body's absorption of the drug. Take a calcium or iron supplement four hours before or after taking your medication (levothyroxine).

PART 7

PELVIC AND URINARY TRACT HEALTH

22
Cervical dysplasia

If you're diagnosed with cervical dysplasia, it means that abnormal changes are beginning to take place in the cells lining the surface of your cervix, the part of your reproductive system that forms the entrance to your uterus. The word *dysplasia* means abnormal cell growth. The cells of your cervix begin to show microscopic changes and start to divide at a faster rate than normal.

If left untreated, cervical dysplasia could progress to become cervical cancer. Despite improvements in diagnosis and treatment over the past fifty years, cancer of the cervix continues to threaten the health of Canadian women. It's the second most common cancer in women, most often striking those between the ages of 35 and 55. It's a cancer that progresses very slowly and may take up to ten years to develop. If detected in the early stages, it can be treated effectively and the long-term prognosis is very good.

There are no warning signs or symptoms for cervical dysplasia. The only reliable way to detect this pre-cancerous condition is to have an annual Pap smear, a laboratory test of a small sample of your cervical tissue.

What causes cervical dysplasia?

Scientists know that specific persistent strains of human papillomavirus (HPV) are linked with cervical cancer. About one-third of HPV strains are sexually transmitted and some types cause genital warts. Two strains, HPV-16 and HPV-18, are linked to cervical dysplasia and cervical cancer. Researchers now believe that most young people who engage in sexual activity carry HPV viruses. In most cases, HPV leaves the body naturally. But some of the strains linked with cervical cancer can persist, especially in women over 30 years of age. It's estimated that about 75 percent of sexually active men and women in Canada will have at least one HPV infection in their lifetime. Young women 20 to 24 years old generally have the highest rates of cancer-causing HPV infection.[1]

There are three stages of cervical dysplasia. If abnormal cells are found only on the surface of the cervix, the condition is considered mild. This is the most common form, and up to 70 percent of mild dysplasia cases regress on their own without treatment. But unfortunately, sometimes these pre-cancerous cells can spread deeper into the tissue of the cervix lining. When this happens, cervical dysplasia is labelled as moderate or severe, depending on the extent of the tissue penetration. Moderate and severe cervical dysplasia are less likely to self-resolve and have a higher risk of progressing to cancer within ten years.

Symptoms

As I mentioned earlier, there are no warning signs of cervical dysplasia. Without the appropriate medical testing, you probably won't realize that anything is wrong until the disease is well advanced. If you have regular medical checkups, your doctor may notice a growth, sore or suspicious area on your cervix during a routine pelvic examination.

In most cases, identifiable symptoms don't appear until the cervical dysplasia has progressed to cervical cancer. At that time, a woman may experience some pain or some intermittent bleeding or spotting between menstrual cycles. To prevent cervical cancer, it's critical that you get tested for cervical dysplasia by having a Pap smear on an annual basis. The Pap smear identifies pre-cancerous changes of cervical cells and also indicates the presence of invasive cancer cells. But an abnormal result doesn't always mean your health is at risk. Sometimes a virus may cause temporary cell changes that will disappear in a short period of time.

Who's at risk?

Although it can develop at any age, cervical dysplasia most often occurs in women between the ages of 25 to 35. Women at greater risk include those who begin having sexual intercourse at an early age (16 years or younger) and those who have multiple sexual partners. Women who have a history of sexually transmitted disease, especially HPV infection, are also at increased risk for cervical dysplasia. Eighty percent to 90 percent of women with cervical dysplasia have an HPV infection. Other conditions that may increase the risk for cervical dysplasia include:

- smoking cigarettes or exposure to secondhand smoke
- using oral contraceptives for more than ten years (oral contraceptives can interfere with folic acid metabolism in the cells around the cervix; women who use oral contraceptives may have increased exposure to sexually transmitted diseases)
- having a history of a gynecological cancer
- following a diet that's low in vitamin A, beta carotene and folate; a poor diet may also result in a weakened immune system, decreasing the body's ability to fight HPV

Women who are sexually active and who don't have regular Pap smears have a greater chance of having cervical dysplasia that then develops into cervical cancer. Two vaccines have been developed to prevent HPV-16 and HPV-18 infections. One is available in Canada; the other is currently being reviewed by Health Canada.

Diagnosis

Ever since the Pap test was introduced in Canada in 1949, we've seen a dramatic decline in the number of deaths caused by cervical cancer. To perform a Pap test, your doctor will conduct a regular pelvic examination. Using a small spatula and a brush, he or she will scrape some cells from the surface of your cervix and smear them on a slide. This tiny tissue sample will then be sent to a laboratory and examined under a microscope for abnormal cells.

The Pap smear identifies pre-cancerous changes in cervical cells and also indicates the presence of invasive cancer cells. But an abnormal result doesn't always mean your health is at risk. Sometimes a virus may cause temporary cell changes that will disappear after a short period of time.

A normal Pap smear result is reassuring because it indicates that you have a very low risk of cervical cancer. However, it's not a guarantee that your cervix is cancer-free. It's possible that cancer cells or abnormal cells can be missed if they're not part of the tissue sample collected for the test. For that reason, doctors recommend that women who are sexually active or who are over 18 years old have a Pap smear once a year.

Conventional treatment

Approximately 8 percent of all Pap smears show abnormal results. The treatment for cervical dysplasia varies, depending on the extent and severity of the dysplasia. Treatment may involve removal of the abnormal cervical tissue.

If you're diagnosed with mild dysplasia and have no other risk factors for cervical cancer, your doctor will probably just monitor your condition and wait to see if the affected cells return to normal. If a second Pap smear in four to six months shows cell growth is normal, no treatment is necessary. With mild dysplasia, it's recommended that you continue to monitor the health of your cervix by returning for a pelvic examination and Pap smear twice a year for at least two years.

A diagnosis of moderate or severe dysplasia is treated a little differently. Your doctor checks the surface of your cervix for abnormalities by performing a *colposcopy:* Using a viewing tube with a magnifying lens, he or she inspects your cervix and takes a *biopsy* of tissue from the abnormal area. There are two types of biopsy used in this procedure: a *punch biopsy* samples a tiny piece of your cervix; *endocervical curettage* is used to scrape tissue from the cervical canal. These samples are sent to a laboratory to determine the extent of changes in cervical cells.

Once the severity of the cervical dysplasia is known, the treatment involves removing all the abnormal growth that can potentially turn into cervical cancer. Your doctor may perform a surgical procedure called a *cervical conization*, which removes a cone-shaped section of tissue. Other ways of removal include cauterizing with heat, freezing with cryosurgery, vaporizing with lasers or excising with an electrified wire loop procedure known as LEEP. These treatments usually don't affect your ability to become pregnant. But because cervical dysplasia can return, it's important to monitor yourself carefully and have Pap smears every three months for the first year after surgery and every six months after that.

In more severe cases, a hysterectomy to remove your uterus may be necessary. This decision prevents you from having children in the future.

The sooner you detect and treat cervical dysplasia, the lower your risk for developing cervical cancer. In the meantime, there are dietary and nutritional strategies that can help prevent cervical dysplasia from developing in the first place. If your recent Pap test has revealed abnormal cervical cells, some of the strategies I discuss below might even reverse the dysplasia.

Preventing and treating cervical dysplasia

The sooner cervical dysplasia is detected and treated, the lower a woman's risk for developing cervical cancer. The following dietary and nutritional strategies may help prevent cervical dysplasia from developing in the first place. Some of these strategies might even reverse the dysplasia.

VITAMINS AND MINERALS
Antioxidants

Many studies have found a link between cervical dysplasia and low blood levels of antioxidant nutrients, especially beta carotene and vitamin C. Women with cervical dysplasia are also more likely to have poor dietary intakes of these and other antioxidants. Antioxidants are vitamins, minerals and natural plant chemicals that protect cells in the body from damage caused by free radicals—highly reactive oxygen molecules that are produced by normal body processes. Excess free radicals can also be formed by pollution, cigarette smoke and heavy exercise. These compounds can damage the genetic material of cells, which, in turn, may lead to cancer development. Antioxidants neutralize free radicals, preventing them from causing damage to cells.

Our body has built-in antioxidant enzymes for keeping free radical activity in check, but levels decline as we age. Scientists are learning that a daily supply of dietary antioxidants is important for reducing the risk of certain cancers (not to mention heart disease, cataracts and possibly Alzheimer's disease).

When it comes to cervical dysplasia (a precursor to cervical cancer), a handful of dietary antioxidants have been identified that may prevent free radical damage to cervical cells. These include beta carotene, lycopene, vitamin C and vitamin E. Below I discuss the antioxidants that have been studied the most with respect to cervical dysplasia. To boost your intake of all these antioxidants, try to eat at least 7 to 10 servings of fruit and vegetables each day. One serving equals a piece of fruit, 1/2 cup (125 ml) of vegetables, 1 cup (250 ml) of green salad or 3/4 cup (175 ml) of unsweetened juice.

Beta carotene

This antioxidant is plentiful in dark-green vegetables and orange fruit and vegetables. It's been hypothesized that beta carotene may protect from cervical dysplasia and cervical cancer in a few ways. First of all, we know that beta carotene is a potent antioxidant and may therefore protect cervical cells from free radical damage. Beta carotene is also used to synthesize some vitamin A in the body. Vitamin A is essential for normal cellular growth and development. A number of laboratory studies have shown the ability of vitamin A to prevent abnormal cell growth. Researchers have found that, compared to women free of cervical dysplasia, those with the condition have significantly lower blood levels and dietary intakes of beta carotene.[2] Despite this consistent finding, studies, including a two-year randomized controlled trial, haven't found that beta carotene supplements are able to enhance the regression of severe cervical dysplasia, especially in women with HPV.[3-5]

Currently, there's no recommended daily intake for beta carotene, but many experts believe that 3 to 6 milligrams per day offers protection from disease. A diet containing plenty of fruit and vegetables—at least 7 to 10 servings per day—helps you consume an adequate amount of beta carotene. Orange and dark-green produce, including carrots, sweet potato, winter squash, broccoli, collard greens, kale, spinach, apricots, cantaloupe, peaches, nectarines, mango and papaya, contain the most beta carotene. Here's a look at the beta carotene content of some of the very best food sources.

Beta Carotene Content of Selected Foods

Food	Beta carotene (milligrams)
Sweet potato, baked, 1 medium	16.8 mg
Carrot juice, 1/2 cup (125 ml)	11.0 mg
Pumpkin, canned, 1/2 cup (125 ml)	8.5 mg
Pumpkin pie, 1 slice	7.4 mg
Carrots, cooked, 1/2 cup (125 ml)	6.5 mg
Carrots, raw, 1/2 cup (125 ml)	4.6 mg
Winter squash, 1/2 cup (125 ml)	2.9 mg

Source: U.S. Department of Agriculture, Agricultural Research Service, USDA Nutrient Database for Standard Reference, Release 19, 2006. Available at: www.ars.usda.gov/nutrientdata.

Your body doesn't absorb the beta carotene in raw foods efficiently. To enhance absorption, cook the vegetables and eat them with a little fat.

Lycopene

Lycopene belongs to the same family of carotenoid compounds as beta carotene—but it's twice as potent an antioxidant as beta carotene. As such, it's yet another dietary defence mechanism against free radical damage to the genetic material of cells.

A few studies have suggested that lycopene protects women from cervical dysplasia. One study from the University of Pennsylvania School of Medicine found that women with the highest intake of lycopene were one-third as likely to have dysplasia compared to those who consumed the least.[6]

Lycopene is found in red-coloured fruit and vegetables. It's the natural chemical that gives these foods their bright colour. Tomatoes are the richest source of lycopene, but you'll also find some in pink grapefruit, watermelon, guava and apricots.

Although more work needs to be done to unravel the precise role lycopene plays in cervical health, there's no reason why you shouldn't be getting a good supply in your daily diet. Based on the research that has been conducted in the area of heart disease, it appears that an intake of 5 to 7 milligrams offers protection. And that's easy to get if you eat heat-processed tomato products.

Lycopene Content of Selected Foods

Food	Lycopene (milligrams)
Tomato, raw, 1 small	0.8–3.8 mg
Tomato juice, 1 cup (250 ml)	23.0 mg
Tomato paste, 2 tbsp (30 ml)	8.0 mg
Tomato sauce, 1/2 cup (125 ml)	3.1 mg
Tomatoes, cooked, 1 cup (250 ml)	9.25 mg
Ketchup, 2 tbsp (30 ml)	3.1–4.2 mg
Apricots, dried, 10 halves	0.3 mg
Grapefruit, pink, 1/2	4.2 mg
Papaya, 1 whole	6.2–16.5 mg
Watermelon, 1 slice (25 cm x 2 cm)	8.5–26.4 mg

Heat-processed tomato products provide a source of lycopene that's much more available to the body. Even though one fresh tomato can pack up to 4 milligrams of lycopene, your body doesn't absorb all of it. And here's another tip to increase the amount of lycopene you absorb—add a little olive oil to your pasta sauce. Lycopene is a fat-soluble compound and is better absorbed in the presence of a little fat.

If you're looking for a boost of lycopene, all you have to do is add a glass of low-sodium tomato juice to your lunch. However, lycopene supplements are available in health food stores and drugstores. If you opt for supplements, I recommend that you choose a brand that's made with the Lyc-O-Mato or LycoRed extract. This source of lycopene comes from Israel and is derived from whole tomatoes. It's also the extract that has been used in clinical studies. Most supplements offer 5 milligrams of lycopene per tablet, so one a day is all you need.

Vitamin C

Much less research has been done on this antioxidant vitamin and its potential role in protection from cervical dysplasia. A few studies have determined that women with low blood levels of vitamin C have a greater risk of cervical dysplasia compared to women with higher levels. Furthermore, cigarette smoke decreases the level of vitamin C in the body. One American study found a strong association between a woman's history of smoking and her level of vitamin C, whether or not she had cervical dysplasia.[7]

Healthy women require 75 milligrams of vitamin C each day; if you smoke you need 110 milligrams. The best food sources include citrus fruit, kiwi, strawberries, broccoli, cauliflower and red pepper. Cantaloupe, grapefruit, mango and tomato juice are also good sources of vitamin C, as well as beta carotene and/or lycopene.

VITAMIN C SUPPLEMENTS. If you don't eat at least two vitamin C–rich foods each day, a supplement is a good idea. Keep in mind, though, that fruit and vegetables contain many other natural chemicals that may work with vitamin C to keep you healthy. So even if you do take a vitamin C pill, I recommend that you still add foods rich in vitamin C to your daily diet. Here's what you need to know about vitamin C supplements.

- If you don't like to swallow pills and prefer a chewable supplement, make sure it contains calcium ascorbate or sodium ascorbate. These forms of vitamin C are less acidic and therefore less harmful to tooth enamel.

- Take a 500 milligram supplement once or twice a day. There's little point in swallowing much more than that at once, since your body can use only about 200 milligrams at one time. If you want to take more, split your dose over the day.

- The daily upper limit for vitamin C has been set at 2000 milligrams, to avoid diarrhea.

Vitamin E

A discussion of dietary antioxidants can't exclude vitamin E. Chances are you've already heard about this heart healthy nutrient (read Chapter 12 for all the facts on vitamin E and heart disease). As with vitamin C, less research has been done in the area of vitamin E and cervical dysplasia. Nevertheless, observational studies have found a link between the risk of dysplasia and blood levels of the vitamin. For instance, one study from the Cancer Research Center of Hawai'i revealed that women with the highest blood–vitamin E levels had a 70 percent lower risk of cervical dysplasia than those with the lowest blood levels.[8] The researchers also noticed what's called a dose-response effect. That means the higher the level of vitamin E, the lower the risk of dysplasia.

Like the antioxidants discussed above, vitamin E is a potent scavenger of harmful free radical molecules and thus may keep cervical cells healthy. Until we learn more about the role of vitamin E in cervical health, strive to meet your daily targets—see the RDA guide in Chapter 1, page 33.

VITAMIN E FOOD SOURCES AND SUPPLEMENTS. Wheat germ, nuts, seeds, soy beans, vegetable oils, corn oil, whole grains and kale are all good sources of vitamin E, so be sure to include a few of these in your daily diet. But when you consider that adding 2 tablespoons (30 ml) of wheat germ to your morning smoothie gives you only 4 international units (IU) of the vitamin—and wheat germ is one of the best sources—it can be a challenge to reach the recommended daily intake of 22 IU. For this reason, many women opt for a daily supplement to help them meet their target intakes. To help you choose the right vitamin E supplement, consider the following suggestions:

- Start taking 100 to 400 IU per day. There's no evidence to warrant taking more.
- Buy a natural source vitamin E supplement (or look for *d-alpha-tocopherol* on the label; synthetic forms are labelled *dl-alpha-tocopherol*). Although the body absorbs both synthetic and natural forms equally well, your liver prefers the natural form, as it incorporates more natural vitamin E into transport molecules. Studies have shown that twice as much vitamin E ends up in the blood of people taking natural E compared with those taking the same amount of synthetic E.
- Consider choosing a vitamin E supplement that's labelled "mixed tocopherols." Preliminary research shows that one form of vitamin E, called gamma-tocopherol, has potent anti-inflammatory effects in addition to its antioxidant properties. This may play a role in cancer prevention.
- If you're taking a blood-thinning medication like Coumadin (warfarin), don't take vitamin E without your doctor's approval, since it has slight anti-clotting properties.
- The daily upper limit for vitamin E is 1500 IU.

Folate

Moving away from the antioxidant connection, let's turn our attention to a vitamin that appears to have a very important role in preventing the development of dysplasia. Research shows that as one's intake of folate-rich foods decreases, the risk of cervical dysplasia increases. An American study found that women consuming less than 400 micrograms of folate each day were 2.6 times more likely to develop dysplasia than women who consumed more than 400 micrograms.[9]

A lack of this B vitamin may promote the development of dysplasia in a number of ways. Folate may act in some way to protect cervical cells. Studies have found that many women with dysplasia have normal blood levels of folate but low levels of the vitamin in cervical tissue. A deficiency of folate may also enhance the harmful effect of human papillomavirus (HPV) infection on cervical cells.

Folate is critical for the synthesis of DNA (deoxyribonucleic acid), the genetic material of cells. Low levels of folate in cervical tissue can make cellular DNA more susceptible to damage. Even a marginal folate deficiency can cause damage to DNA in cells, damage that resembles cervical dysplasia. It's possible that this alteration to DNA is an early step in the progression of cervical dysplasia and cervical cancer. Furthermore, this damage to a cell's genetic material may be stopped or reversed if you're given supplements of the B vitamin. In fact, two trials have found that folic acid supplements improved dysplasia in women taking birth control pills.[10-13] However, trials conducted in women not taking oral contraceptives didn't find that folic acid supplements altered the course of dysplasia. The researchers concluded that a deficiency of the B vitamin may be involved in the initiation of dysplasia, but once you have the disease, supplements don't appear to reverse it.

What these studies suggest is that getting enough folate every day is an important strategy in the prevention of cervical dysplasia. See the RDA guide in Chapter 1, page 33, for how much folate women should strive for every day. Be sure to choose whole-grain breads, cereals and pasta more often than refined grain foods. Although refined grain products are enriched with folic acid in Canada and the United States, whole grains provide more. For a list of selected foods rich in folate, see Chapter 1, page 19.

FOLIC ACID SUPPLEMENTS. For some women, consuming 400 micrograms of folate every day can be challenging. As you can see from the list in Chapter 1, you pretty much have to make sure your daily diet includes beans, spinach and orange juice. Some of you might want to take a multivitamin and mineral supplement to ensure you're reaching your target. Look for a supplement that gives 0.4 to 1.0 milligrams of folic acid (check the ingredient list for this information).

By the way, you may have noticed that I've been using the terms folate and folic acid throughout this section. Folate refers to the B vitamin as it's found naturally in foods. Folic acid refers to the synthetic form—whether it's in a supplement or added back to foods, like enriched breakfast cereals.

If you take a separate folic acid supplement, be sure to buy one that has vitamin B12 added. High doses of folic acid taken over a period of time can hide a B12 deficiency and result in progressive nerve damage. The daily upper limit for folic acid intake from a supplement is 1000 micrograms (1 milligram).

THE BOTTOM LINE...
Leslie's recommendations for preventing and managing cervical dysplasia

1. First things first: If you're sexually active, make sure you get an annual Pap test.
2. Whether or not you're sexually active, don't smoke cigarettes.
3. Boost your antioxidant intake by eating a diet that's loaded with fruit and vegetables. Strive for at least 7 to 10 servings of fruit and vegetables each day.
4. To get more beta carotene, reach for bright orange and dark-green produce. The best choices are sweet potato, carrots, winter squash, mango, cantaloupe, kale and collard greens.
5. If you're a non-smoker and want to increase your daily intake of beta carotene, buy a multivitamin and mineral supplement with added beta carotene. Most brands offer 5000 to 10,000 international units (IU). If your multivitamin doesn't include this antioxidant, consider taking a separate beta carotene supplement.
6. If you're a smoker, avoid taking a beta carotene supplement. Increase your daily intake of beta carotene from foods only.
7. Boost your intake of lycopene, found in red-coloured fruit and vegetables. The best sources are heat-processed tomato products such as tomato sauce, stewed tomatoes, tomato juice and ketchup. Other foods to add to your diet include pink grapefruit, guava juice, apricots and papaya.
8. If you opt for a lycopene supplement, choose one that has Lyc-O-Mato or LycoRed on the label.
9. Try to get more vitamin C into your diet. If you take a daily vitamin C pill, take 500 milligrams once or twice daily.
10. Be sure vitamin E is included in your daily antioxidant regime. Vegetable oils, corn oil, nuts, seeds, wheat germ and kale are good sources. Consider taking a separate vitamin E supplement that's natural source and offers "mixed tocopherols."
11. Eat more foods rich in folate. Foods that offer the most folate and that should be eaten on a regular basis include asparagus, spinach, broccoli, lentils, kidney beans, unsweetened orange juice and whole-grain enriched breakfast cereals.

12. To meet the RDA for folate, make sure your multivitamin and mineral supplement contains 0.4 to 1.0 milligrams (400 to 1000 micrograms) of the vitamin (look for folic acid on the ingredient list). If you decide to take a separate folic acid supplement, buy one with vitamin B12 added, since high doses of folic acid can hide a B12 deficiency.

23
Endometriosis

Endometriosis is a poorly understood disease that afflicts as many as 18 percent of women. The condition develops in women when uterine-type cells grow outside the uterus. These cells may travel throughout the body and attach to a number of different areas, including the intestines. The misplaced cells develop into nodules, lesions, implants or growths that are affected by the hormonal fluctuations of the menstrual cycle. These growths cause pelvic pain, pain during intercourse, infertility and other problems.

What causes endometriosis?

The uterus, a reproductive organ located within the abdominal cavity, is lined with a type of tissue called *endometrium*. When you have endometriosis, tissue that looks and acts like endometrium is found living outside your uterus. In most cases, the misplaced tissue is discovered growing somewhere within the abdominal cavity. It may be found attached to your ovaries, bowel, bladder, Fallopian tubes or cervix. Although rare, the appearance of endometrial tissue in other sites around the body, including the lung, arm and thigh, is possible. Endometrial growths can vary in size and penetration of the surrounding tissue. Rest assured that endometrial growths are generally not cancerous—they're normal tissue found growing outside the normal location.

During the course of a normal menstrual cycle, the endometrial lining of your uterus gradually builds up in preparation for pregnancy. If you don't become pregnant, the lining breaks down, bleeds and is discharged from your body during your period. Unfortunately, the endometrial tissue living outside your uterus responds to the hormonal cycles of menstruation in exactly the same way. But, unlike the menstrual flow from the uterus, the blood from the misplaced tissue has no place to go. This causes episodes of internal bleeding and inflammation that can result in internal scarring, severe pain and infertility.

Scientists still don't know what causes endometriosis. The most commonly held view is the *retrograde menstruation theory*. This theory suggests that menstrual tissue occasionally flows backwards through the Fallopian tubes during menstruation. The tissue is discharged from the Fallopian tubes into the abdomen, where it becomes implanted and develops into endometrial growths. Another theory proposes that endometrial tissue may be distributed from the uterus to other parts of the body through the lymph glands or blood vessels. In some cases, endometrial tissue may be accidentally transplanted into distant sites through surgical procedures. It's possible that hereditary factors are involved, making some families more susceptible to the disease. Eventually, scientists may discover that endometriosis is caused by a combination of factors.

Women with endometriosis have a slightly increased risk for certain types of cancer of the ovary known as epithelial ovarian cancer. The risk seems to be highest in women with endometriosis and primary infertility (women who have never given birth to a child), but the use of oral contraceptives appears to significantly reduce the risk of cancer.

Symptoms

The most common symptom of endometriosis is pain before and during menstruation. Symptoms include:

- severe menstrual cramps
- irregular vaginal bleeding
- pelvic pain
- painful sexual intercourse
- painful bowel movements
- pain during exercise
- painful and frequent urination
- backache
- constipation or diarrhea
- fatigue

The pain intensity of endometriosis can change from month to month and varies greatly among affected women. Some women experience progressive worsening of pain while others find their symptoms resolve without treatment. Pelvic pain depends partly on where the implants of endometriosis are located. If they're deep or in areas with many pain-sensing nerves, the pain is likely to be more intense. Endometrial implants can also produce substances that circulate in the bloodstream and cause pain. As well, pain can result when implants form scar tissue. Symptoms usually start after the onset of menstruation and subside after menopause, when the growths tend to shrink or disappear.

Many women with endometriosis experience ongoing gastrointestinal discomfort, including diarrhea, painful bowel movements and general intestinal distress. Studies have revealed that endometriosis is associated with changes to the intestinal tract, such as altered motility and bacterial overgrowth. Women with endometriosis experience bowel problems as a result of endometrial growths that develop directly on the bowel, usually the latter part of the large intestine. Most specialists carefully check the bowel for the presence of endometriosis, but because the intestine is so long, it's possible for growths to be missed. Also, adhesions, resulting from the endometriosis itself or from past surgeries, can cause bowel symptoms (adhesions are fibrous bands of tissue that bind organs together). The adhesions pull on the bowel and cause pain.

Women with endometriosis are often told by their doctor that they have irritable bowel syndrome (IBS). Unfortunately that diagnosis isn't very helpful, because it doesn't indicate the underlying problem. IBS is an umbrella term used to describe gastrointestinal distress when no other diagnosis can be made. Having your doctor thoroughly investigate the cause of your bowel problems is important for effective treatment.

Who's at risk?

It's estimated that 3 percent to 18 percent of North American women and teenaged girls have endometriosis.[1] The disease generally appears between the ages of 15 and 50; however, it has been diagnosed in girls as young as 11. The disease is believed to run in families; you're at higher risk if you have a first-degree relative (e.g., mother or sister) with endometriosis. Other risk factors include being of Caucasian descent, having your first child after the age of 30, having a low body mass index and having an abnormal uterus.

Diagnosis

If you're suffering from the symptoms listed above, or you're having difficulty becoming pregnant, your doctor may suspect that you have endometriosis. He or she will evaluate your medical history and conduct a complete physical examination, including a pelvic exam. It's sometimes possible to actually feel an endometrial growth during the pelvic exam.

Most often, an accurate diagnosis can be made only if patches of endometrial tissue can be seen. To determine the presence of misplaced tissue, your doctor will conduct a minor surgical procedure called a laparoscopy. A small surgical tube with a light attached is inserted through a small incision in your abdomen. This allows your doctor to examine your abdominal organs and to evaluate the size and extent of any endometrial growths. In some cases, tissue samples may be removed and sent to a laboratory for microscopic examination.

Conventional treatment

The choice of treatment is guided by the extent of your symptoms, your age and your plans to have a family. For mild cases, your doctor may wish to simply wait and see how the disease progresses. The only treatment may be pain relief medication such as Aspirin or ibuprofen. Exercise, heat from a bath or heating pad, massage and relaxation may also help ease painful symptoms.

If a woman with endometriosis isn't planning to have children, hormone suppression treatment may be recommended. This involves taking a combination of drugs to prevent ovulation and limit the amount of estrogen that stimulates the endometrial growths. This will hopefully slow the growth of the misplaced tissue and minimize injury to surrounding organs. Drugs commonly prescribed include:

- **Birth control pills** to control irregular vaginal bleeding and diminish pain with a regulated, low-dose combination of estrogen and progesterone.

- **Progestins** to prevent ovulation and reduce estrogen levels.
- **Gonadotropin-releasing hormone (GnRH) agonists** (such as Lupron or Synarel) to create a temporary and reversible menopause by suppressing estrogen production by the ovaries. (Side effects include hot flashes, mood swings, headache, vaginal dryness and some bone loss.)
- **Danazol (danocrine)**, a synthetic testosterone, to reduce the production of estrogen from the ovaries and stop menstruation. (Possible side effects include water retention, weight gain, oily skin, muscle cramps, mood changes and hot flashes. Occasionally a rash, facial hair or deepening of the voice may occur, in which case this treatment should be stopped.)

For cases of moderate or severe endometriosis, surgery may be necessary. As much misplaced tissue as possible is removed, while preserving the woman's ability to have children by retaining the ovaries and uterus. This type of surgery usually provides only temporary relief of symptoms, since endometriosis recurs in most women.

A complete hysterectomy, which removes all reproductive organs, is considered only for women not planning to become pregnant and those who have severe pelvic pain that's not relieved by medication. After surgery, estrogen replacement therapy may be prescribed to counteract the menopausal symptoms that will develop.

Managing endometriosis

There's some evidence that diet therapy is as effective as hormonal suppression and more effective than surgery in reducing endometrial pelvic pain.[2] The nutritional approaches listed below are aimed at easing endometriosis-associated pain, improving fertility and minimizing the side effects of certain medications. Although these are neither cures for endometriosis nor stand-alone treatments for the condition, they can help women feel better.

DIETARY STRATEGIES
Essential fatty acids and omega-3 fats
Dietary fats are made up of building blocks called fatty acids. These fatty acids are incorporated into cell membranes, where they affect the integrity

and fluidity of the membrane. The body is able to make all but two fatty acids: linoleic and alpha-linolenic. Because these two are indispensable to health, they must be obtained from food and, therefore, are called essential fatty acids. The body uses these two essential fatty acids to produce hormone-like compounds called prostaglandins (PGs), which are sometimes referred to as eicosanoids.

Prostaglandins regulate our blood pressure, blood-clot formation, blood fats, immune compounds and hormones. They're produced by the lining of the uterus, by endometrial lesions and by immune compounds called macrophages. Researchers have learned that prostaglandin formation is altered in women with endometriosis. Studies have revealed that these women have significantly higher levels of prostaglandins compared to women who are free of endometriosis.[3-8] A high level of prostaglandins can alter the contractility of the uterus and Fallopian tubes, resulting in painful menstrual periods and infertility. Some of these PGs can enter the bloodstream and affect smooth muscle in other parts of the body. PGs can stimulate the gastrointestinal tract, causing it to contract in an uncontrolled manner.

The body makes different types of prostaglandins, which can either increase or decrease inflammation. In the case of endometriosis, two inflammatory prostaglandins called PGE and PGF appear to be involved. A diet that's high in fatty acids from animal foods and processed fat favours the production of prostaglandins that cause inflammation. A diet that's high in omega-3 fatty acids, such as those found in flaxseed oil, canola oil, walnuts, soybeans and fish, favours the formation of anti-inflammatory prostaglandins.

The balance of omega-6 to omega-3 oils in the diet is important for proper prostaglandin formation. The optimal ratio is thought to be 4:1, or four times the amount of omega-6 oils to omega-3 oils. It's estimated that we currently follow a diet that has over twenty times more omega-6 oils than omega-3 oils. That kind of imbalance will lead to a greater production of inflammatory PGs.

To achieve a better balance of omega-6 oils to omega-3 oils, practise the following:

- **Reduce the amount of animal fat in your diet.** Findings from Italian researchers revealed that women with the highest intakes of red meat are twice as likely to have endometriosis as women who consume the least.[9] Limit your intake of meat to once per week. Choose lean cuts of meat and poultry (e.g., flank steak, inside round, sirloin, eye of round, extra-lean ground beef, venison, centre-cut pork chops, pork tenderloin, skinless chicken breast, turkey breast, lean ground turkey). Choose 1% or skim milk, cheeses made with less than 20% milk fat and yogurt with less than 2% milk fat.

- **Avoid foods with trans fat.** This unhealthy fat is formed when manufacturers partially hydrogenate vegetable oils for commercial foods such as certain margarines, baked goods, snack foods and deep-fried fast foods. Read nutrition labels on food packages and choose foods that don't contain trans fat.
- **Add 1 to 2 tablespoons (15 to 30 ml) of flaxseed oil to your daily diet.** This oil is one of the richest sources of the omega-3 fatty acid called alpha-linolenic acid (ALA). Flaxseed oil is easily broken down by heat, so don't cook with it. If you want to add it to a hot dish such as pasta sauce, stir it in at the end of cooking. Use the oil in salad dressing and dip recipes. Store flaxseed oil in the fridge. You'll find flaxseed oil in the refrigerator section of health food stores and supermarkets. Supplements of flaxseed oil are also available. Keep in mind that it takes four capsules (4 grams) to give you a teaspoon of oil. It may be more convenient—and less expensive—to use the bottled oil.
- **Eat fatty fish at least two times a week.** Salmon, trout, sardines, Arctic char, herring and mackerel are the richest sources of the omega-3 fatty acids called DHA and EPA.

Fruit and vegetables

Women who report higher intakes of fruit and green vegetables have a lower risk of developing endometriosis.[10] It's speculated that natural compounds in fruit and vegetables, called flavonoids, might be responsible. These plant compounds have been shown to suppress a process called angiogenesis, the formation of new blood vessels from existing blood vessels. Uncontrolled angiogenesis is a major contributor to a number of diseases, including endometriosis.[11]

To increase your intake of flavonoids, include 7 to 10 daily servings of fruit and vegetables combined in your diet. (One serving is equivalent to 1 medium fruit, 1/4 cup/60 ml of dried fruit, 1/2 cup/125 ml of cooked or raw vegetables or 1 cup/250 ml of salad greens.) The best sources of flavonoids include berries, cherries, red grapes, apples, citrus fruit, broccoli, kale and onions.

Dietary fibre

Getting enough fibre each day is an important way to help regulate bowel habits and ease gastrointestinal symptoms of endometriosis. It's estimated that Canadians are getting roughly 14 grams of fibre each day, only one-half of the daily recommendation. Experts agree that a daily intake of 25 to 38 grams of dietary fibre is needed to reap its health benefits. Good food choices include whole-grain breads, breakfast cereals with at least 5 grams of fibre per serving (check the Nutrition Facts box), dried fruit, nuts and legumes. To add higher-fibre foods to your daily diet, see Chapter 1, page 29.

When adding fibre to your diet, gradually build up to the recommended 25 grams. Too much too soon can cause bloating, gas and diarrhea. Spread high-fibre foods out over the course of the day. And aim to drink a minimum of 8 ounces (250 ml) of fluid with each high-fibre meal and snack. To help you add more fibre to your daily diet, try the following:

- Strive for 7 or more servings of fruit and vegetables each day.
- Eat at least 5 servings of whole-grain foods each day.
- Buy high-fibre breakfast cereals. Aim for at least 5 grams of fibre per serving (check the nutrition information panel).
- Top your breakfast cereal with banana, berries or raisins.
- Add 2 tablespoons (30 ml) of natural wheat bran, oat bran or ground flaxseed to cereals, yogurt, casseroles and soup.
- Eat legumes more often—add white kidney beans to pasta sauce, black beans to tacos, chickpeas to salads, lentils to soup. Start with small portions to minimize gas.
- Add a few tablespoons of walnuts, soy nuts, sunflower seeds or raisins to salads.
- Reach for high-fibre snacks like popcorn, dried apricots or dates.

Probiotics

Research suggests that women with endometriosis may have bacterial or yeast overgrowth in their gastrointestinal tract, which may aggravate bloating, stomach pain, early satiety, diarrhea and/or constipation. In one study conducted at the Woman's Hospital of Texas in Houston, 40 out of 50 women studied had excessive levels of bacteria.[12]

The term *probiotic* literally means "to promote life" and refers to living organisms that, upon ingestion in certain numbers, improve microbial balance in the intestine and exert health benefits. Such friendly bacteria are known collectively as lactic acid bacteria and include *L. acidophilus, L. bulgaricus, L. casei, S. thermophilus* and bifidobacteria. The human digestive tract contains hundreds of strains of bacteria making up what is called the normal intestinal flora. Among the intestinal flora are lactic acid bacteria, which inhibit the growth of unfriendly, or disease-causing, bacteria by preventing their attachment to the intestine and by producing lactic acid and other antibacterial substances that suppress harmful bacteria. Numerous studies have shown that consuming probiotic foods or supplements increases the number of lactic acid bacteria in the intestinal tract. Lactic acid bacteria have been shown to help treat diarrhea and constipation and also to inhibit the growth of *Candida albicans*, the organism that causes yeast infections.

Lactic acid bacteria are found in fermented milk products. Include 1 serving of yogurt or kefir in your daily diet. See the section on probiotic supplements below.

PREBIOTICS. It's possible to eat foods that promote the growth of protective lactic acid bacteria in your intestinal tract. These foods are called prebiotics and contain components called fructo-oligosaccharides (FOSs). The human intestine doesn't digest FOSs; instead, they remain in the intestinal tract and feed lactic acid bacteria, supporting their growth. Good food sources include Jerusalem artichokes, asparagus, onions and garlic. A number of commercial food products found in grocery stores, such as breads, pasta and fruit and vegetable juices, contain inulin, a prebiotic isolated from chicory root.

Food sensitivities

Certain foods and spices may aggravate the bowel discomfort of endometriosis. To help you determine food sensitivities, keep a food and symptom diary over the course of at least one menstrual cycle. Record everything you eat, how much of the food you eat, when you eat and any symptoms you feel. If you're working with a consulting dietitian, he or she will use this tool to identify potential food culprits.

It can be difficult to detect foods that are causing you grief because a particular food may not bother you all the time. Sometimes it isn't what you ate but how much of the food or how quickly you ate, or how many aggravating foods you ate in one day or how much stress you were under at the time. Use your food diary to look for patterns, not just specific foods.

The following foods may cause intestinal problems in women with endometriosis:

- **Caffeine and alcohol.**
- **Artificial sweeteners.**
- **High-fat and/or high-calorie meals.** Both dietary fat and large meals have a greater stimulating effect on colon contractions.
- **Excessive sugar** from soft drinks, fruit drinks, candy and sweets.
- **Dairy products.** Some women don't produce enough of an enzyme called lactase in the intestinal tract. Lactase breaks down natural milk sugar or lactose. If lactose remains undigested in the intestinal tract, it causes bloating, gas and diarrhea. Women who have moderate lactose intolerance can usually tolerate yogurt, since it has less lactose than milk. Hard cheeses contain even less lactose. If you're symptomatic, try lactose-free milk or low-lactose yogurt. Alternatively, you can purchase Lactaid enzyme pills at the pharmacy; take a pill before a meal that contains dairy. Alternatives to dairy include calcium-fortified soy beverages.
- **Wheat.** In some women with endometriosis, bloating, distension and gas is caused by intolerance to wheat-based foods such as bread, bagels, muffins, pasta, ready-to-eat breakfast cereals and crackers, as well as baked goods made from wheat flour. If you're unsure whether wheat is causing your gas and bloating, try eliminating it from your diet for one month to see if your symptoms improve. Then, slowly add wheat back to your diet. As long as you have no adverse reaction, add one new wheat food every two days. If your symptoms recur, consider alternatives to wheat such as rice, rice pasta, rice crackers, quinoa, quinoa pasta, millet, potato, sweet potato, corn, 100% rye breads and oats. Natural food stores and many large grocery stores often stock many products—breakfast cereals, pasta, crackers, cookies and breads—that are made from wheat-free grains.
- **Raw vegetables.** Be sure to cook your vegetables; cooked vegetables are less likely to cause gas than raw vegetables. Vegetables that have a

414 Pelvic and Urinary Tract Health

greater potential to cause gas include bok choy, broccoli, Brussels sprouts, cabbage, cauliflower, kale, radishes, rutabaga, onions and raw garlic.

- **Legumes** such as kidney beans, chickpeas and black beans. Natural sugars called ogliosaccharides, found in dried peas, beans and lentils, often cause gas and bloating. To reduce potential symptoms, rinse canned beans before adding them to recipes and eat a smaller portion. You may also want to try Beano; available at pharmacies and health food stores, this natural enzyme breaks down ogliosaccharides so they can be absorbed in the intestinal tract.
- **Certain fruit**, such as berries, apple with the peel, melon and prunes.
- **Nuts and seeds.**
- **Spices** such as chili powder, curry, ginger, garlic and hot sauce.

Caffeinated beverages

A study from the Harvard School of Public Health found that women with endometriosis who consumed 5 to 7 grams of caffeine per month (one to two cups of coffee per day) had almost double the risk of not conceiving compared to women who didn't drink any caffeinated beverages.[13] This study suggests that caffeine may delay conception and therefore further aggravate fertility in women with endometriosis.

Women taking a gonadotropin-releasing hormone (GnRH) drug like Lupron (leuprolide) or Synarel (nafarelin) should limit their consumption of caffeine, because these drugs cause bone loss, as does caffeine. If you don't want to eliminate caffeine completely from your diet, ensure you're meeting your daily requirement of 1000 to 1500 milligrams of calcium.

Caffeine can also aggravate gastrointestinal symptoms. It can stimulate the intestinal tract and cause more frequent bowel movements and diarrhea.

Assess your current caffeine intake using the list of caffeine-containing beverages and foods in Chapter 1, page 11. Gradually cut back over a period of two to three weeks to minimize withdrawal symptoms such as headaches, tiredness or muscle pain. Switch to low-caffeine beverages like tea or hot chocolate or caffeine-free alternatives such as decaf coffee, herbal tea, cereal coffee, juice, milk or water.

Alcoholic beverages

When it comes to fertility, alcohol consumption should be minimized or avoided altogether. The same researchers from the Harvard School of

Public Health who investigated caffeine and conception in women with endometriosis examined the effect of alcohol.[14] They determined that women who consumed one or two drinks a day had a 60 percent higher risk of infertility compared to non-drinkers. And like caffeine, alcohol can also increase bowel discomfort.

VITAMINS AND MINERALS
Vitamin E
Some researchers theorize that oxidative damage caused by free radical molecules contributes to endometriosis by promoting the growth of endometrial tissue. Free radicals are highly reactive oxygen molecules produced by normal body processes, including the body's own inflammatory immune response. It's thought that damaged red blood cells and misplaced endometrial tissue signal the recruitment and activity of immune compounds in the abdominal cavity. In the process of engulfing foreign particles and protecting the body, these activated immune compounds generate harmful free radicals, which cause oxidation.

Studies conducted in women with endometriosis have shown that, in the fluid of the abdominal cavity, compounds called lipoproteins do indeed have lower levels of vitamin E, an important antioxidant.[15] Certain vitamins, minerals and natural plant chemicals have antioxidant properties that can protect cells in the body from damage caused by free radicals.

The best food sources of vitamin E include vegetable oils, nuts, seeds, soybeans, olives, wheat germ, whole grains and leafy green vegetables like kale. To supplement, take 200 to 400 international units (IU) of natural source vitamin E per day. If you have diabetes or coronary heart disease, avoid taking single supplements of vitamin E.

Calcium
If you're taking a GnRH drug such as Lupron (leuprolide) or Synarel (nafarelin), bone health is a concern. These drugs suppress estrogen production, resulting in accelerated bone loss. A review of studies of women taking GnRH drugs determined the average bone loss to be 1 percent per month or 6 percent in total.[16] If you compare that with an average bone loss of 3 percent in the first year of menopause, it seems considerable. Due to the negative effect of GnRH drugs on bone density, Health Canada limits its continuous use to six months. Ensure that you're meeting your daily requirement of 1000 to 1500 milligrams of calcium by choosing foods

listed in Chapter 1, page 15. If you're not meeting your daily targets for calcium, take a supplement. One serving of milk or calcium-fortified beverage (1 cup/250 ml) or plain yogurt (3/4 cup/175 ml) or cheese (1-1/2 ounces/45 g) supplies roughly 300 milligrams of calcium. If you require 1000 milligrams, your diet should provide 3 milk or milk alternative servings. For every serving you're missing and not making up with other calcium-rich foods, take a 300 milligram calcium citrate supplement. See Chapter 1 for information on calcium supplements.

Vitamin D

This nutrient is also critical for bone health. As well, vitamin D has anti-inflammatory effects in the body. The current recommended intake for adults is 1000 international units (IU) per day, an amount that can be achieved only by taking a supplement. (Many experts recommend 2000 IU per day.) To determine the dose of vitamin D you need to take, calculate how much you're already consuming from a multivitamin and calcium supplement and then make up the difference to reach your RDA. Vitamin D comes in 400 IU or 1000 IU doses. Choose a supplement made with vitamin D3 rather than vitamin D2; the former is more biologically active in the body. You'll find more information about vitamin D recommendations and supplements in Chapter 1, page 13.

OTHER NATURAL HEALTH PRODUCTS

Fish oil supplements

There's some evidence that taking fish oil reduces menstrual pain in women who suffer from endometriosis and dysmenorrhea.[17,18] (Dysmenorrhea is pain and discomfort associated with menstruation.) It's well established that the two omega-3 fatty acids found in fish oil, DHA and EPA, have anti-inflammatory effects in the body. To treat painful menstruation, a daily dose of fish oil supplying 1080 milligrams of EPA and 720 milligrams of DHA has been used. This dose of omega-3 fatty acids is best achieved by using a high-potency liquid fish oil supplement such as Carlson's MedOmega Fish Oil (1 teaspoon/5 ml provides 1200 milligrams of EPA and 1200 milligrams of DHA).

Probiotic supplements

If you don't eat dairy products, probiotic capsules or tablets are a good alternative. In fact, many health experts believe that taking a high-quality supplement is the only way to ensure that you're getting a sufficient number of friendly bacteria to the intestinal tract. Use the following guide when choosing a product:

- **Buy a product that offers 1 billion to 10 billion live cells per dose.** Taking more than this may result in gastrointestinal discomfort.
- **Choose a product that's stable at room temperature.** It's more convenient and, since it doesn't require refrigeration, you can continue taking your supplement while travelling.
- **Always take your supplement with food.** When eating a meal, the stomach contents become less acidic due to the presence of food. This allows live bacteria to withstand stomach acids and reach their final destination in the intestinal tract.

THE BOTTOM LINE...
Leslie's recommendations for managing endometriosis

1. To help your body produce friendly, non-inflammatory prostaglandins, choose healthy fats and oils in your diet. Reduce the amount of animal fat in your diet by selecting lean cuts of beef, poultry breast and low-fat dairy products. As much as possible, avoid foods with partially hydrogenated vegetable oils, a major source of trans fat. To boost your intake of omega-3 oils, supplement your diet with 1 or 2 tablespoons (15 to 30 ml) of flaxseed oil daily. For additional omega-3, eat fish two times a week and take a daily fish oil supplement.
2. To help ease bowel discomfort, gradually increase your intake of dietary fibre. Aim for a daily intake of 25 grams. Be sure to increase your water intake, too, since fibre needs fluid to work properly.
3. Eat 3/4 cup (175 ml) of yogurt each day for a dose of friendly lactic acid bacteria. If you don't eat fermented dairy products, consider taking a probiotic supplement each day. Look for a product that's stable at room temperature and provides 1 billion to 10 billion live cells per dose.
4. If you're trying to get pregnant, avoid caffeine-containing beverages, foods and medications. Cutting back on your caffeine intake may also reduce bowel discomfort.
5. Eliminate alcoholic beverages, as alcohol may reduce your chances of conceiving and aggravate diarrhea.

6. Keep a food and symptom diary to pinpoint trigger foods that you might be sensitive to.

7. Increase your intake of vitamin E, an antioxidant vitamin. Food sources include vegetable oils, nuts, seeds, soybeans, wheat germ, whole grains and leafy green vegetables. Consider supplementing your diet with 200 or 400 IU of a natural source vitamin E.

8. If you take a GnRH drug, make an extra effort to boost your intake of calcium and vitamin D. Aim for 1000 to 1500 milligrams of calcium and 1000 IU of vitamin D.

24
Interstitial cystitis (IC)

This chronic inflammatory condition of the bladder is very much a woman's disease—the vast majority of people who suffer with interstitial cystitis (IC) are female. Interstitial cystitis causes bladder pain, bladder pressure, the need to urinate urgently and frequently and, sometimes, pelvic pain. Some women with the disease feel only mild discomfort, while others suffer intense pain.

Although the symptoms are similar, interstitial cystitis is not a true urinary tract infection. Unlike common urinary tract infections, IC is resistant to conventional antibiotic therapy. Treatment usually involves medication to ease pain and reduce inflammation. Unfortunately, long-term therapy has had limited success in achieving a cure.

What causes interstitial cystitis?

The bladder, an important part of the urinary tract, is connected to the kidneys by two small tubes called ureters. The kidneys produce urine, and as urine accumulates, it flows through the ureters into the bladder, which acts as a storage tank for the fluid waste. The bladder gradually expands to hold a larger quantity of urine. When maximum bladder capacity is reached, urine is released into another tube, the urethra, where it flows out of the body in a process called urination.

In interstitial cystitis, small areas on the walls of the bladder become irritated by constant inflammation. This causes the bladder wall to become scarred and stiff, impairing its normal function. The inflammation can also cause the bladder to spasm, which can reduce its capacity to store urine, causing an urgent need to urinate. As the irritation becomes more pronounced, small spots of pinpoint bleeding, called glomerulations, develop on the bladder walls. In rare cases, ulcers appear behind the bladder lining.

The exact cause of this disabling disorder remains a mystery. Because the symptoms are varied, most experts believe interstitial cystitis represents a spectrum of disorders rather than one single disease. One theory suggests a defective defence barrier in the bladder lining is responsible. It's thought this protective layer of the bladder is "leaky," allowing toxins or infective agents in the urine to permeate the lining and irritate the bladder wall, triggering interstitial cystitis. Some researchers are investigating the possibility that reduced levels of protective compounds called glycosaminoglycans in the bladder wall cause this condition. It has also been speculated that interstitial cystitis is an autoimmune disorder and that the chronic inflammation is the body's response to an earlier bladder infection.

Symptoms

Fortunately, interstitial cystitis isn't a progressive disease and symptoms don't usually become worse over time. They may go into remission for extended periods, only to recur months or years later. Symptoms vary among individuals and even in the same person. The most common symptoms of interstitial cystitis include

- **Frequent urination.** Women with IC feel the urge to urinate more often, both during the day and at night. In mild cases, this may be the only symptom of the disorder. In severe cases, people with IC have been known to urinate up to sixty times a day.
- **Urgent urination.** Another symptom is the pressure to urinate immediately; this sensation may be accompanied by pain and bladder spasms.
- **Pain.** Women with IC feel mild to severe discomfort in the lower abdomen or vaginal area. IC makes sexual intercourse quite painful and sex drive may be reduced as a result.
- **Other disorders.** Muscle and joint pain, gastrointestinal discomfort, allergies and migraine headaches may also occur in some people with IC. There appears to be some unknown connection between IC and other chronic disease and pain disorders, such as fibromyalgia, lupus, endometriosis and irritable bowel syndrome.

Who's at risk?

Very little is known about the risk factors of interstitial cystitis, but research indicates that it's much more prevalent than was previously reported. Ninety percent of people with interstitial cystitis are women. Although the average age of onset is 40, interstitial cystitis can attack people at any age. It can affect men and children as well as women.

Diagnosis

The earlier a diagnosis is made, the better one's chances are of responding to medical treatment. Fortunately, IC isn't a progressive disease and symptoms don't usually become worse over time.

There's no definitive test that will identify IC. Because symptoms such as frequent, urgent urination and pelvic pain are similar to other urinary tract disorders, your doctor will rely on a process of elimination to arrive at a diagnosis of IC. He or she must first rule out the possibility that your symptoms are caused by another disorder, such as a urinary tract infection, bladder cancer, kidney disease, vaginal infection, sexually transmitted disease or endometriosis, to name just a few.

After taking a medical history and discussing your symptoms, your doctor will take a urine culture to determine if a bacterial infection exists. If your urine tests positive for bacteria, then you probably don't have IC; you're likely suffering from a urinary tract infection that can be treated with an antibiotic.

If no bacteria are found in your urine and you don't have any other disorder that could be causing your symptoms, your doctor will perform more tests to confirm a diagnosis of IC. The most reliable test for IC is a cystoscopy. Because this procedure can be quite uncomfortable, it's normally conducted under general anesthesia. Your doctor uses a cysto-scope, a hollow tube with a light and several lenses, to look inside your bladder and urethra. Your bladder is also stretched or distended with gas or some type of liquid. A cystoscopy detects bladder inflammation, a stiff, thick bladder wall and pinpoint bleeding.

In some instances, a biopsy of your bladder may be necessary. If this is the case, a sample of bladder tissue is removed during the cystoscopy and examined under a microscope. A biopsy helps your doctor confirm that you have IC and rules out the possibility of bladder cancer.

The very process of diagnosing IC can be therapeutic for some people. Distending the bladder to perform a cystoscopy occasionally improves symptoms, possibly because the process increases bladder capacity and interrupts pain signals.

Conventional treatment

At this time there's no cure for IC. Nor is there a single treatment that works effectively in all people who have the disease. Symptoms vary from individual to individual and may appear or disappear at random. Because scientists don't yet know what causes the disorder, treatment is aimed mainly at relieving symptoms.

One of the more effective treatments is the oral drug Elmiron (pentosan polysulphate sodium or PPS). This medication provides a protective lining to the bladder wall and is believed to repair the bladder wall's defence barrier. Symptoms may continue for some time after therapy with Elmiron has begun. Because sensory nerves in the bladder have been hyperactive, it takes time for the nerves to return to their normal state of activation—which is why doctors recommend continuing the drug for one year in cases of mild interstitial cystitis and for two years in severe cases before deciding if treatment is effective. Most people taking the medication improve within three months. Side effects of Elmiron may include upset stomach, diarrhea and hair loss, which disappear when the medication is discontinued.

Pain medications such as Aspirin and ibuprofen are helpful in treating the discomfort of IC. Sometimes antidepressants and antihistamines are prescribed to ease the chronic pain and psychological stress associated with IC. If pain is quite severe, narcotic drugs may be necessary to control symptoms.

Another treatment that can be effective is a bladder installation, or bladder wash. A solution of PPS, heparin or dimethyl sulphoxide (DMSO) is passed into the bladder and held for a few seconds or up to 15 minutes before being expelled. The washes are done regularly for six to eight weeks, usually in the doctor's office. They're thought to be effective because they reach the bladder tissue more directly, reducing inflammation and pain.

If all treatment methods have failed and your pain is severe, surgery may be considered. Various procedures, including removing bladder ulcers with a laser, enlarging the bladder with a piece of bowel or removing the bladder altogether, may help improve symptoms. Unfortunately, the results of these procedures can be unpredictable and many people continue to have symptoms even after the surgery.

Several alternative treatments have proven to ease the chronic pain of IC. Transcutaneous electrical nerve stimulators (TENS), which use mild electrical pulses to relieve daily discomfort, have produced good results for a small percentage of IC sufferers. TENS may work by increasing blood flow to the bladder, strengthening the pelvic muscles that control the bladder or triggering substances that block pain. Self-help techniques such as exercise, bladder retraining, biofeedback and stress reduction may reduce the severity and frequency of symptom flare-ups. Many people with IC have achieved success in controlling their symptoms with a program of diet modification.

Managing interstitial cystitis

DIETARY STRATEGIES

Food triggers

Many women with IC develop painful symptoms after eating certain foods. Once you know your trigger foods, eliminating them from the diet can help control symptoms and flare-ups. If you have IC, you've probably read through many lists of problematic foods that can cause you grief. The problem is that no two IC sufferers are alike when it comes to food sensitivities. Some of these foods may pose no problem at all for you, while others not on the list may irritate your bladder wall. Doctors compile food avoidance lists based on patient case histories. They should be used as a general guideline to help you pinpoint your triggers.

Below is a list of foods that have been reported as triggering pain in women with IC. Many of these foods are acidic and can irritate the bladder.

Food List for Women with Interstitial Cystitis (IC)

Preservatives & Additives
Avoid: artificial colours, aspartame (NutraSweet), benzol alcohol, citric acid, monosodium glutamate (MSG), saccharin, tyramine-containing foods including aged cheese, bananas, beer, brewer's yeast, chocolate, nuts, soy sauce, wine, yogurt

Fruit
Avoid: apples, citrus fruit, cantaloupe, cranberries, figs, grapes, guava, mango, nectarines, peaches, pineapple, plums, prunes, rhubarb, strawberries
Okay: melons (except cantaloupe), pears

Vegetables
Avoid: artichokes, asparagus, beet greens, beets, corn, dandelion greens, eggplant, mushrooms, parsley, peppers, pickles, purslane, raw onion, sauerkraut, spinach, sweet potato, Swiss chard, tomatoes, tomato-based sauces, turnip greens
Okay: homegrown tomatoes (tend to be less acidic), other vegetables

Meats & Fish
Avoid: aged, canned, cured, processed or smoked meats and fish; anchovies, caviar, chicken livers, corned beef, meats that contain nitrates or nitrites
Okay: Other meats, poultry, fish

Dairy products
Avoid: aged and natural cheeses, goat's milk, sour cream, yogurt
Okay: cottage cheese, frozen yogurt, milk

Grain foods
Avoid: yeast-based products such as leavened bread; barley, corn, oats, rye, wheat. Grain products are usually not well tolerated so try them in small quantities.
Okay: pasta, potatoes, rice, rice pasta

Legumes
Avoid: fava beans, lentils, lima beans, soybeans, tofu
Okay: all other beans

Nuts & Seeds
Avoid: most nuts
Okay: almonds, cashews, pine nuts

Eggs
Eggs may aggravate symptoms.

Herbs, Spices & Condiments
Avoid: BBQ sauce, cocktail sauce, hot sauce, ketchup, mayonnaise, miso, relish, salad dressing, salsa, soy sauce, spicy foods, vinegar, Worcestershire sauce
Okay: garlic and other seasonings

Beverages
Avoid: alcohol (especially beer and wine), carbonated drinks, coffee, cranberry juice, tea
Okay: bottled still (flat) water, decaffeinated coffee or tea, some herbal teas

Other
Avoid: caffeine (chocolate, especially dark chocolate; certain medications), diet pills, junk foods, tobacco, all vitamins that contain starch fillers

Painful symptoms often occur within four hours after eating, making it relatively easy to pinpoint problem foods. But sometimes symptoms don't appear until the following day. In these cases, identifying foods that trigger your condition can be challenging and frustrating.

Elimination/Challenge diet

The steps below outline an elimination diet for identifying food sensitivities:

1. ELIMINATION PHASE. For a period of two weeks, eat only foods identified above as Okay, unless you already know that one of these foods causes you bladder or pelvic pain.

   At the same time, keep a food and symptom diary. Record everything you eat, amounts eaten and what time you ate the food or meal. Document any symptoms, including the time of day you started to feel the symptom and its duration. You might want to grade your symptoms: 1 = mild, 2 = moderate, 3 = severe.

2. CHALLENGE PHASE. After two weeks, start introducing foods from the Avoid section. Do this gradually, introducing them one at a time. I recommend the following procedure for testing foods:

   Day 1: Introduce the food in the morning, at or after breakfast. If you don't experience symptoms, try that food again in the afternoon or with dinner.

   Day 2: Don't eat any of the test food. Follow your elimination diet. If you don't experience a reaction today, the food is considered safe and can be included in your diet. If you do experience a reaction to a tested food on Day 1 or 2, don't continue eating it and don't reintroduce any other foods until your symptoms have resolved.

   Day 3: If no symptoms occurred on Day 1 or 2, try the next food on your list, according to the above schedule.

   You may find that you can tolerate some foods if you eat them once every few days, but not if you eat them every day. You may also learn that some troublesome foods are better tolerated if eaten in small portions.

   Some people with interstitial cystitis have food allergies that contribute to their symptoms.[1] Allergies to wheat, corn, rye, oats and barley are common. If you suspect you have a food allergy, speak to your family doctor about allergy testing. The elimination diet outlined above will also help determine allergenic foods.

Determining which foods you need to stay away from can take time. I recommend you consult a registered dietitian in your community. Visit www.dietitians.ca to find a nutritionist in private practice who can work with you to plan a healthy diet for your condition.

Low-acid foods

Many of the foods in the Avoid section of the food list above are acidic and can cause bladder pain and urinary urgency in people with interstitial cystitis. If your list of troublesome foods leaves you little to eat, you might want to try a dietary supplement called Prelief (manufactured by AkPharma in the United States). This supplement reduces the acid in foods and beverages so that they don't have to be excluded from your diet. Two studies of more than 200 interstitial cystitis sufferers found that Prelief reduced the pain and discomfort associated with consuming foods such as pizza, tomatoes, spicy foods, coffee, fruit juices, alcohol and chocolate.[2,3]

The supplement is made of calcium glycerophosphate. It's available in tablet form to be taken with food or as granules that can be mixed into foods. The supplement isn't available in Canada but can be ordered directly from the manufacturer by calling 1-800-994-4711 or visiting www.akpharma.com. In the United Sates, it's sold in the antacid section of drugstores. It's important to use the correct amount of Prelief for the respective food; the company offers a free pocket guide to help you do this.

If eating a certain food brings on bladder symptoms, you can neutralize the acid in your urine by drinking a glass of water mixed with 1 teaspoon (5 ml) of baking soda. Practicing this as a precautionary measure—for example, when you're dining out and don't know all the ingredients in a dish—may also help prevent bladder irritation. To prevent a flare-up after eating, drink plenty of water to help dilute the urine.

OTHER NATURAL HEALTH PRODUCTS
L-arginine

Supplementing your diet with the amino acid L-arginine can help lessen symptoms of interstitial cystitis. Amino acids are the building blocks of protein. Twenty amino acids exist in high-protein foods like meat, poultry, fish, eggs and dairy products. L-arginine is considered a nonessential amino acid; that means we don't have to consume it from food because the body is usually able to make enough on its own. L-arginine is used to make an enzyme necessary for the formation of nitric oxide, a compound that relaxes the smooth muscle of the bladder. Research suggests that patients with interstitial cystitis have reduced levels of nitric oxide in their urine.[4] Women with a larger bladder capacity and/or a history of recurrent urinary infections may respond more favourably to this amino acid.

A handful of studies have found that 500 to 1500 milligrams of L-arginine taken orally can significantly reduce voiding discomfort, urinary frequency, lower abdominal pain and pelvic pain in as little as five weeks of treatment.[5–8]

Although our bodies make L-arginine and we consume it from protein-rich foods in our diet, a supplement is required to achieve an intake of 500 to 1500 milligrams per day.

L-arginine is available in certain health food and supplement stores. Pregnant and breastfeeding women are advised not to take L-arginine, as we lack information about its use during these times.

THE BOTTOM LINE...
Leslie's recommendations for managing interstitial cystitis

1. Determine which foods trigger symptoms and/or which foods you may be allergic to. Start by following an elimination diet for two weeks. Next, add potential trigger foods back to your diet one at a time. Keep a detailed food and symptom diary during the elimination and challenge phases of your diet.
2. If you find your list of comfortable foods is limited, or you really crave a food that brings on symptoms, try using Prelief, a dietary supplement that neutralizes the acid content of foods.
3. If you're dining out and aren't sure about ingredients used, take along Prelief or a little baking soda. Dissolve 1 teaspoon (5 ml) of baking soda in a glass of water and drink it right before you eat.
4. If you eat a food that triggers bladder pain and/or urinary frequency, drink plenty of water to dilute your urine.
5. Try L-arginine, an amino acid supplement. Take 500 to 1500 milligrams per day.

25

Urinary tract infections (UTIs)

Women experience the symptoms of a urinary tract infection (UTI) far more often than men. In fact, one in every two adult women will have a urinary tract infection at some time in her life. A UTI occurs in the urinary system, which is made up of the kidneys, ureters, bladder and urethra. An infection can occur in any part of the tract, but the majority arise in the bladder and urethra. Although distressing and uncomfortable, UTIs are easily cured and rarely have lasting complications if treated promptly. However, if left untreated, they can lead to potentially life-threatening problems. Early detection and treatment are essential to prevent a serious health risk.

What causes a urinary tract infection?

The role of the urinary system is to help the body eliminate waste products in the form of urine. The urinary process begins with the kidneys, which filter and remove waste products from the bloodstream. These waste products become urine, which flows from the kidneys through small tubes called ureters into the bladder. The bladder serves as a storage tank, collecting the urine until it can be eliminated. During urination, muscles in the bladder push urine out through the urethra, which has an opening on the outside of your body to discharge this fluid waste.

Normally, the urine that flows through the urinary tract system is sterile, which means that it doesn't contain bacteria. UTIs usually begin when bacteria enter the urethra and travel upwards through the urinary tract, producing inflammation and irritation. Most UTIs are caused by

Escherichia coli (E. coli) bacteria, which migrate into the urinary tract from the rectum or the vagina. On rare occasions, bacteria may enter the urinary tract through the bloodstream.

Subtle differences in the anatomy of the male and female urinary tract make women more prone than men to develop UTIs. In women, the opening of the urethra is very close to the opening of the rectum, or anus. Because of the close proximity of these two openings, bacteria can be easily transferred from the rectum into the urinary tract, causing infection. Also, the urethra is considerably shorter in women than in men, which allows the bacteria to reach the bladder much more easily. The final difference is that the female urethra is purely a urinary duct, whereas the male urethra also carries semen. It's thought that the male prostate gland secretes a bacteria-killing fluid into the urethra to protect the semen as it travels through this multifunctional passageway. This fluid may help prevent men from contracting UTIs.

The most common type of UTI is *cystitis*, which is an infection of the bladder. Cystitis may be accompanied by an inflammation of the urethra, a condition known as *urethritis*. Sexually transmitted diseases, such as herpes, chlamydia and gonorrhea, often cause urethritis in both men and women. If the infection is left untreated, bacteria travel farther into the urinary tract. In some cases, the infection may even attack the kidneys, which can cause permanent kidney damage if not treated promptly.

Symptoms

Any woman who has suffered through a UTI will tell you that it's a very uncomfortable condition and can make you feel quite miserable. One of the most recognizable symptoms of a UTI is a burning sensation when you urinate. You'll feel the burning either when you begin to urinate or when you're in the middle of urination. As the condition progresses, your urge to urinate may become stronger and more frequent. You may also notice that your urine has a strange odour and is cloudy, dark and even a little blood-tinged.

Sometimes a UTI may produce fever, chills and vomiting, or may cause pain in your back or in your lower abdominal area. It's very important that you not ignore these symptoms because they may indicate the beginning of a kidney infection, a serious complication of a UTI. Young children and elderly women are particularly prone to developing kidney infections.

Fortunately, most UTIs are uncomplicated and, if treated promptly, are easily cured in just a few days.

Who's at risk?

Sexually active girls and women are most often at risk for developing a UTI. During intercourse, friction can push bacteria from the anus into the urethra, initiating the cycle of infection. Women who use diaphragms or spermicidal agents for birth control are also at increased risk of UTIs.

Pregnant women are at high risk for developing a UTI. Approximately 4 percent to 7 percent of pregnant women contract a urinary tract infection, often in the first trimester. Pregnancy produces hormonal changes that affect the urinary system, increasing the likelihood of infection. The urinary tract is often dislodged from its normal position by pressure from the growing fetus, which further increases susceptibility. If you're pregnant and develop a UTI, especially during your third trimester, you should be treated promptly to prevent premature delivery, high blood pressure and other serious complications.

Urinary tract infections are also a common concern for elderly women. As women approach menopause, falling estrogen levels leave them prone to infections and irritations of the vagina and urinary tract. In rare cases, UTIs may be the result of anatomical problems, causing obstructions within the urinary tract.

Diagnosis

Because the symptoms are so well defined, most doctors are able to identify a UTI fairly easily. To confirm the diagnosis, a urine test will usually be required. An uncontaminated sample of your urine is collected and tested for bacteria. Persistent UTIs may require further testing with ultrasound, X-ray, bladder examination or dye testing to identify any underlying conditions that may prevent a full recovery from the infection.

Conventional treatment

In some cases, UTIs will clear up spontaneously, without any treatment. However, most are treated with antibiotics. The drugs may be given in a single, large dose or may be spread over three to seven days. A repeat infection is treated with a second round of antibiotics. Treatment normally continues until symptoms disappear and a urine test shows no bacteria.

Statistics indicate that the vast majority of women who have a UTI will get another one within eighteen months. Low daily doses of antibiotics for a six-month period or a single dose of antibiotic after sexual activity may prevent long-term problems. Post-menopausal women with recurrent UTIs may find some relief through estrogen replacement therapy, particularly estrogen creams that are applied to the vagina.

Preventing and managing urinary tract infections

PERSONAL HYGIENE

One of the most important methods of preventing a UTI is to practice good personal hygiene. To avoid spreading bacteria from the rectum into the urethra, wipe gently from front to back whenever you urinate or have a bowel movement. When you feel the urge to urinate, try not to resist. A regular release of fresh, sterile urine often washes harmful bacteria out of the urethra before it has a chance to travel into the urinary tract.

It's also a wise idea to clean your genital area before having intercourse, as this removes harmful bacteria that might be accidentally transferred into the urethra. Urinating before and after intercourse helps wash out any bacteria that have migrated into the urinary tract.

Bacteria grow best in a warm, moist environment. Wear cotton underwear or pantyhose with cotton liners for good ventilation. Avoid tight-fitting pants or other types of clothing that may trap heat, irritate tissues and promote bacterial growth. Washing your undergarments in strong soaps or bleach may cause irritations that could lead to a UTI. Avoid chemical irritants such as bubble bath, perfumed soaps, douches, feminine hygiene deodorants and deodorant tampons and pads.

DIETARY STRATEGIES

Aggravating foods

During your recovery period, avoid coffee, alcohol and spicy foods, which may aggravate the urinary tract. You may find that other foods can also exacerbate discomfort. See Chapter 24, Interstitial Cystitis, page 424, for a list of condiments and spices that can irritate the bladder; some of these may also aggravate UTIs.

Cranberry juice

The anti-infective properties of cranberries are attributed to compounds called anthocyanins. These phytochemicals "wrap" around the UTI *Escherichia coli* (*E. coli*) bacteria and prevent it from adhering to the urinary tract wall. However, cranberry doesn't seem to have the ability to release bacteria that have already adhered to urinary tract cells. Studies in the lab suggest that fructose in cranberries might also contribute to the berry's anti-infective action.

Clinical research has demonstrated that, compared to a placebo, drinking 300 millilitres of (Ocean Spray) cranberry juice cocktail daily significantly reduced the risk of recurrent urinary tract infections in elderly women. Studies have also found that drinking 16 ounces (500 ml) of cranberry juice cocktail daily reduces the amount of bacteria found in the urine and urinary tract infections in pregnant women.[1-4]

For preventing UTIs, drink 10 to 16 ounces (300 to 500 ml) of cranberry juice cocktail daily. To avoid the extra sugar calories, use 2 tablespoons (30 ml) of pure cranberry juice once or twice daily. Alternatively, a cranberry capsule can be taken (see below).

Cranberry is usually well tolerated. However, in very large doses, for example, 12 to 16 cups (3 to 4 L) of juice per day, cranberry can cause stomach upset and diarrhea. Nausea, vomiting and diarrhea have also been reported in pregnant women who drank 16 ounces (500 ml) of cranberry juice cocktail daily, the equivalent of about 1/2 cup (125 ml) of pure cranberry juice.

Blueberries

Anthocyanins, the same compounds found in cranberries that prevent *E. coli* bacteria from adhering to the wall of the urinary tract, are also abundant in blueberries. Reports from Rutgers, The State University of New Jersey suggest that blueberries also promote urinary tract health. If you don't like cranberry juice, or you want variety, add 1/2 to 1 cup (125 to 250 ml) of fresh, frozen or dried blueberries to your daily diet. Blueberry concentrate is also available in grocery and natural food stores and can be added to water.

Blueberries are available fresh, frozen and dried year-round. Here are a few tips to add blueberries to your diet:

- Add frozen blueberries to a breakfast smoothie.
- Toss dried blueberries into your morning bowl of cold cereal, or mix them into oatmeal.
- Add dried blueberries to a green salad, then toss with a raspberry vinaigrette.
- Thaw frozen berries and mix into yogurt, or use them to top a scoop of low-fat ice cream.
- Use dried or frozen blueberries in baked goods like muffins and loaves.

Water
Drink at least 9 cups (2.2 L) of water each day to help flush bacteria out of your system. Women who engage in vigorous exercise should drink 12 to 16 cups (3 to 4 L) per day. Drink 1 to 2 cups (250 to 500 ml) with each meal and snack. If you engage in moderate or vigorous exercise, drink an additional 4 cups (1 L) of water each day. Carry a water bottle with you when you travel.

HERBAL REMEDIES
Cranberry extract
If you don't want to consume the sugar and calories found in cranberry cocktail, you might consider taking capsules of dried cranberry, available at health food stores and pharmacies. Take a 400 milligram capsule twice daily—the equivalent of 300 ml or a little over 1 cup of cranberry juice.

Garlic (Allium sativum)
A daily intake of garlic can help the body fight bacterial infection. Studies have shown that garlic, in particular the allyl sulphur compounds in aged garlic extract, stimulates the body's immune system by increasing the activity of white blood cells that fight infection.[5-7]

Scientists agree that one-half to one clove of fresh garlic consumed each day offers health benefits. And most people can take one or two cloves a day without any side effects such as gastrointestinal upset. Add fresh garlic to salad dressings, pasta sauces and stir-fries.

The oil-soluble compounds in fresh garlic account for its odour and its potential to cause stomach upset. If you decide to supplement instead of eating fresh garlic, buy an aged garlic extract. This form of garlic has the highest concentration of the sulphur compounds that boost the immune system. Aged garlic extract is also odourless and gentler on the stomach. Take two to six capsules per day, in divided doses. Since both fresh garlic and garlic supplements can thin the blood, consult your physician if you're taking blood-thinning medication such as warfarin (Coumadin).

OTHER NATURAL HEALTH PRODUCTS
Probiotic supplements

Once consumed, friendly bacteria such as *Lactobacillus* and *Bifidobacterium* produce lactic acid and hydrogen peroxide, compounds that suppress the growth of *E. coli* in the intestinal tract. Research has demonstrated that these bacteria prevent *E. coli* from attaching to the lining of the intestine and of the vagina.[8-10] Studies have also found that probiotics, especially strains of *Lactobacillus*, can reduce the recurrence of UTIs in women.[11,12] As well, probiotics have been demonstrated to enhance the body's immune system.

If you're taking an antibiotic for your UTI, consider adding a probiotic supplement to your treatment regime. Antibiotics kill all bacteria—friendly and disease-causing. Taking a probiotic supplement while on antibiotic therapy may lessen the chances of a repeat infection and decrease gastrointestinal upset caused by the drug. To prevent antibiotic medication from killing a significant number of probiotic bacteria in the supplement, take antibiotics and probiotic supplements two hours apart.

The strength of a probiotic supplement is expressed in the number of live bacteria cells per capsule. To treat a UTI, take 1 billion to 10 billion live cells daily, in three divided doses. Take your supplement with a meal. Probiotic supplements may cause flatulence, which usually subsides as you continue treatment. There are no safety issues associated with taking these supplements.

In addition to taking a supplement, add probiotic foods such as yogurt and kefir to your daily diet.

THE BOTTOM LINE...

Leslie's recommendations for managing urinary tract infections (UTIs)

1. If you're experiencing a UTI, avoid foods and beverages that can irritate your urinary tract—coffee, alcoholic beverages and spicy foods are a few examples.
2. To prevent or treat an existing UTI, drink at least 10 to 16 ounces (300 to 500 ml) of cranberry juice each day.
3. If you want a change from cranberry juice, add 1/2 to 1 cup (125 to 250 ml) of blueberries to your diet.
4. If you're leery about the sugar, excess calories or artificial sweeteners in cranberry juice, try capsules of cranberry extract. Take 400 milligrams twice daily.
5. To help flush bacteria from your urinary tract, drink at least 9 cups (2.2 L) of water each day. If you exercise regularly, add an extra 4 cups (1 L) of fluid to your daily intake.
6. To give your immune system a hand in fighting off a UTI, add garlic to your nutrition regime. If you decide to supplement, take one or two aged garlic extract capsules with meals.
7. If you're looking for added protection from infection-causing *E. coli* bacteria, take a probiotic supplement with your meals. Take 1 billion to 10 billion live cells daily, in three divided doses. Add probiotic foods such as yogurt and kefir to your daily diet.

26
Ovarian cancer

Ovarian cancer is the seventh most common cancer among women world-wide. In Canada, 2500 women were diagnosed with it in 2009. Over her lifetime, a woman has a 1.4 percent chance of developing ovarian cancer, a disease that's usually fatal. Sadly, an estimated 1750 Canadian women died from the disease in 2009.

Until recently, a diagnosis of ovarian cancer was akin to a death sentence because the disease typically wasn't found until it had spread to other parts of the body. Although only one in five women are diagnosed before the cancer has spread, recent studies indicate that women may experience symptoms early in the disease, prompting earlier detection and treatment. If diagnosed at an early stage, the chances of survival are much improved.

What causes ovarian cancer?

The ovaries are two small reproductive organs located in a woman's pelvis. The ovaries make the female hormones estrogen and progesterone and each month release an egg that travels down one of the two Fallopian tubes to the uterus where it may be fertilized by a sperm. If the egg isn't fertilized, it's shed as part of your monthly period. At menopause, a woman's ovaries stop releasing eggs and produce significantly lower levels of female hormones.

Ovarian cancer begins in the cells that make up the ovary or ovaries. When cells grow out of control, they can form a mass of tissue called a tumour, which can be benign (non-cancerous) or malignant (cancerous). There are three main types of ovarian cancer.

1. **Epithelial cancer**, the most common type, starts in the cells that line the ovaries.
2. **Germ cell tumours** occur in the egg-producing cells of the ovary and typically strike younger women.
3. **Stromal tumours** develop in the estrogen- and progesterone-producing connective tissue that holds the ovaries together.

Malignant ovarian tumours can spread, or metastasize, to other areas of the body. An ovarian tumour can grow and invade organs next to the ovaries, such as the uterus and Fallopian tubes. Cancer cells can also break off, or shed, from the main ovarian tumour and cause new tumours to develop on the surface of nearby organs and tissues. As well, cancer cells can spread through the body's lymphatic system to lymph nodes in the pelvis, abdomen and chest. (Your lymphatic system is an interconnected system of spaces and vessels between tissues and organs through which lymph—a body fluid containing mainly white blood cells—circulates throughout the body.) Finally, cancer cells may spread through the blood-stream to the liver and lungs.

The exact cause of ovarian cancer remains unclear. It's thought a defect in the tissue-repair process that follows the monthly release of an egg from the ovary into the Fallopian tube may be responsible. Faulty repair of ovarian tissue over the years of a woman's reproductive cycle may initiate the formation of a tumour. It's also possible that rising hormone levels before and during ovulation may stimulate the growth of abnormal cells.

Another theory proposes that cancer-causing substances enter the body through the vagina and pass through the uterus and Fallopian tubes to reach the ovaries. This might explain the finding that tubal ligation and hysterectomy reduce the risk of ovarian cancer; removing the uterus or blocking the Fallopian tubes prevents harmful substances from reaching the ovaries.

Other researchers speculate that male hormones (androgens) can cause ovarian cancer.

Who's at risk?

Women with certain risk factors may be more likely than others to develop ovarian cancer. Current evidence suggests the following factors may increase a woman's risk of getting ovarian cancer:

- **Inherited gene mutations.** The most predictive risk factor for developing ovarian cancer is having an inherited (hereditary) mutation in one of two genes—breast cancer gene 1 (BRCA1) or breast cancer gene 2 (BRCA2). Women with the BRCA1 mutation have a 35 percent to 70 percent higher risk of ovarian cancer compared to women without this mutation. For women with the BRCA2 mutation, the risk of ovarian cancer is increased by up to 30 percent. Keep in mind, however, that inherited gene mutations account for a very, very small proportion of ovarian cancer cases.
- **Family history.** Women who have a mother, daughter or sister with ovarian cancer have a 10 percent to 15 percent increased risk for the disease. Women with a family history of breast, uterine or colorectal cancer may also have a higher risk of ovarian cancer.
- **Personal history of cancer.** If you have had breast cancer, you have a higher likelihood of developing ovarian cancer.
- **Age.** Ovarian cancer is rare in women under 40 years of age. It typically occurs after menopause and is most often diagnosed in women over the age of 55.
- **Never pregnant.** Older women who have never been pregnant have an increased risk for the cancer. Women who have had at least one pregnancy are thought to have a lower risk.
- **Hormone replacement therapy (HRT).** Some research suggests that use of estrogen only (estrogen without progesterone) for more than five years increases the risk of ovarian cancer.
- **Use of fertility drugs.** Some research indicates that use of the fertility drug clomiphene citrate (Clomid) for longer than one year may increase the risk of ovarian tumours. Fertility drugs appear to increase the risk of a type of tumour called "low malignant potential." The risk seems to be highest for women who didn't get pregnant while on the drug.
- **Obesity.** Evidence indicates that women who are obese have a greater risk of developing ovarian cancer. Obesity is also associated with more aggressive ovarian cancers.

Symptoms

Warning signs in the early stages of ovarian cancer are often vague and very mild. Symptoms, which usually develop as the cancer advances, may include

- abdominal discomfort or pain: swelling or bloating; a sense of pressure in the pelvic area
- pain in the lower back or legs
- digestive discomfort: bloating; feeling full after a small meal; heartburn; gas; belching; indigestion; nausea
- change in bowel habits: constipation; a sense that the bowel hasn't completely emptied after a bowel movement

Less common symptoms include fatigue, feeling the need to urinate frequently, abnormal menstrual periods and bleeding after menopause. Recognizing the symptoms of ovarian cancer and getting regular checkups are the best ways to detect ovarian cancer as early as possible. The sooner symptoms are reported to your doctor, the sooner a diagnosis and treatment plan can be made.

Diagnosis

If you have a symptom that suggests ovarian cancer, your doctor will discuss your personal health and family medical history with you and will conduct a physical exam of your abdomen and pelvis. Your doctor may also order a blood test for CA-125, a substance found on the surface of ovarian cancer cells and some normal cells. An elevated CA-125 level indicates a greater likelihood of ovarian cancer; other tests will be conducted to confirm a diagnosis.

Your doctor may order a pelvic ultrasound, which aims sound waves at the pelvis to create a picture that may show an ovarian tumour. For a better picture, the ultrasound device may be inserted into the vagina (transvaginal ultrasound).

If the blood test and ultrasound results suggest the possibility of cancer, surgery is usually necessary for a biopsy in order to make a definite diagnosis. (A biopsy involves removing cells from the body and checking them under a microscope.) Samples of tissue and fluid are removed during a laparoscopy or laparotomy. In a laparoscopy, a thin, flexible tube equipped with a light and camera is inserted through a small cut near the belly button. A laparotomy is used both to diagnose and treat ovarian cancer. If cancer is found during a biopsy procedure, your doctor will remove as much of the cancer as possible.

An imaging test, such as a CT scan or MRI, may also be ordered to determine whether the cancer has spread.

Treatment

A woman's overall health and the stage of her cancer determines the best treatment plan. Your doctor will describe your treatment options and the expected outcome for each. Treatment for ovarian cancer may include a combination of surgery, chemotherapy and radiation. Most women have surgery and chemotherapy; rarely is radiation used. Chemotherapy kills cancer cells in the pelvis, in the abdomen or throughout the body. Since cancer treatments often damage healthy cells and tissues, side effects are common. Before treatment starts, it's important to be informed about possible side effects and how to manage them.

Preventing ovarian cancer

DIETARY STRATEGIES

Weight control

Growing evidence indicates that maintaining a healthy weight after menopause helps lower the risk of developing ovarian cancer, particularly if you never used hormone replacement therapy (HRT). In a study published in 2009, researchers from the U.S. National Cancer Institute followed 94,525 healthy women aged 50 to 71 over a seven-year period and found a strong link between obesity and ovarian cancer. Among women who had never taken HRT, having a body mass index (BMI) of 30 or greater was associated with an almost 80 percent greater risk of ovarian cancer.[1] Scientists believe that obesity may enhance ovarian cancer risk through a hormonal mechanism. Excess body fat in post-menopausal women leads to an increased production of estrogen, which in turn may stimulate the growth of ovarian cells.

Research also suggests that carrying excess weight may increase the risk of aggressive forms of ovarian cancer. In a study conducted among 300,537 post-menopausal women who were followed for sixteen years, women who were overweight (BMI of 25 to 29.9) and obese (BMI of 30 or greater) were significantly more likely to die from ovarian cancer than were women with a BMI of less than 25. The increased the risk of ovarian cancer associated with obesity was limited to women who had never used HRT.[2]

Although most cases of ovarian cancer occur in women over the age of 55, it's still critical to control your weight before menopause. A study from the Netherlands found that premenopausal women considered obese had a 28 percent increased risk of ovarian cancer compared to their healthy-weight peers.[3]

Cancer experts advise maintaining your weight within a healthy body mass index throughout adulthood to reduce your risk for a number of cancers. Steps should be taken to avoid adult weight gain, especially after menopause. If you are overweight or have gained excess weight since menopause, I strongly advise that you take action to lose weight. Start by determining your body mass index (see Chapter 2, page 37). You'll also find plenty of strategies in that chapter that will help you successfully lose excess weight.

Carbohydrates: Low glycemic index

Research suggests that high-glycemic diets increase the risk of ovarian cancer, and the risk may be even greater among obese women.[4] The glycemic index (GI) is a scale that ranks carbohydrate-rich foods by how quickly they are digested and raise blood sugar compared to pure glucose. Foods that are ranked high on the GI scale are fast acting—they're digested quickly and, as a result, cause sharp rises in blood sugar and insulin, the hormone that removes sugar from the blood and stores it in cells. Examples include white bread, whole-wheat bread, baked potatoes, refined breakfast cereals, instant oatmeal, cereal bars, raisins, ripe bananas, carrots, honey and sugar. It's thought that high insulin levels may increase the risk of ovarian cancer; insulin may affect ovarian cells directly or stimulate the growth of cancerous cells.

Foods with a low GI release sugar more slowly into the bloodstream and don't produce an outpouring of insulin. Examples include grainy breads with seeds, steel-cut oats, 100% bran cereals, oat bran, brown rice, sweet potato, pasta, apples, citrus fruit, grapes, pears, legumes, nuts, milk, yogurt and soy milk.

In general, whole grains, bran cereals, legumes, fruit and vegetables have a low glycemic index. Include at least one low-GI food per meal, or base two of your meals on low-GI choices. Use salad dressings made from vinegar or lemon juice—the acidity results in a further reduction in the GI of your meal. Choose fruit that's more acidic (e.g., oranges, grapefruit, cherries, strawberries, green apples) as these have a low GI.

See Chapter 5, page 93, for a list of selected foods and their corresponding glycemic-index value.

Dairy products and lactose

Based on the observation that ovarian cancer rates are higher in parts of the
world that consume the most milk, researchers have proposed that lactose,
the natural sugar in dairy products, may increase the risk of ovarian cancer.
Findings from studies have been varied but do suggest that high intakes of
dairy foods are linked with a greater risk of ovarian cancer. In a study of
61,084 post-menopausal women living in Sweden, those who consumed
4 or more daily servings of dairy products had twice the risk of ovarian
cancer compared to women who consumed less than 2 servings per day. A
high dairy intake increased the risk of serous ovarian cancer, but not other
subtypes. (Serous tumours are the most common type of epithelial ovarian
tumour and typically occur in women aged 40 to 60. Roughly 50 percent
of serous tumours are malignant.) Milk was the dairy product that had the
strongest association with ovarian cancer.[5]

Another study revealed that women who consumed the most lactose had
a twofold higher risk of serous ovarian cancer than women who consumed
the least. For each 11 gram increase in lactose consumed (the amount in an
8 ounce/250 ml glass of milk), the researchers observed a 20 percent increase
in risk of the cancer. Skim and low-fat milk were the biggest contributors to
lactose in the diet of these women. Women who consumed 1 or more
servings of milk daily had a 32 percent higher risk of developing any type of
ovarian cancer.[6] When researchers combined the results of three large
studies, they found a significant positive association between all dairy foods,
low-fat milk and lactose and the risk of ovarian cancer.[7]

It's thought that the breakdown product of lactose, a sugar called galactose, may impact the ovaries. Galactose, whose main food source is lactose,
may be toxic to the ovaries. Galactose also stimulates the secretion of
certain hormones that may lead to ovarian cancer.

If you're at increased risk for ovarian cancer, avoid consuming large
quantities of milk. Although studies haven't proven that milk increases
ovarian cancer risk, the findings suggest it's wise to limit your intake of
low-fat milk to less than 2 servings (2 cups/500 ml) per day. Be sure,
however, to make up for any calcium you'll be missing from your diet.
Replace milk with a calcium-fortified soy beverage. Take a calcium supplement once or twice daily to ensure you're meeting your daily calcium

requirements of 1000 or 1500 milligrams, depending on your age. See Chapter 1, page 15, for more information about calcium in foods and calcium supplements.

Flavonoids

Emerging evidence suggests that a high intake of these naturally occurring plant chemicals is protective from ovarian cancer. It's thought that flavonoids help reduce the risk of ovarian cancer by altering reactions inside cells that lead to cancer development. Flavonoids also act as antioxidants in the body and protect cells from the harmful effect of free radicals.

There are many different flavonoids in foods, and studies have linked a few with protection from ovarian cancer. In one study, women who had the highest intake of a flavonoid called apigenin had a 21 percent lower risk of the cancer than women with the lowest intake.[8] Another study found that isoflavones and flavonols were protective.[9] A study of 66,940 American women revealed that those who had the highest intake of a particular flavonol called kaempferol were 40 percent less likely to develop ovarian cancer compared to women who consumed the least.[10]

To help reduce your risk of ovarian cancer, add the following flavonoid-rich foods to your diet:

Apigenin	Isoflavones	Flavonols & Kaempferol
Celery	Legumes	Broccoli
Hot peppers	Soy foods	Green onions
Parsley	Soybeans	Kale
Thyme		Yellow onions
		Apples
		Berries
		Tea

VITAMINS AND MINERALS

Folate

Meeting your daily requirement for the B vitamin folate may lower the risk of ovarian cancer, especially if you drink alcohol. A Canadian study of 49,613 women found that a high intake of folate was associated with a

25 percent lower risk of ovarian cancer. Folate-rich foods were also protective from cancer in women who consumed at least one alcoholic drink per day.[11] Another study reported that, overall, dietary folate was weakly protective from ovarian cancer. But when the researchers factored alcohol intake into their analysis, they found that folate offered a strong protective effect. Among women who consumed more than one drink per day, those whose diets provided the most folate were 73 percent less likely to develop ovarian cancer compared to women who consumed the least folate.[12]

Folate's critical role in repairing DNA, the genetic material inside every cell, makes it a cancer-fighting nutrient. Alcohol interferes with the metabolism of folate in the body, inhibiting the ability of cells to repair faulty genes.

Your daily requirement for folate is 400 micrograms. The richest food sources include cooked spinach, lentils, black beans, asparagus, avocados and oranges. In Canada, white flour, white pasta and enriched cornmeal are fortified with folic acid, the synthetic form of this B vitamin. Use the table in Chapter 1, page 19, to increase your intake of folate-rich foods.

THE BOTTOM LINE...
Leslie's recommendations for preventing ovarian cancer

1. Follow a healthy diet, practice portion control and exercise regularly to prevent adult weight gain, especially after menopause. If you're overweight, take action to lose weight. Aim for a body mass index of between 20 and 25.

2. Make sure your diet emphasizes low-glycemic carbohydrates such as grainy bread, large-flake oatmeal, brown rice, pasta, legumes, sweet potato, apples, pears and citrus fruit. Limit your intake of refined flour products that spike your blood glucose and insulin.

3. If you're at an increased risk for ovarian cancer, limit your intake of low-fat milk to less than 2 daily servings. Replace milk on cereal and in smoothies and lattes with calcium-fortified soy milk. Supplement your diet with calcium to ensure that you're meeting your daily requirements for the mineral.

4. Add foods rich in cancer-fighting flavonoids, like legumes, kale, broccoli, celery, berries and tea, to your daily diet.

5. Eat foods every day that are a good source of the B vitamin folate to help keep the DNA of your cells in good repair. Make a special effort to increase your folate intake if you drink alcohol.

References

Introduction

1. Kuhnlein, HV, et al. Dietary nutrient profiles of Canadian Baffin Island Inuit differ by food source, season, and age. *J Am Diet Assoc* Feb 1996; 96(2):155–162.
2. Godel, JC, et al. Iron status and pregnancy in a northern Canadian population: Relationship to diet and iron supplementation. *Can J Public Health* Sept–Oct 1992; 83(5):339–343.
3. Adult obesity in Canada: Measured height and weight. Statistics Canada, November 2008. Available at www.statcan.gc.ca/pub/82-620-m/2005001/article/adults-adultes/8060-eng.htm.
4. Gray-MacDonald, K, et al. Food habits of Canadians: Reduction of fat intake over a generation. *Can J Public Health* Sept–Oct 2000; 91(5):381–385.

Part 1: Nutrition Essentials for Women

2   Strategies for Weight Control

1. Hollis, JF, CM Gullion, VJ Stevens, PJ Brantley, LJ Appel, JD Ard, CM Champagne, A Dalcin, TP Erlinger, K Funk, D Laferriere, PH Lin, CM Loria, C Samuel-Hodge, WM Vollmer, LP Svetkey; Weight Loss Maintenance Trial Research Group. Weight loss during the intensive intervention phase of the weight-loss maintenance trial. *Am J Prev Med* 2008; 35(2):118–126.
2. McGuire, MT, et al. Behavioural strategies of individuals who have maintained long-term weight losses. *Obes Research* 1999; 7(4):334–341.
3. Ibid.

Part 2: Low Energy Levels, Fatigue and Pain

3   Anemia

1. Cole, BF, JA Baron, RS Sandler, RW Haile, DJ Ahnen, RS Bresalier, G McKeown-Eyssen, RW Summers, RI Rothstein, CA Burke, DC Snover, TR Church, JI Allen, DJ Robertson, GJ Beck, JH Bond, T Byers, JS Mandel, LA Mott, LH Pearson, EL Barry, JR Rees, N Marcon, F Saibil, PM Ueland, ER Greenberg; Polyp Prevention Study Group. Folic acid for the prevention of colorectal adenomas: A randomized clinical trial. *JAMA* 2007; 297(21):2351–2359.
2. Figueiredo, JC, MV Grau, RW Haile, et al. Folic acid and risk of prostate cancer: Results from a randomized clinical trial. *J Natl Cancer Inst* 2009; 101(6):432–435.
3. Kuzminski, AM, et al. Effective treatment of cobalamin deficiency with oral cobalamin. *Blood* Aug 15, 1998; 92(4):1191–1198.

4   Chronic Fatigue Syndrome (CFS)

1. Schluederberg, A, et al. NIH conference. Chronic fatigue syndrome research: Definition and medical outcome assessment. *Ann Intern Med* Aug 15, 1992; 117(4):325–331.
2. Sibbald, B. Chronic Fatigue Syndrome comes out of the closet. *CMAJ* 1998; 159:537–541.
3. U.S. Department of Health and Human Services. *The Facts about Chronic Fatigue Syndrome* (Atlanta, GA: March 1995).
4. Hobday, RA, S Thomas, A O'Donovan, et al. Dietary intervention in chronic fatigue syndrome. *J Hum Nutr Diet* 2008; 21(2):141–149.
5. Gray, JB, and AM Martinovic. Eicosanoids and essential fatty acid modulation in chronic disease and the chronic fatigue syndrome. *Med Hypotheses* 1994; 43(1):32–42.
6. Puri, BK, J Holmes, and G Hamilton. Eicosapentaenoic acid-rich essential fatty acid supplementation in chronic fatigue syndrome associated with symptom remission and structural brain changes. *Int J Clin Prac* 2004; 58(3):297–299.
7. Puri, BK. The use of eicosapentaenoic acid in the treatment of chronic fatigue syndrome. *Prostaglandins Leukot Essent Fatty Acids* 2004; 70(4):399–401.
8. Heap, LC, et al. Vitamin B status in patients with chronic fatigue syndrome. *J R Soc Med* 1999; 92(4):183–185.
9. Regland, B, et al. Increased concentrations of homocysteine in the cerebrospinal fluid in patients with fibromyalgia and chronic fatigue syndrome. *Scand J Rheumatol* 1997; 26(4):301–307.
10. Werbach, MR. Nutritional strategies for treating chronic fatigue syndrome. *Altern Med Rev* 2000; 5(2):93–108.

11. Jacobson, W, et al. Serum folate and chronic fatigue syndrome. *Neurology* 1993; 43(12):2645–2647.

12. Moorkens, G, et al. Magnesium deficit in a sample of the Belgian population presenting with chronic fatigue syndrome. *Magnes Res* 1997; 10(4):329–337.

13. Cox, IM, et al. Red blood cell magnesium and chronic fatigue syndrome. *Lancet* 1991; 337(8744):757–760.

14. Manuel y Keenoy, B, G Moorkens, J Vertommen, et al. Magnesium status and parameters of the oxidant-antioxidant balance in patients with chronic fatigue: Effects of supplementation with magnesium. *J Am Col Nutr* 2000; 19(3):374–382.

15. See, DM, et al. In vitro effects of Echinacea and ginseng on natural killer and antibody-dependent cell cytotoxicity in healthy subjects and chronic fatigue syndrome or acquired immunodeficiency syndrome patients. *Immunopharmacology* 1997; 35(3):229–235.

16. Scaglione, F, et al. Immunodulatory effects of two extracts of Panax ginseng C.A. Meyer. *Drugs Exp Clin Res* 1990; 16(10):537–542.

17. Hartz, AJ, S Bentler, R Noyes, et al. Randomized controlled trial of Siberian ginseng for chronic fatigue. *Psychol Med* 2004; 34(1):51–61.

18. Behan, PO, et al. Effects of high doses of essential fatty acids on the postviral fatigue syndrome. *Acta Neurol Scand* 1990; 82(3):209–216.

19. Warren, G, et al. The role of essential fatty acids in chronic fatigue syndrome: A case-controlled study of red-cell membrane essential fatty acids (EFA) and a placebo-controlled treatment study with high dose of EFA. *Acta Neurol Scand* 1999; 99(2):112–116.

20. Plioplys, AV, and S Plioplys. Serum levels of carnitine in chronic fatigue syndrome: Clinical correlates. *Neuropsychobiology* 1995; 32(3):132–138.

21. Kuratsune, H, et al. Acylcarnitine deficiency in chronic fatigue syndrome. *Clin Infec Dis* 1994; 18(Suppl 1):S62–S67.

22. Malaguarnera, M, MP Garganet, E Cristaldi, et al. Acetyl-L-carnitine (ALC) treatment in elderly patients with fatigue. *Arch Gerontol Geriatr* 2008; 46(2):181–190.

23. Vermeulen, RC, and HR Scholte. Exploratory open label, randomized study of acetyl- and propionylcarnitine in chronic fatigue syndrome. *Psychosom Med* 2004; 66(2):276–282.

24. van Heukelom, RO, JB Prins, MG Smits, and G Bleijenberg. Influence of melatonin on fatigue severity in patients with chronic fatigue syndrome and late melatonin secretion. *Eur J Neurol* 2006; 13(1):55–60.

5   Hypoglycemia

1. Kerr, D, et al. Effect of caffeine on the recognition of and response to hypoglycemia in humans. *Ann Intern Med* 1993; 119(8):799–804.

2. Anderson, RA, et al. Effects of supplemental chromium on patients with symptoms of reactive hypoglycemia. *Metabolism* 1987; 36(4):351–355.

3. Clausen, J. Chromium induced clinical improvement in symptomatic hypoglycemia. *Biol Trace Elem Res* 1988; 17:229–236.

6   Insomnia

1. Study: Insomnia. Statistics Canada, 2002. Available at www.statcan.gc.ca/daily-quotidien/051116/dq051116a-eng.htm.

2. Curless, R, et al. Is caffeine a factor in subjective insomnia of elderly people? *Age Ageing* 1993; 22(10):41–45.

3. Bliwise, NG. Factors related to sleep quality in healthy elderly women. *Psychol Aging* 1992; 7(1):83–88.

4. Paterson, LM, SJ Wilson, DJ Nutt, et al. A transitional, caffeine-induced model of onset insomnia in rats and healthy volunteers. *Psychopharmacology* 2007; 191(4):943–950.

5. Bonnett, MH, TJ Balkin, DF Dinges, et al. The use of stimulants to modify performance during sleep loss: A review by the Sleep Deprivation and Stimulant Task Force of the American Academy of Sleep Medicine. *Sleep* 2005; 28(9):1163–1187.

6. Bonnett, MH, and DL Arand. Situational insomnia: Consistency, predictors, and outcomes. *Sleep* 2003; 26(8):1029–1036.

7. Shirlow, MJ, and CD Mathers. A study of caffeine consumption and symptoms: Indigestion, palpitations, tremor, headache and insomnia. *Int J Epidemiol* 1985; 14(2):239–248.

8. Landolt, HP, et al. Caffeine intake (200 mg) in the morning affects human sleep and EEG power spectra at night. *Brain Research* 1995; 675(1–2):67–74.

9. Landolt, HP, et al. Caffeine reduces low-frequency delta activity in the human sleep EEG. *Neuropsychopharmacology* 1995; 12(3):229–238.

10. Stein, MD, and PD Friedmann. Disturbed sleep and its relationship to alcohol use. *Subst Abus* 2005; 26(1):1–13.

11. Okawa, M, et al. Vitamin B12 treatment for sleep-wake rhythm disorders. *Sleep* 1990; 13(1):15–23.

12. Mayer, G, et al. Effects of vitamin B12 on performance and circadian rhythm in normal subjects. *Neuropsychopharmacology* 1996; 15(5):456–464.

13. Lindahl, O, et al. Double blind study of a valerian preparation. *Pharmacology Biochemistry and Behaviour* 1989; 32:1065–1066.

14. Leathwood, PD, et al. Aqueous extract of valerian root improves sleep quality in man. *Pharmacol Biochem and Behav* 1982; 17:65–71.

15. Leathwood, PD, et al. Aqueous extract of valerian root reduces latency to fall asleep in man. *Planta Medica* 1985; 51:144–148.

7 Migraine Headaches

1. William, EM, et al. Guidelines for the diagnosis and management of migraine in clinical practice. *CMAJ* 1997; 156:1273–1287.

2. Wobber, C, J Holzhammer, J Zeitlhofer, et al. Trigger factors of migraine and tension-type headache: Experience and knowledge of the patients. *J Headache Pain* 2006; 7(4):188–195.

3. Millichap, JG, and MM Yee. The diet factor in pediatric and adolescent migraine. *Pediatr Neurol* 2003; 28(1):9–15.

4. Savi, L, I Rainero, W Valfre, et al. Food and headache attacks: A comparison of patients with migraine and tension-type headaches. *Panminerva Med* 2002; 44(1):27–31.

5. Littlewood, JT, et al. Red wine as a cause of migraine. *Lancet* 1988; 1(8585):558–559.

6. Monro, J, et al. Food allergy in migraine: Study of dietary exclusion and RAST. *Lancet* 1980; 2(8184):1–4.

7. Grant, EC. Food allergies and migraine. *Lancet* 1979; 1(8123):966–969.

8. Mansfield, LE, et al. Food allergy and adult migraine: Double-blind and mediator confirmation of an allergic etiology. *Ann Allergy* 1985; 55(2):126–129.

9. Boehnke, C, U Reuter, U Flach, et al. High-dose riboflavin treatment is efficacious in migraine prophylaxis: An open study in a tertiary care centre. *Eur J Neurol* 2004; 11(7):475–477.

10. Schoenen, J, et al. Effectiveness of high-dose riboflavin in migraine prophylaxis: A randomized controlled trial. *Neurology* 1998; 50(2):466–470.

11. Maizels, M, A Blumenfeld, and R Burchette. A combination of riboflavin, magnesium and ferverfew for migraine prophylaxis: A randomized trial. *Headache* 2004; 44(9):885–890.

12. Peikert, A, et al. Prophylaxis of migraine with oral magnesium: Results from a prospective, multi-center, placebo-controlled and double-
blind randomized study. *Cephalalgia* 1996; 16(4):257–263.

13. Wang, F, SK Van Den Eeden, LM Ackerson, et al. Oral magnesium oxide prophylaxis of frequent migrainous headache in children: A randomized, double-blind, placebo-controlled trial. *Headache* 2003; 43(6):601–610.

14. Murphy, JJ, et al. Randomised double-blind placebo-controlled trial of feverfew in migraine prevention. *Lancet* 1988; 2(8604):189–192.

8 Lupus

1. Lupus. The Arthritis Society, April 29, 2009. Available at www.arthritis.ca/types%20 of%20arthritis/lupus/default.asp?s=1.

2. Morimoto, I. A study on immunological effects of L-canavanine. *Kobe J Med Sci* 1989; 35(5–6):287–298.

3. Alcocer-Varela, J, et al. Effects of L-canavanine on T cells may explain the induction of systemic lupus erythematosus by alfalfa. *Arth Rheum* 1985; 28(1):52–57.

4. Akaogi, J, T Barker, Y Kuroda, et al. Role of non-protein amino acid L-canavanine in autoimmunity. *Autoimmun Rev* 2006; 5(6):429–435.

5. Vasoo, S. Drug-induced lupus: An update. *Lupus* 2006; 15(11):757–761.

6. Philbrick, DJ, and BJ Holub. Flaxseed: A potential treatment for lupus nephritis. *Kidney Int* 1995; 48(2):475–480.

7. Clark, WF, C Kortas, AP Heidenheim, et al. Flaxseed in lupus nephritis: A two-year nonplacebo-controlled crossover study. *J AM Coll Nutr* 2001; 20(2 Suppl):143–148.

8. Minami, Y, T Sasaki, Y Arai, et al. Diet and symptomatic lupus erythematosus: A 4 year prospective study of Japanese patients. *J Rheumatol* 2003; 30(4):747–754.

9. Ruiz-Irastorza, G, MV Egurbide, N Olivares, et al. Vitamin D deficiency in systemic lupus erythematosus: Prevalence, predictors and clinical consequences. *Rheumatology* (Oxford) 2008; 47(6):920–923.

10. Cutolo, M, and K Otsa. Review: Vitamin D, immunity and lupus. *Lupus* 2008; 17(1):6–10.

11. Kamen, DL, GS Cooper, H Bouali, et al. Vitamin D deficiency in systemic lupus erythemaosus. *Autoimmun Rev* 2006; 5(2):114–117.

12. Serban, MG, et al. Lipid peroxidase and erythrocyte redox system in systemic vasculitides treated with corticoids: Effect of vitamin E administration. *Rom J Intern Med* 1994; 32(4):283–289.

13. Comstock, GW, et al. Serum concentrations of alpha tocopherol, beta carotene, and retinal preceding the diagnosis of rheumatoid arthritis

and systemic lupus erythematosus. *Ann Rheum Dis* 1997; 56(5):323–325.

14. Weinmann, BJ, and D Hermann. Inhibition of autoimmune deterioration in MRL/lpr mice by vitamin E. *Int J Vitam Nutr Res* 1999; 69(4):255–261.

15. Maeshima, E, XM Liang, M Goda, et al. The efficacy of vitamin E against oxidative damage and autoantibody production in systemic lupus erythematosus: A preliminary study. *Clin Rheumatol* 2007; 26(3):401–404.

16. Compeyrot-Lacassange, S, PN Tyrrell, E Atenafu, et al. Prevalance and etiology of low bone mineral density in juvenile systemic lupus erythematosus. *Arthritis Rheum* 2007; 56(6):1966–1973.

17. Bhattoa, HP, P Bettembuk, A Balogh, et al. Bone mineral density in women with systemic lupus erythematosus. *Clin Rheumatol* 2002; 21(2):135–141.

18. Crosbie, D, C Black, L McIntyre, et al. Dehydroepiandrosterone for systemic lupus erythematosus. *Cochrane Database Syst Rev* Oct 2007; 17(4):CD005114.

19. Mease, PJ, EM Ginzler, OS Gluck, et al. Effects of prasterone on bone mineral density in women with systemic lupus erythematosus receiving chronic glucocorticoid therapy. *J Rheumatol* 2005; 32(4):616–621.

20. Nordmark, G, C Bengtsson, A Larsson, et al. Effects of dehydroepiandrosterone supplement on health-related quality of life in glucocorticoid treated female patients with systemic lupus erythematosus. *Autoimmunity* 2005; 38(7):531–540.

21. Barry, NN, et al. Dehydroepiandrosterone in systemic lupus erythematosus: Relationship between dosage, serum levels, and clinical response. *J Rheumatol* 1998; 25(12):2352–2356.

22. van Vollenhoven, RF, et al. A double-blind, placebo-controlled, clinical trial of dehydroepiandrosterone in severe systemic lupus erythematosus. *Lupus* 1999; 8(3):181–187.

23. van Vollenhoven, RF, et al. Treatment of systemic lupus erythematosus with dehydro-epiandrosterone: 50 patients treated up to 12 months. *J Rheumatol* 1998; 25(2):285–289.

24. van Vollenhoven, RF, et al. Dehydroepiandro-sterone in systemic lupus erythematosus: Results of a double-blind, placebo-controlled, randomized clinical trial. *Arth Rheum* 1995; 38(12):1826–1831.

25. van Vollenhoven, RF, et al. An open trial of dehydroepiandrosterone in systemic lupus erythematosus. *Arth Rheum* 1994; 37(9):1305–1310.

26. Wright, SA, FM O'Prey, MT McHenry, et al. A randomized interventional trial of omega-3 polyunsaturated fatty acids on endothelial function and disease activity in systemic lupus erythematosus. *Ann Rheum Dis* 2008; 67(6):841–848.

27. Duffy, EM, GK Meenagh, SA McMillan, et al. The clinical effect of dietary supplementation with omega-3 fish oils and/or copper in systemic lupus erythematosus. *J Rheumatol* 2004; 31(8):1551–1558.

28. Das, UN. Beneficial effect of eicosapentanoic and docosahexaenoic acids in the management of systemic lupus erythematosus and its relationship to the cytokine network. *Prostaglandins Leukot Essent Fatty Acids* 1994; 51(3):207–213.

29. Clark, WF, and A Parbtani. Omega-3 fatty acid supplementation in clinical and experimental lupus nephritis. *Am J Kidney Dis* 1994; 23(5):644–647.

30. Clark, WF, et al. Fish oil in lupus nephritis: Clinical findings and methodological implica-tions. *Kidney Int* 1993; 44(1):75–86.

31. Walton, AJ, et al. Dietary fish oil and the severity of symptoms in patients with systemic lupus erythematosus. *Ann Rheum Dis* 1991; 50(7):463–466.

32. Mohan IK, and UN Das. Oxidant stress, anti-oxidants and essential fatty acids in systemic lupus erythematosus. *Prostaglandins Leukot Essent Fatty Acids* 1997; 56(3):193–198.

Part 3: Breast, Bone and Heart Health

9 Breast Cancer

1. Breast cancer stats. The Canadian Cancer Society, April 9, 2009. Available at www.cancer.ca/canadawide/about%20cancer/cancer%20statistics/stats%20at%20a%20glance/breast%20cancer.aspx?sc_lang=en.

2. Ibid.

3. Holmes, MD, et al. Association of dietary fat and fatty acids with risk of breast cancer. *JAMA* 1999; 281(10):914–920.

4. Boyd, NF, et al. Effects of a low-fat high-carbo-hydrate diet on plasma sex hormones in premenopausal women: Results from a randomized controlled trial. Canadian Diet and Breast Cancer Prevention Study Group. *Br J Cancer* 1997; 76(1):127–135.

5. Prentice, RL, B Caan, RT Chlebowski, et al. Low fat dietary pattern and risk of invasive breast cancer: The Women's Health Initiative Randomized Controlled Dietary Modification Trial. *JAMA* 2006; 295(6):629–642.

6. Chlebowski, RT, GL Blackburn, CA Thomson, et al. Dietary fat reduction and breast cancer outcome: Interim efficacy results from the Women's Intervention Nutrition Study. *J Natl Cancer Inst* 2006; 98(24):1767–1776.

7. Zheng, W, et al. Well-done meat intake and the risk of breast cancer. *JNCI* 1998; 90(22): 1724–1729.

8. Rose, DP, et al. Effect of omega-3 fatty acids on the progression of metastases after surgical excision of human breast cancer cell solid tumors growing in nude mice. *Clin Cancer Res* 1996; 2(10):1751–1756.

9. MacLean, CH, SJ Newberry, WA Mojica, et al. Effects of omega-3 fatty acids on cancer risk: A systematic review. *JAMA* 2006; 295(4): 403–415.

10. Silvera, SA, M Jain, GR Howe, et al. Dietary carbohydrates and breast cancer risk: A prospective study of the roles of overall glycemic index and glycemic load. *Int J Cancer* 2005; 114(4):653–658.

11. Shu, XO, F Jin, Q Dai, W Wen, JD Potter, LH Kushi, Z Ruan, YT Gao, and W Zheng. Soyfood intake during adolescence and subsequent risk of breast cancer among Chinese women. *Cancer Epidemiol Biomarkers Prev* 2001; 10(5):483–488.

12. Korde, LA, AH Wu, T Fears, AM Nomura, DW West, LN Kolonel, MC Pike, RN Hoover, and RG Ziegler. Childhood soy intake and breast cancer risk in Asian American women. *Cancer Epidemiol Biomarkers Prev* 2009; 18(4):1050–1059.

13. Thompson, LU, et al. Flaxseed and its lignan and oil components reduce mammary tumor growth at a late stage of carcinogenesis. *Carcinogenesis* 1996; 17(6):1373–1376.

14. Thompson, LU, et al. Antitumorigenic effect of a mammalian lignan precurser from flaxseed. *Nutr Cancer* 1996; 26(2):159–165.

15. Flaxseed's role in breast cancer prevention suggested. August 31, 2001. Available at www.nutraingredients-usa.com/news/ng.asp?n=20958-flaxseed-s-role.

16. Thompson, LU, JM Chen, T Li, K Strasser-Weippl, and PE Goss. Dietary flaxseed alters tumor biological markers in postmenopausal breast cancer. *Clin Cancer Res* 2005; 11(10):3828–3835.

17. Hunter, DJ, et al. A prospective study of intake of vitamin C, E and A and the risk of breast cancer. *N Engl J Med* 1993; 329:234–240.

18. Freudenheim, JL, et al. Premenopausal breast cancer risk and intake of vegetables, fruits and related nutrients. *JNCI* 1996; 88(6):340–348.

19. Sauerkraut consumption may fight off breast cancer. Dominic Patton, November 4, 2005. Available at www.nutraingredients.com/Research/Sauerkraut-consumption-may-fight-off-breast-cancer.

20. Howe, GR, et al. Dietary factors and risk of breast cancer: Combined analysis of 12 case-control studies. *JNCI* 1990; 82:561–569.

21. Sun, CL, JM Yuan, WP Koh, and MC Yu. Green tea, black tea and breast cancer risk: A meta-analysis of epidemiological studies. *Carcinogenesis* 2006; 27(7):1310–5. Epub 2005 Nov 25.

22. Nakachi, K, K Suemasu, K Suga, et al. Influence of drinking green tea on breast cancer malignancy among Japanese patients. *Jpn J Cancer Res* 1998; 89(3):254–261.

23. Key, J, S Hodgson, RZ Omar, et al. Meta-analyis of alcohol and breast cancer with consideration of the methodological issues. *Cancer Causes Control* 2006; 17(6):759–770.

24. Allen, NE, V Beral, D Casabonne, SW Kan, GK Reeves, A Brown, J Green; Million Women Study Collaborators. Moderate alcohol intake and cancer incidence in women. *J Natl Cancer Inst* 2009; 101(5):296–305.

25. Hankinson, SE, et al. Alcohol, height, and adiposity in relation to estrogen and prolactin levels in postmenopausal women. *JNCI* 1995; 87(17):1297–1302.

26. Hirose, K, et al. Effect of body size on breast cancer risk among Japanese women. *Int J Cancer* 1999; 80(3):349–355.

27. Huang, Z, et al. Dual effects of weight and weight gain on breast cancer risk. *JAMA* 1997; 278(17):1407–1411.

28. La Vecchia, C, et al. Body mass index and post-menopausal breast cancer: An age-specific analysis. *Br J Cancer* 1997; 75(3):441–444.

29. Silvera, SA, M Jain, GR Howe, et al. Energy balance and breast cancer risk: A prospective cohort study. *Breast Cancer Res Treat* 2006; 97(1):97–106.

30. Chang, SC, RG Ziegler, B Dunn, et al. Association of energy intake and energy balance with postmenopausal breast cancer in the prostate, lung, colorectal, and ovarian cancer screening trial. *Cancer Epidemiol Biomarkers Prev* 2006; 15(2):334–341.

31. Reeves, GK, K Pirie, V Beral, et al. Cancer incidence and mortality in relation to body mass index in the Million Women Study: Cohort study. *BMJ* 2007; 335(7630): 1134.

32. Zhang, S, et al. Dietary carotenoids and vitamins A, C, and E and risk of breast cancer. *JNCI* 1999; 91(6):547–556.

33. Cui, Y, JM Shikany, S Liu, et al. Selected antioxidants and risk of hormone receptor-defined invasive breast cancers among postmenopausal women in the Women's Health Initiative Observational Study. *Am J Clin Nutr* 2008; 87(4):1009–1018.

34. Sato, R, KJ Helzlsouer, AJ Alberg, et al. Prospective study of carotenoids, tocopherols, and retinoid concentrations and the risk of breast cancer. *Cancer Epidemiol Biomarkers Prev* 2002; 11(5):451–457.

35. Robien, K, GJ Cutler, and D Lazovich. Vitamin D intake and breast cancer risk in postmenopausal women: The Iowa Women's Healthy Study. *Cancer Causes Control* 2007; 18(7):775–782.

36. Lappe, JM, D Travers-Gustafson, KM Davies, et al. Vitamin D and calcium supplementation reduces cancer risk: Results of a randomized trial. *Am J Clin Nutr* 2007; 85(6):1586–1591.

37. Zhang, S, et al. A prospective study of folate intake and the risk of breast cancer. *JAMA* 1999; 281(17):1632–1637.

10   Fibrocystic Breast Conditions

1. Boyd, NF, et al. Clinical trial of a low-fat, high-carbohydrate diet in subjects with mammographic breast dysplasia: Report of early outcomes. *JNCI* 1988; 80(15):1244–1248.

2. Rose, DP, et al. Effect of a low-fat diet on hormone levels in women with cystic breast disease: I. Serum steroids and gonodotropins. *JNCI* 1987; 78(4):623–626.

3. Rose, DP, et al. Effect of a low-fat diet on hormone levels in women with cystic breast disease: II. Serum radioimmunoassayable prolactin and growth hormone and bioactive lactogenic hormones. *JNCI* 1987; 78(4):627–631.

4. Rose, DP, et al. Effects of diet supplementation with wheat bran on serum estrogen levels in the follicular and luteal phases of the menstrual cycle. *Nutrition* 1997; 13:535–539.

5. Rose, DP, et al. High-fiber diet reduces serum estrogen concentrations in premenopausal women. *Am J Clin Nutr* 1991; 24:520–524.

6. Xu, X, et al. Effects of soy isoflavones on estrogen and phytoestrogens metabolism in premenopausal women. *Cancer Epidemiol Biomarkers Prev* 1998; 7:1101–1108.

7. Nagata, C, et al. Decreased serum estradiol concentration associated with high dietary intake of soy products in premenopausal Japanese women. *Nutr Cancer* 1997; 29:228–233.

8. Cassidy, A, et al. Biological effects of a diet of soy protein rich in isoflavones on the menstrual cycle of premenopausal women. *Am J Clin Nutr* 1994; 60:333–340.

9. Petrakis, NL, et al. Stimulatory influence of soy protein isolate on breast secretion in pre- and postmenopausal women. *Cancer Epidemiol Biomarkers Prev* 1996; 5:785–794.

10. Bryant, M, A Cassidy, C Hill, et al. Effect of consumption of soy isoflavones on behavioural, somatic and affective symptoms in women with premenstrual syndrome. *Br J Nutr* 2005; 93(5):731–739.

11. Fleming, RM. What effect, if any, does soy protein have on breast tissue? *Integr Cancer Ther* 2003; 2(3):225–228.

12. Rosolowich, V, E Saettler, B Szuck, et al. Mastalgia. *J Obstet Gynaecol Can* 2006; 28(1): 49–71.

13. Russell, LC. Caffeine restriction as initial treatment of breast pain. *Nurse Pract* 1989; 14(2):36–37.

14. Meyer, EC, et al. Vitamin E and benign breast disease. *Surgery* 1990; 107(5):549–551.

15. Ernster, VL, et al. Vitamin E and benign breast disease: A double-blind, randomized clinical trial. *Surgery* 1985; 97(4):490–494.

16. Pye, JK, et al. Clinical experience of drug treatments for mastalgia. *Lancet* 1985; 2(8451): 373–377.

17. Tamborini, A, and R Taurelle. Value of standardized Ginkgo biloba extract (EGb 761) in the management of congestive symptoms of premenstrual syndrome. *Rev Fr Gynecol Obstet* Jul–Sep 1993; 88(7–9):447–457. [French]

11   Osteoporosis

1. Cauley, JA, et al. The effect of HRT on fracture risk: Results of a 4-year randomized trial of 2,763 postmenopausal women. American Society for Bone and Mineral Research, June 1998. [Abstract T394]

2. Alekel, D, et al. Isoflavone-rich soy protein isolate exerts significant bone sparing effect in the lumbar spine of perimenopausal women. Third International Symposium on the Role of Soy in Preventing and Treating Chronic Disease, October 1999. [Abstract]

3. Schieber, MD, et al. Dietary soy isoflavones favorably influence lipids and bone turnover in healthy postmenopausal women. Third International Symposium on the Role of Soy in Preventing and Treating Chronic Disease, October 1999. [Abstract]

4. Ma, DF, LQ Qin, PY Wang, and R Katoh. Soy isoflavone intake inhibits bone resorption and stimulates bone formation in menopausal women: Meta-analysis of randomized controlled trials. *Eur J Clin Nutr* 2008; 62(2):155–161.

5. Ma, DF, LQ Qin, PY Wang, and R Katoh. Soy isoflavone intake increases bone mineral density in the spine of menopausal women: Meta-analysis of randomized controlled trials. *Clin Nutr* 2008; 27(1):57–64.

6. Brink, E, V Coxam, S Robins, et al. Long-term consumption of isoflavone-enriched foods does not affect bone mineral density, bone metabolism, or hormonal status in early postmenopausal women: A randomized, double-blind, placebo controlled study. *Am J Clin Nutr* 2008; 87(3):761–770.

7. Munger, RG, et al. Prospective study of dietary protein intake and risk of hip fracture in postmenopausal women. *Am J Clin Nutr* 1999; 69(1):147–152.

8. Rapuri, PB, JC Gallagher, and V Haynatzka. Protein intake: Effects on bone mineral density and the rate of bone loss in elderly women. *Am J Clin Nutr* 2003; 77(6):1517–1525.

9. Schurch, MA, et al. Protein supplements increase serum insulin-like growth factor-I levels and attenuate proximal femur bone loss in patients with recent hip fracture: A randomized, double-blind, placebo-controlled trial. *Ann Intern Med* 1998; 128(10):801–809.

10. Tengstrand, B, T Cederholm, A Soderqvist, and J Tidermark. Effects of protein-rich supplementation and nandrolone on bone tissue after a hip fracture. *Clin Nutr* 2007; 26(4):460–465.

11. Lloyd, T, et al. Dietary caffeine intake and bone status of postmenopausal women. *Am J Clin Nutr* 1997; 65(6):1826–1830.

12. Harris, SS, and B Dawson-Hughes. Caffeine and bone loss in healthy menopausal women. *Am J Clin Nutr* 1994; 60(4): 573–578.

13. Wetmore, CM, J Ichikawa, AZ LaCroix, et al. Association between caffeine intake and bone mass among young women: Potential effect. *Osteoporos Int* 2008; 19(4):519–527.

14. Sakhaee, K, et al. The effect of calcium citrate on bone density in the early and mid-postmenopausal period: A randomized, placebo-controlled study. The Second Joint Meeting of the American Society for Bone and Mineral Research and the International Bone and Mineral Society, 1998. Mission Pharmacal Company. [Abstract]

15. Tang, BM, GD Eslick, C Nowson, et al. Use of calcium or calcium in combination with vitamin D supplementation to prevent fractures and bone loss in people aged 50 years and older: A meta-analysis. *Lancet* 2007; 370(9588):657–666.

16. Baran, DT, et al. A placebo-controlled study of pre-menopausal women: Calcium supplementation and bone density. Annual Meeting of the American Society for Bone and Mineral Research, 1999. [Abstract]

17. Harris, SS, and B Dawson-Hughes. Seasonal changes in plasma 25-hydroxyvitamin D concentrations of young American black and white women. *Am J Clin Nutr* 1998; 67(6): 1232–1236.

18. Crandell, C. Vitamin A intake and osteoporosis: A clinical update. *J Womens Health* 2004; 13(8):939–953.

19. Jackson, HA, and AH Sheehan. Effect of vitamin A on fracture risk. *Ann Pharmacother* 2005; 39(12):2086–2090.

20. Feskanich, D, V Singh, WC Willett, and GA Colditz. Vitamin A intake and hip fractures among postmenopausal women. *JAMA* 2002; 287(1):47–54.

21. Melhus, H, K Michaëlsson, A Kindmark, et al. Excessive dietary intake of vitamin A is associated with reduced bone mineral density and increased risk for hip fracture. *Ann Intern Med* 1998; 129(10):770–778.

22. Leveille, SG, et al. Dietary vitamin C and bone mineral density: Results from the PEPI study. *Calcif Tissue Int* 1998; (63)3:183–189.

23. Feskanich, D, et al. Vitamin K intake and hip fractures in women: A prospective study. *Am J Clin Nutr* 1999; 69(1):74–79.

24. Booth, SL, KL Tucker, H Chen, et al. Dietary vitamin K intakes are associated with hip fracture but not with bone mineral density in elderly men and women. *Am J Clin Nutr* 2000; 71(5):1201–1208.

25. Ryder, KM, RI Shorr, AJ Bush, et al. Magnesium intake from food and supplements is associated with bone mineral density in healthy older white subjects. *J Am Geriatr Soc* 2005; 53(11):1875–1880.

26. Strause, L, et al. Spinal bone loss in postmenopausal women supplemented with calcium and trace minerals. *J Nutr* 1994; 124(7):1060–1064.

27. Devine, A, et al. A longitudinal study of the effect of sodium and calcium intakes on regional bone density in postmenopausal women. *Am J Clin Nutr* 1995; 62(4):740–745.

28. Salari, P, A Rezaie, B Larijani, and M Abdollahi. A systematic review of the impact of n-3 fatty acids in bone health and osteoporosis. *Med Sci Monit* 2008; (3):RA37–RA44.

29. Rousseau, JH, A Kleppinger, and AM Kenny. Self-reported dietary intake of omega-3 fatty acids and association with bone and lower extremity function. *J Am Geriatr Soc* Aug 22, 2008. [Epub ahead of print.]

30. Högström, M, P Nordström, and A Nordström. n-3 Fatty acids are positively associated with peak bone mineral density and bone accrual in healthy men: The NO2 Study. *Am J Clin Nutr* 2007; 85(3):803–807.

31. Dalsky, GP, et al. Weight-bearing exercise training and lumbar bone mineral content in postmenopausal women. *Ann Intern Med* Jun 1988; 108(6):824–828

32. Wolff, I, JJ van Croonenborg, HC Kemper, et al. The effect of exercise training programs on

bone mass: A meta-analysis of published controlled trials in pre- and postmenopausal women. *Osteoporos Int* 1999; 9(1):1–12.

12 Heart Disease and High LDL Cholesterol

1. Pietinen, P, A Ascherio, P Korhonen, AM Hartman, et al. Intake of fatty acids and risk of coronary heart disease in a cohort of Finnish men: The Alpha-Tocopherol, Beta-Carotene Cancer Prevention Study. *Am J Epidemiol* 1997; 145(10):876–887.

2. Ascherio, A, EB Rimm, EL Giovannucci, D Spiegelman, et al. Dietary fat intake and risk of coronary heart diseae in men: Cohort follow up study in the United States. *BMJ* 1996; 13(7049):84–90.

3. Hu, FB, MJ Stampfer, JE Manson, E Rimm, et al. Dietary fat intake and the risk of coronary heart disease in women. *N Eng J Med* 1997; 337(21):1491–1499.

4. Albert, CM, O Kyungwon, W Whang, JE Manson, et al. Dietary a-linolenic acid intake and risk of sudden cardiac death and coronary heart disease. *Circulation* 2005; 112(21):3232–3238.

5. Herron, KL, IE Lofgren, M Sharman, JS Volek, and ML Fernandez. High intake of cholesterol results in less atherogenic low-density lipoprotein particles in men and women independent of response classification. *Metabolism* 2004; 53(6):823–830.

6. Mutungi, G, J Ratliff, M Puglisi, M Torres-Gonzalez, et al. Dietary cholesterol from eggs increases plasma HDL cholesterol in overweight men consuming a carbohydrate-restricted diet. *J Nutr* 2008; 138(2):272–276.

7. Greene, CM, D Waters, RM Clark, JH Contois, and ML Fernandez. Plasma LDL and HDL characteristics and carotenoid content are positively influenced by egg consumption in an elderly population. *Nutr Metab* (London) 2006; 3(6):1–10.

8. Goodrow, EF, TA Wilson, SC Houde, R Vishwanathan, et al. Consumption of one egg per day increases serum lutein and zeaxanthin concentrations in older adults without altering serum lipid and lipoprotein cholesterol concentrations. *J Nutr* 2006; 136(10):2519–2524.

9. Hu, FB, MJ Stampfer, EB Rimm, JE Manson, et al. A prospective study of egg consumption and risk of cardiovascular disease in men and women. *JAMA* 1999; 281(15):1387–1394.

10. Albert, CM, JM Gaziano, WC Willett, and JE Manson. Nut consumption and decreased risk of sudden cardiac death in the Physicians' Health Study. *Arch Intern Med* 2002; 162(12):1382–1387.

11. Hu, FB, MJ Stampfer, JE Manson, EB Rimm, et al. Frequent nut consumption and risk of coronary heart disease in women: Prospective cohort study. *BMJ* 1998; 317(7169): 1341–1345.

12. Ellsworth, JL, LH Kushi, and AR Folsom. Frequent nut intake and risk of death from coronary heart disease and all causes in postmenopausal women: The Iowa Women's Health Study. *Nutr Metab Cardiovasc Dis* 2001; 11(6):372–377.

13. Fraser, GE, J Sabaté, WL Beeson, and TM Strahan. A possible protective effect of nut consumption on risk of coronary heart disease: The Adventist Health Study. *Arch Intern Med* Jul 1992; 152(7):1416–24.

14. Brown, L, B Rosner, WW Willett, and FM Sacks. Cholesterol-lowering effects of dietary fiber: A meta-analysis. *Am J Clin Nutr* 1999; 69(1):30–42.

15. Anderson, JW, LD Allgood, A Lawrence, LA Altringer, et al. Cholesterol-lowering effects of psyllium intake adjunctive to diet therapy in men and women with hypercholesterolemia: Meta-analysis of 8 controlled trials. *Am J Clin Nutr* 2000; 71(2):472–479.

16. Keenan, JM, JB Wenz, S Myers, C Ripsan, and ZQ Huang. Randomized, controlled, crossover trial of oat bran in hypercholesterolemic subjects. *J Fam Prac* 1991; 33(6):60–608.

17. Peters, U, C Poole, and L Arab. Does tea affect cardiovascular disease? A meta-analysis. *Am J Epidemiol* 2001; 154(6):495–503.

18. Sesso, HD, JM Gaziano, S Liu, and JE Buring. Flavonoid intake and the risk of cardiovascular disease in women. *Am J Clin Nutr* 2003; 77(6):1400–1408.

19. Geleijnse, JM, LJ Launer, DA Van der Kuip, et al. Inverse association of tea and flavonoid intakes with incident myocardial infarction: The Rotterdam Study. *Am J Clin Nutr* 2002; 75(5):880–886.

20. Mukamal, KJ, M Maclure, JE Muller, et al. Tea consumption and mortality after acute myocardial infarction. *Circulation* 2002; 105(21):2476–2481.

21. Simon, JA, et al. Serum ascorbic acid and cardiovascular disease prevalence. *Epidemiology* 1998; 9(3):316–321.

22. Lopes, C, et al. Diet and risk of myocardial infarction: A case-control community-based study. *Acta Med Port* 1998; 11(4):311–317.

23. Giovannucci, E, Y Liu, BW Hollis, and EB Rimm. 25-hydroxyvitamin D and risk of myocardial infarction in men. *Arch Intern Med* 2008; 168(11):1174–1180.

24. Lee, IM, NR Cook, JM Gaziano, D Gordon, et al. Vitamin E in the primary prevention of cardiovascular disease and cancer: The Women's Health Study: A randomized controlled trial. *JAMA* 2005; 294(1):56–65.

25. Yusuf, S, G Dagenais, J Pogue, J Bosch, and P Sleight. Vitamin E supplementation and cardiovascular events in high-risk patients. The Heart Outcomes Prevention Evaluation Study Investigators. *N Engl J Med* 2000; 342(3):154–160.

26. Dietary supplementation with n-3 polyunsaturated fatty acids and vitamin E after myocardial infarction: Results of the GISSI-Prevenzione trial. Gruppo Italiano per lo Studio della Sopravvivenza nell'Infarto miocardico. *Lancet* 1999; 354(9177):447–455.

27. Lonn, E, J Bosch, S Yusuf, P Sheridan, J Pogue, JM Arnold, C Ross, A Arnold, P Sleight, J Probstfield, GR Dagenais; HOPE and HOPE-TOO Trial Investigators. Effects of long-term vitamin E supplementation on cardiovascular events and cancer: A randomized controlled trial. *JAMA* 2005; 293(11):1338–1347.

28. Miller 3rd, ER, R Pastor-Barriuso, D Dalal, RA Riemersma, et al. Meta-analysis: High-dosage vitamin E supplementation may increase all-cause mortality. *Ann Intern Med* 2005; 142(1):37–46.

29. Lopez-Ridaura, R, WC Willett, EB Rimm, S Liu, et al. Magnesium intake and risk of type 2 diabetes in men and women. *Diabetes Care* 2004; 27(1):134–140.

30. Meyer, KA, LH Kishi, DR Jacobs Jr., J Slavin, et al. Carbohydrates, dietary fiber, and incident type 2 diabetes in older women. *Am J Clin Nutr* 1999; 71(4):921–930.

31. Song, V, JE Manson, JE Buring, and S Liu. Dietary magnesium intake in relation to plasma insulin levels and risk of type 2 diabetes in women. *Diabetes Care* 2003; 27(1):59–65.

32. Larsson, SC, and A Wolk. Magnesium intake and risk of type 2 diabetes: A meta-analysis. *J Intern Med* 2007; 262(2):208–214.

33. Rodriguez-Moran, M, and F Guerrero-Romero. Oral magnesium supplementation improves insulin sensitivity and metabolic control in type 2 diabetic subjects. *Diabetes Care* 2003; 26(4):1147–1152.

34. Shechter, M, CN Bairey Merz, HG Stuehlinger, et al. Effects of oral magnesium therapy on exercise tolerance, exercise-induced chest pain, and quality of life in patients with coronary artery disease. *Am J Cardiol* 2003; 91(5): 517–521.

35. Tran, MT, TM Mitchell, DT Kennedy, and JT Giles. Role of coenzyme Q10 in chronic heart failure, angina, and hypertension. *Pharmacotherapy* 2001; 21(7):797–806.

36. Singh, RB, MA Niaz, SS Rastogi, PK Shukla, and AS Thakur. Effect of hydrosoluble coenzyme Q10 on blood pressures and insulin resistance in hypertensive patients with coronary artery disease. *J Hum Hypertens* 1999; 13(3):203–208.

37. Burke, BE, R Neuenschwander, and RD Olson. Randomized, double-blind, placebo-controlled trial of coenzyme Q10 in isolated systolic hypertension. *South Med J* 2001; 94(11):1112–1117.

38. Watts, GF, DA Playford, KD Croft, NC Ward, et al. Coenzyme Q(10) improves endothelial dysfunction of the brachial artery in Type II diabetes mellitus. *Diabetologia* 2002; 45(3): 420–426.

39. Hill, AM, JD Buckley, KJ Murphy, and PR Howe. Combining fish-oil supplements with regular aerobic exercise improves body composition and cardiovascular disease risk factors. *Am J Clin Nutr* 2007; 85(5):1267–1274.

40. Wang, C, WS Harris, M Chung, AH Lichtenstein, et al. n-3 Fatty acids from fish or fish-oil supplements, but not alpha-linolenic acid, benefit cardiovascular disease outcomes in primary- and secondary-prevention studies: A systematic review. *Am J Clin Nutr* 2006; 84(1):5–17.

Part 4: Emotional Health

13 Depression

1. Mood Disorders. The Canadian Mental Health Association, 2009. Available at www.cmha.ca/bins/content_page.asp?cid=3-86-92&lang=1.

2. Su, KP, SY Huang, TH Chiu, et al. Omega-3 fatty acids for major depressive disorder during pregnancy: Results from a randomized, double-blind, placebo controlled trial. *J Clin Psychiatry* 2008; 69(4): 644–651.

3. Lin, PY, and KP Su. A meta-analytic review of double-blind, placebo-controlled trials of antidepressant efficacy of omega-3 fatty acids. *J Clin Psychiatry* 2007; 68(7):1056–1061.

4. Montgomery, P, and AJ Richardson. Omega-3 fatty acids for bipolar disorder. *Cochrane Database Syst Rev* Apr 16, 2008; (2):CD005169.

5. Su, KP, WW Shen, and SY Huang. Are omega3 fatty acids beneficial in depression but not mania? *Arch Gen Psychiatry* 2000; 57(7): 716–717.

6. Kinrys, G. Hypomania associated with omega3 fatty acids. *Arch Gen Psychiatry* 2000; 57(7):715–716.

7. Stoll, AL, et al. Omega 3 fatty acids in bipolar disorder: A preliminary double-blind, placebo-controlled trial. *Arch Gen Psychiatry* 1999; 56:407–412.

8. Wyatt, KM, et al. Efficacy of vitamin B6 in the treatment of premenstrual syndrome: systematic review. *Br J Med* 1999; 318(7195): 1375–1381.

9. Morris, DW, MH Trivedi, and AJ Rush. Folate and unipolar depression. *J Altern Complement Med* 2008; 14(3):277–285.

10. Fava, M. Augmenting antidepressants with folate: A clinical perspective. *J Clin Psychiatry* 2007; 68(Suppl 10):4–7.

11. Young, SN. Folate and depression: A neglected problem. *Rev Psychiatr Neurosci* 2007; 32(2):80–82.

12. Roberts, SH, E Bedson, D Hughes, et al. Folate augmentation of treatment—evaluation for depression (FolATED): Protocol of a randomized controlled trial. *BMC Psychiatry* Nov 2007; 7:65.

13. Pennix, BW, et al. Vitamin B(12) deficiency and depression in physically disabled older women: Epidemiologic evidence from the Women's Health and Aging Study. *Am J Psychiatry* 2000; 157(5):715–721.

14. Ebly, EM, et al. Folate status, vascular disease and cognition in elderly Canadians. *Age Ageing* 1998; 27(4):485–491.

15. Fava, M, et al. Folate, vitamin B12, and homocysteine in major depressive disorder. *Am J Psychiatry* 1997; 154(3):426–428.

16. Bell, IR, et al. B complex vitamin patterns in geriatric and young adult inpatients with major depression. *J Am Geriatr Soc* 1991; 39(3):252–257.

17. Docherty, JP, DA Sack, M Roffman, et al. A double-blind, placebo-controlled, exploratory trial of chromium picinolate in atypical depression: Effect on carbohydrate craving. *J Psychiatr Practice* 2005; 11(5):302–314.

18. Davidson, JR, K Abraham, KM Connor, and MN McLeod. Effectiveness of chromium in atypical depression: A placebo-controlled trial. *Biol Psychiatry* 2003; 53(3):261–264.

19. Marcellini, F, C Giuli, R Papa, et al. Zinc in elderly people: Effects of zinc supplementation on psychological dimensions in dependence of IL-6-174 polymorphisms: A Zincage study. *Rejuvenation Res* 2008; 11(2):479–483.

20. Marcellini, F, C Giuli, R Papa, et al. Zinc status, psychological and nutritional assessment in old people recruited in five European countries: Zincage study. *Biogerontology* 2006; 7(5–6):339–345.

21. Nowak, G, B Szewczyk, and A Pilc. Zinc and depression: An update. *Pharmaceutical Reports* 2005; 57:713–718.

22. Nowak, G, M Siwek, D Dudek, et al. Effect of zinc supplementation on antidepressant therapy in unipolar depression: A preliminary placebo-controlled study. *Pol J Pharamacol* 2003; 55(6):1143–1147.

23. Kasper, S, M Gastpar, WE Müller, HP Volz, A Dienel, M Kieser, and HJ Möller. Efficacy of St. John's wort extract WS 5570 in acute treatment of mild depression: A reanalysis of data from controlled clinical trials. *Eur Arch Psychiatry Clin Neurosci* 2008; 258(1):59–63.

24. Linde, K, et al. St. John's wort for depression: An overview and meta-analysis of randomized clinical trials. *Br Med J* 1996; 313:253–258.

25. Janicak, PG, J Lipinski, JM Davis, et al. S-adenosylmethionine in depression: A literature review and preliminary report. *Ala J Med Sci* 1988; 25(3):306–313.

26. Bressa, GM. S-adenosyl-l-methionine (SAMe) as antidepressant: Meta-analysis of clinical studies. *Acta Neurol Scand* 1994; 154(Suppl): S7–S14.

27. Bell, KM, SG Potkin, D Carreon, and L Plon. S-adenosylmethionine blood levels in major depression: Changes with drug treatment. *Acta Neurol Scand* 1994; 154(Suppl):S15–S18.

28. Bell, KM, L Plon, WE Bunney Jr, and SG Potkin. S-adenosylmethionine treatment of depression: A controlled clinical trial. *Am J Psychiatry* 1988; 145(9):1110–1114.

29. Salmaggi, P, GM Bressa, G Nicchia, et al. Double-blind, placebo-controlled study of S-adenosyl-L-methionine in depressed postmenopausal women. *Psychother Psychosom* 1993; 59(1):34–40.

30. De Vanna, M, and R Rigamonti. Oral S-adenosyl-L-methionine in depression. *Curr Ther Res* 1992; 52(3):478–485.

31. Rosenbaum, JF, M Fava, WE Falk, et al. The antidepressant potential of oral S-adenosyl-l-methionine. *Acta Psychiatr Scand* 1990; 81(5):432–36.

32. Delle Chiaie, R, P Pancheri, and P Scapicchio. Efficacy and tolerability of oral and intramuscular S-adenosyl-L-methionine 1,4-butanedisulfonate (SAMe) in the treatment of major depression: Comparison with imipramine in multicenter studies. *Am J Clin Nutr* 2002; 76(5):1172S–1176S.

Part 5: Conception, Pregnancy and Motherhood

15 Infertility

1. Stoppard MD, Miriam, and Catherine Younger-Lewis MD, eds. *Woman's Body* (Montreal: The

Reader's Digest Association [Canada] Ltd., 1995: 162.

2. Hammoud, AO, M Gibson, CM Peterson, et al. Obesity and male reproductive potential. *J Androl* 2006; 27(5):619–626.

3. Stanton, CK and RH Gray. Effects of caffeine consumption on delayed conception. *Am J Epidemiol* 1995; 142(12):1322–1329.

4. Wilcox, A, et al. Caffeinated beverages and decreased fertility. *Lancet* 1988; 2(8626–8627): 1453–1456.

5. Bolumar, F, et al. Caffeine and delayed conception: A European multicenter study on infertility and subfecundity. European Study Group on Infertility. *Subfecundity Am J Epidemiol* 1997; 145(4):324–334.

6. Grodstein, F, et al. Infertility in women and moderate alcohol use. *Am J Epidemiol* 1994; 84(9):1429–1432.

7. Forges, T, P Monneir-Barbarino, JM Alberto, et al. Impact of folate and homocysteine metabolism on human reproductive health. *Hum Reprod Update* 2007; 13(3):225–238.

8. Gulden, KD. Pernicious anemia, vitiligo and infertility. *J Am Board Fam Pract* 1990; 3(3):217–220.

9. Sanfilippo, JS, and YK Liu. Vitamin B12 deficiency and infertility: A case report. *Int J Fertil* 1991; 36(1):36–38.

10. Kumamoto, Y, et al. Clinical efficacy of mecobalamin in treatment of oligozoospermia: Results of a double-blind comparative clinical study. *Acta Urol Jpn* 1998; 34:1109–1132.

11. Song, GJ, EP Norkus, and V Lewis. Relationship between seminal ascorbic acid and sperm DNA integrity in infertile men. *Int J Androl* 2006; 29(6):569–575.

12. Mostafa, T, G Tawadrous, MM Roaia, et al. Effect of smoking on seminal plasma ascorbic acid in infertile and fertile males. *Andrologia* 2006; 38(6):221–224.

13. Hansen, JC, and Y Deguchi. Selenium and fertility in animals and man: A review. *Acta Vet Scand* 1996; 37(1):19–30.

14. Scott, R, et al. The effect of oral selenium supplementation on human sperm motility. *Br J Urol* 1998; 82(1):76–80.

15. Suleiman, SA, et al. Lipid peroxidation and human sperm motility: Protective role of vitamin E. *J Androl* 1996; 17(5):530–537.

16. Geva, E, et al. The effect of antioxidant treatment on human spermatozoa and fertilization rate in an in vitro fertilization program. *Fertil Steril* 1996; 66(3):430–434.

17. Omu, AE, MK Al-Azemi, EO Kehinde, et al. Indications of the mechanisms involved in improved sperm parameters by zinc therapy. *Med Princ Pract* 2008; 17(2):108–116.

18. Netter, A, et al. Effect of zinc administration on plasma testosterone, dihydrotestosterone, and sperm count. *Arch Androl* 1981; 7:69–73.

19. Westphal, LM, ML Polan, and AS Trant. Double-blind, placebo-controlled study of FertilityBlend: A nutritional supplement for improving fertility in women. *Clin Exp Obstet Gynecol* 2006; 33(4):205–208.

20. Matalliotakis, I, et al. L-carnitine levels in the seminal fluid of fertile and infertile men: Correlation with sperm quality. *Int J Fertil Womens Med* 2000; 45(3):236–240.

21. Vitali, G, et al. Carnitine supplementation in human idiopathic asthenospermia: Clinical results. *Drugs Exp Clin Res* 1995; 21(4): 157–159.

22. Zhou, X, F Liu, and S Zhai. Effect of L-carnitine and/or L-acetyl-carnitine in nutrition treatment for male infertility: A systematic review. *Asia Pac J Clin Nutr* 2007; 16(Suppl 1):383–390.

23. El-Nemr, A, et al. Effect of smoking on ovarian reserve and ovarian stimulation in-vitro fertilization and embryo transfer. *Hum Reprod* 1998; 13(8):2192–2198.

24. Joesoef, MR, et al. Fertility and use of cigarettes, alcohol, marijuana, and cocaine. *Ann Epidemiol* 1993; 3(6):592–594.

16 Pregnancy

1. Nausea and vomiting during pregnancy. Society of Obstetricians and Gynaecologists of Canada, October 19, 2006. Available at www.sogc.org/health/pregnancy-nausea_e.asp.

2. Vutyavanich, T, et al. Pyridoxine for nausea and vomiting of pregnancy: A randomized, double-blind, placebo-controlled trial. *Am J Obstet Gynecol* 1995; 173(3 Pt 1):881–884.

3. Sahakian, V, et al. Vitamin B6 is effective therapy for nausea and vomiting of pregnancy: A randomized, double-blind, placebo-controlled study. *Obstet Gynecol* 1991; 78(1):33–36.

4. Fischer-Rasmussen, W, et al. Ginger treatment of hyperemesis gravidarum. *Eur J Obstet Gynecol Reprod Biol* 1991; 38(1):19–24.

5. Vutyavanich, T, et al. Ginger for nausea and vomiting in pregnancy: Randomized, double-masked, placebo-controlled trial. *Obstet Gynecol* 2001; 97(4):577–582.

6. Luke, B, et al. Critical periods of maternal weight gain: Effect on twin birth weight. *Am J Obstet Gynecol* 1997; 177(5):1055–1062.

7. Lantz, ME, et al. Maternal weight gain patterns and birth weight outcomes in twin gestation. *Obstet Gynecol* 1996; 87(4):551–556.

8. Screening Tests. Women's Health Matters, Sunnybrook and Women's College Health

Sciences Centre, 2002. Available at www.womenshealthmatters.ca/centres/pregnancy/pregnancy/screening.html.

9. Hilton, E, HD Isenberg, P Alperstein, et al. Ingestion of yogurt containing Lactobacillus acidophilus as prophylaxis for candidal vaginitis. *Ann Intern Med* 1992; 116(5): 353–357.

10. Shalev, E, S Battino, E Weiner, et al. Ingestion of yogurt containing Lactobacillus acidophilus compared with pasteurized yogurt as prophylaxis for recurrent candidal vaginitis and bacterial vaginosis. *Arch Fam Med* 1996; 5(10): 593–596.

11. Duley, L. Routine calcium supplementation in pregnancy: Review no. 05938, June 23, 1993, in Enkin, MW, MJNC Keirse, MJ Renfrew, JP Neilson, eds. Cochrane database of systematic reviews. Issue 1 (Oxford, UK: Update Software, 1994).

12. Bucher, HC, et al. Effect of calcium supplementation and pregnancy-induced hypertension and pre-eclampsia: A meta-analysis of randomized controlled trials. *JAMA* 1996; 275(14):1113–1119.

13. Zhang, C, et al. Vitamin C and the risk of pre-eclampsia: Results from dietary questionnaire and plasma assay. *Epidemiology* 2002; 13(4):409–416.

14. Chappell, LC, et al. Effect of antioxidants on the occurrence of pre-eclampsia in women at increased risk: A randomized trial. Lancet 1999; 354(9181):810–816.

15. Klebanoff, MA, et al. Maternal serum paraxanthine, a caffeine metabolite, and the risk of spontaneous abortion. *N Eng J Med* 1999 Neilson 341(22):1639–1644.

16. Fernandes, O, et al. Moderate to heavy caffeine consumption during pregnancy and relationship to spontaneous abortion and abnormal fetal growth: A meta-analysis. *Reprod Toxicol* 1998 Neilson 12(4):435–444.

17 Breastfeeding

1. McNally, E, et al. A look at breastfeeding trends in Canada (1963–1982). *Can J Public Health* 1985; 76:101–107.

2. Breastfeeding. Table I—Breastfeeding initiation rates by selected maternal characteristics, Canada excluding territories, 1994/1995. Canadian Perinatal Surveillance System. Available at www.hc-sc.gc.ca.

3. Hanson, LA. Breastfeeding provides passive and likely long-lasting active immunity. *Ann Allergy Asthma Immunol* 1998; 81(6): 523–533.

4. Schoetazau, A, et al. Effect of exclusive breastfeeding and early solid food avoidance on the incidence of atopic dermatitis in high-risk infants at 1 year of age. *Pediatr Allergy Immunol* 2002; 13(4):234–242.

5. Oddy, WH, et al. Maternal asthma, infant feeding, and the risk of asthma in childhood. *J Allergy Clin Immunol* 2002; 110(1):65–67.

6. Oddy, WH, et al. The effect of respiratory infections, atopy, and breastfeeding on childhood asthma. *Eur Respir J* 2002; 19(5):899–905.

7. Oddy, WH, et al. Association between breast feeding and asthma in 6 year old children: Findings of a prospective birth cohort study. *BMJ* 1999; 319(7213):815–819.

8. Gdalvevih, M, et al. Breast-feeding and the risk of bronchial asthma in childhood: A systematic review with meta-analysis of prospective studies. *J Pediatr* 2001; 139(2):261–266.

9. Oddy, WH, et al. Breast feeding and cognitive development in childhood: A prospective birth cohort study. *Paediatr Perinat Epidemiol* 2003; 17(1): 81–90.

10. Mortensen, EL, et al. Breast feeding and intelligence. *Ugeskr Laeger* 2003; 165(13): 1361–1366. [Danish]

11. Gomez-Sanchiz, M, et al. Influence of breast-feeding on mental and psychomotor development. *Clin Pediatr* (Phila) 2003; 42(1):35–42.

12. Horwood, LJ, et al. Breast milk feeding and cognitive ability at 7–8 years. *Arch Dis Child Fetal Neonatal Ed* 2001; 84(1):F23–27.

13. Anderson, JW, et al. Breast-feeding and cognitive development: A meta-analysis. *Am J Clin Nutr* 1999; 70(4):525–535.

14. Jain, A, et al. How good is the evidence linking breastfeeding and intelligence? *Pediatrics* 2002; 109(6):1044–1053.

15. Mortensen, EL, et al. The association between duration of breastfeeding and adult intelligence. *JAMA* 2002; 287(18):2365–2371.

16. McVea, KL, et al. The role of breastfeeding in sudden infant death syndrome. *J Hum Lact* 2000; 16(1):13–20.

17. Wilson, AC, et al. Relation of infant diet to childhood health: Seven year follow up of cohort in Dundee infant feeding study. *BMJ* 1998; 316(7124):21–25.

18. Taittonen, L, et al. Prenatal and postnatal factors in predicting later blood pressure among children: Cardiovascular risk factors in young Finns. *Pediatr Res* 1996; 40(4): 627–632.

19. Bergmann, KE, et al. Early determinants of childhood overweight and adiposity in a birth cohort study: Role of breast-feeding. *Int J Obes Relat Metab Disord* 2003; 27(2):162–172.

20. Toschke, AM, et al. Overweight and obesity in 6- to 14-year-old Czech children in 1991:

Protective effect of breast-feeding. *J Pediatr* 2002; 141(6):764–769.

21. Armstrong, J, JJ Reilly; Child Health Information Team. Breastfeeding and lowering the risk of childhood obesity. *Lancet* 2002; 359(9322):2003–2004.

22. Liese, AD, et al. Inverse association of overweight and breast feeding in 9- to 10-y-old children in Germany. *Int J Obes Relat Metab Disord* 2001; 25(11):1644–1650.

23. Gillman, MW, et al. Risk of overweight among adolescents who were breastfed as infants. *JAMA* 2001; 285(19):2461–2467.

24. Bener, A, et al. Longer breast-feeding and protection against childhood leukaemia and lymphomas. *Eur J Cancer* 2001; 37(2):234–238.

25. Infante-Rivard, C, et al. Markers of infections, breast-feeding and childhood acute lymphoblastic leukaemia. *Br J Cancer* 2000; 83(11): 1559–1564.

26. Shu, XO, et al. Breast-feeding and risk of childhood acute leukemia. *J Natl Cancer Inst* 1999; 92(20):1765–1772.

27. Collaborative Group on Hormonal Factors in Breast Cancer. Breast cancer and breastfeeding: Collaborative reanalysis of individual data from 47 epidemiological studies in 30 countries, including 50302 women with breast cancer and 96973 women without the disease. *Lancet* 2002; 360(9328):187–195.

28. Mennella, JA, and GK Beauchamp. The transfer of alcohol to human milk: Effects on flavor and the infant's behavior. *N Engl J Med* 1991; 325(14):981–985.

29. Kramer, MS, and R Kakuma. Maternal dietary antigen avoidance during pregnancy and/or lactation for preventing or treating atopic disease in the child (Cochrane Methodology Review), in *The Cochrane Library*, Issue 4 (Chichester, UK: John Wiley & Sons, Ltd., 2003).

Part 6: Hormonal Health

18   Premenstrual Syndrome (PMS)

1. Premenstrual Syndrome (PMS). MedicineNet, Inc., 2009. Available at www.medicinenet.com/premenstrual_syndrome/article.htm.

2. Deuster, PA, et al. Biological, social, and behavioural factors associated with premenstrual syndrome. *Arch Fam Med* 1999; 8:122–128.

3. Blum, I, et al. The influence of meal composition on plasma serotonin and norepinephrine concentrations. *Metabolism* 1992; 41(2): 137–140.

4. Sayegh, R, et al. The effect of a carbohydrate-rich beverage on mood, appetite, and cognitive function in women with premenstrual syndrome. *Obstet Gynecol* 1995; 86(4 pt 1):520–528.

5. Jones, DY. Influence of dietary fat on self-reported menstrual symptoms. *Physiol Behav* 1987; 40(4):483–487.

6. Boyd, NF, et al. Effect of a low-fat high-carbohydrate diet on symptoms of cyclical mastopathy. *Lancet* 1988; 2(8603):128–132.

7. Barnard, ND, et al. Diet and sex-hormone globulin, dysmenorrhea, and premenstrual symptoms. *Obstet Gynecol* 2000; 95(2):245–250.

8. Wyatt, KM, et al. Efficacy of vitamin B6 in the treatment of premenstrual syndrome: Systematic review. *Br J of Med* 1999; 318(7195):1375–1381.

9. De Souza, MC, et al. A synergistic effect of a daily supplement for 1 month of 200 mg magnesium plus 50 mg vitamin B6 for the relief of anxiety-related premenstrual symptoms: A randomized, double-blind, crossover study. *J Women's Health Gend Based Med* 2000; 9(2):131–139.

10. Sharma, P, S Kulshreshtha, GM Singh, and A Bhagoliwal. Role of bromocripitine and pyridoxine in premenstrual tension syndrome. *Indian J Physiol Pharmacol* 2007; 51(4): 368–374.

11. London, RS, et al. Efficacy of alpha-tocopherol on premenstrual symptomology: A double-blind study: II Endocrine correlates. *J Am Coll Nutr* 1984; 3:351–356.

12. London, RS, et al. Efficacy of alpha-tocopherol on premenstrual symptomology: A double-blind study. *J Reprod Med* 1987; 32(6): 400–404.

13. London, RS, et al. Efficacy of alpha-tocopherol on premenstrual symptomology: A double-blind study. *J Am Coll Nutr* 1983; 2:115–122.

14. Thys-Jacobs, S, et al. Calcium carbonate and the premenstrual syndrome: Effects on premenstrual and menstrual symptoms. Premenstrual Syndrome Study Group. *Am J Obstet Gynecol* 1998; 179(2):444–452.

15. Bertone-Johnson, ER, SE Hankinson, A Bendich, et al. Calcium and vitamin D intake and risk of incident premenstrual syndrome. *Arch Intern Med* 2005; 165(11):1246–1252.

16. Posaci, C, et al. Plasma copper, zinc and magnesium levels in patients with premenstrual tension syndrome. *Acta Obstet Gynecol Scand* 1994; 73(6):452–455.

17. Rosenstein, DL, et al. Magnesium measures across the menstrual cycle in premenstrual syndrome. *Biol Psychiatry* 1994; 35(8): 557–561.

18. Walker, AF, et al. Magnesium supplementation alleviates premenstrual symptoms of fluid retention. *J Women's Health* 1998; 7(9):1157–1165.

19. Facchinetti, F, et al. Oral magnesium successfully relieves premenstrual mood changes. *Obstet Gynecol* 1991; 78(2):177–181.

20. Quartanta, S, MA Buscaglia, MG Meroni, et al. Pilot study of the efficacy and safety of a modified-release magnesium 250 mg tablet (Sincromag) for the treatment of premenstrual syndrome. *Clin Drug Investig* 2007; 27(1):51–58.

21. Prilepskaya, VN, AV Ledina, AV Tagiyeva, and FS Revazova. Vitex agnus castus: Successful treatment of moderate to severe premenstrual syndrome. *Maturitas* 2006; 55(1) Suppl 1:S55–S63.

22. Loch, EG, et al. Treatment of premenstrual syndrome with a phytopharmaceutical formulation containing Vitex agnus castus. *J Women's Health Gend Based Med* 2000; 9(3):315–320.

23. Schellenberg, R. Treatment for the premenstrual syndrome with agnus castus fruit extract: Prospective, randomized, placebo-controlled study. *Br Med J* 2001; 322(7279): 134–137.

24. Berger, D, W Schaffner, E Schrader, et al. Efficacy of Vitex agnus castus L. extract Ze 440 in patients with premenstrual syndrome (PMS). *Arch Gynecol Obstet* 2000; 264(3): 150–153.

25. Lauritzen, CH, HD Reuter, R Repges, et al. Treatment of premenstrual tension syndrome with Vitex agnus castus: Controlled-double blind versus pyridoxine. *Phytomedicine* 1997; 4:183–189.

26. Atmaca, M, S Kumru, and E Tezcan. Fluoxetine versus Vitex agnus castus extract in the treatment of premenstrual dysphoric disorder. *Hum Psychopharmacol Clin Exp* 2003; 18(3):191–195.

27. Gateley, CA, et al. Drug treatments for mastalgia: 17 years experience in the Cardiff Mastalgia Clinic. *J R Soc Med* 1992; 85(1):12–15.

28. Pye, JK, RE Mansel, and LE Hughes. Clinical experience of drug treatments for mastalgia. *Lancet* 1985; 2(8451):373–377.

29. Cheung, KL. Management of cyclical mastalgia in oriental women: Pioneer experience of using gamolenic acid (Efamast) in Asia. *Aust N Z J Surg* 1999; 69(7):492–494.

30. Tamborini, A, and R Taurelle. Value of standardized Ginkgo biloba extract (EGb 761) in the management of congestive symptoms of premenstrual syndrome. *Rev Fr Gynecol Obstet* 1993; 88(7–9):447–457. [French]

31. Kasper, S, M Gastpar, WE Müller, HP Volz, A Dienel, M Kieser, and HJ Möller. Efficacy of St. John's wort extract WS 5570 in acute treatment of mild depression: A reanalysis of data from controlled clinical trials. *Eur Arch Psychiatry Clin Neurosci* 2008; 258(1):59–63.

32. Stevison, C, and E Ernst. A pilot study of Hypericum perforatum for the treatment of premenstrual syndrome. *BJOG* 2000; 107(7):870–876.

33. Sampalis, F, R Bunea, MF Pelland, et al. Evaluation of the effects of Neptune Krill Oil on the management of premenstrual syndrome and dysmenorrhea. *Altern Med Rev* 2003; 8(2):171–179.

19 Perimenopause

1. McKinlay, SM, et al. The menopausal syndrome. *Br J Prev Soc Med* 1974; 28: 108–115.

2. Thompsom, B, et al. Menopausal age and symptomatology in a general practice. *J Biosoc Sci* 1973; 5:71–82.

3. Tang, GWK. The climacteric of Chinese factory workers. *Maturitas* 1994; 19:177–182.

4. Murkies, AL, et al. Dietary flour supplementation decreases postmenopausal hot flushes: Effect of soy and wheat. *Maturitas* 1995; 21:189–195.

5. Brzezinski, A, et al. Short-term effects of phytoestrogens-rich diet on postmenopausal women. *Menopause* 1997; 4:89–94.

6. Albertazzi, P, et al. The effect of dietary soy supplementation on hot flushes. *Obstet Gynecol* 1998; 91(1):6–11.

7. Greenwood, S, et al. The role of isoflavones in menopausal health: Consensus opinion of The North American Menopause Society. *Menopause* 2000; 7(2):215–229.

8. Nicklas, TA, et al. Breakfast consumption with and without vitamin-mineral supplement use favorably impacts daily nutrient intake of ninth-grade students. *J Adolesc Health* 2000; 27(5):314–321.

9. Smith, AP, et al. Breakfast cereal and caffeinated coffee: Effects on working memory, attention, mood, and cardiovascular function. *Physiol Behav* 1999; 67(1):9–17.

10. Benton, D, and PY Parker. Breakfast, blood glucose, and cognition. *Am J Clin Nutr* 1998; 67(4):772S–778S.

11. Akata, T, et al. Successful combined treatment with vitamin B12 and bright artificial light of one case with delayed sleep phase syndrome. *Jpn J Psychiatry Neurol* 1993; 47(2):439–440.

12. Maeda, K, et al. A multicenter study of the effects of vitamin B12 on sleep-waking rhythm

disorders: In Shizuoka Prefecture. *Jpn J Psychiatry Neurol* 1992; 46(1):229–230.

13. Ohta, T, et al. Treatment of persistent sleep-wake schedule disorders in adolescents with methylcobalamin (vitamin B12). *Sleep* 1991; 14(5):414–418.

14. Okawa, M, et al. Vitamin B12 treatment for sleep-wake rhythm disorders. *Sleep* 1990; 13(1):15–23.

15. Liske, E, W Hanggi, HH Henneicke-von Zepelin, et al. Physiological investigation of a unique extract of black cohosh (Cimicifugae racemosae rhizoma): A 6-month clinical study demonstrates no systemic estrogenic effect. *J Women's Health Gend Based Med* 2002; 11(2):163–174.

16. Osmers, R, M Friede, E Liske, et al. Efficacy and safety of isopropanolic black cohosh extract for climacteric symptoms. *Obstet Gynecol* 2005; 105 (5 Pt. 1):1074–1083.

17. Nappi, RE, B Malavasi, B Brundu, and F Facchinetti. Efficacy of Cimicifuga racemosa on climacteric complaints: A randomized study versus low-dose transdermal estradiol. *Gynecol Endocrinol* 2005; 20(1):30–35.

18. Lindahl, O, et al. Double blind study of a valerian preparation. *Pharmacol Biochem Behav* 1989; 32:1065–1066.

19. Leathwood, PD, et al. Aqueous extract of valerian root improves sleep quality in man. *Pharmacol Biochem Behav* 1982; 17:65–71.

20. Leathwood, PD, et al. Aqueous extract of valerian root reduces latency to fall asleep in man. *Planta Medica* 1985; 51:144–148.

21. Donath, F, S Quispe, K Diefenbach, et al. Critical evaluation of the effect of valerian extract on sleep structure and sleep quality. *Pharmacopsych* 2000; 33(2):47–53.

22. Bent, S, M Patterson, and D Garvin. Valerian for sleep: A systematic review and meta-analysis. *Alternative Therapies* 2001; 7:S4.

20 Polycystic Ovary Syndrome (PCOS)

1. Lau, D. Screening for diabetes in women with polycystic ovary syndrome. *CMAJ* 2007; 176(7):951–952.

2. Legro, RS. Polycystic ovary syndrome: Current and future treatment paradigms. *Am J Obstet Gynecol* 1998; 179(6 Pt 2):S101–S108.

3. Taylor, AE. Systemic adversities of ovarian failure. *J Soc Gynecol Investig* 2001; (1 Suppl Proceedings):S7–S9.

4. Wahrenberg, H, et al. Divergent effects of weight reduction and oral anticonception treatment on adrenergic lipolysis in obese women with the polycystic ovary syndrome. *J Clin Endocrinol Metab* 1999; 84(6): 2182–2187.

5. Jakubowicz, DJ, and JE Nestler. 17 alpha-Hydroxyprogesterone response to leuprolide and serum androgens in obese women with and without polycystic ovary syndrome after dietary weight loss. *J Clin Endocrinol Metab* 1997; 82(2):556–560.

6. Andersen, P, et al. Increased insulin sensitivity and fibrinolytic capacity after dietary intervention in obese women with polycystic ovary syndrome. *Metabolism* 1995; 44(5):611–616.

7. Franks, S, et al. The role of nutrition and insulin in the regulation of sex hormone binding globulin. *J Steroid Biochem Mol Biol* 1991; 39(5B):835–838.

8. Hoeger, KM, L Kochman, N Wixom, et al. A randomized, 48-week, placebo-controlled trial of intensive lifestyle modification and/or metformin therapy in overweight women with polycystic ovary syndrome: A pilot study. *Fertil Steril* 2004; 82(2):421–429.

9. Tang, T, J Glanville, CJ Hayden, et al. Combined lifestyle modification and metformin in obese patients with polycystic ovary syndrome: A randomized, placebo-controled, double-blind multicentre study. *Hum Reprod* 2006; 21(1):90–89.

10. Panidis, D, D Farmakiotis, D Rousso, et al. Obesity, weight loss, and the polycystic ovary syndrome: Effect of treatment with diet and orlistat for 24 weeks on insulin resistance and androgen levels. *Fertil Steril* 2008; 89(4): 899–906.

11. Franks, S, et al. Obesity and polycystic ovary syndrome. *Ann NY Acad Sci* 1991; 626: 201–206.

12. Kiddy, DS, et al. Improvement in endocrine and ovarian function during dietary treatment of obese women with polycystic ovary syndrome. *Clin Endocrinol (Oxford)* 1992; 36(10):105–111.

13. Moran, LJ, M Noakes, PM Clifton, et al. Dietary composition in restoring reproductive and metabolic physiology in overweight women with polycystic ovary syndrome. *J Clin Endocrinol Metal* 2003; 88(2):812–819.

14. Douglas, CC, BA Gower, BE Darnell, et al. Role of diet in the treatment of polycystic ovary syndrome. *Fertil Steril* 2006; 85(3): 679–688.

15. Qublan, HS, EK Yannakoula, MA AL-Qudah, and FI El-Uri. Dietary intervention versus metformin to improve the reproductive outcome in women with polycystic ovary syndrome: A prospective comparative study. *Saudi Med J* 2007; 28(11):1694–1699.

16. Moghetti, P, et al. Spironolactone, but not flutamide, administration prevents bone loss in hyperandrogenic women treated with gonadotropin-releasing hormone agonist. *J Clin Endocrinol Metab* 1999; 84(4): 1250–1254.

17. Lucidi, RS, AC Thyer, CA Easten, et al. Effect of chromium supplementation on insulin resistance and ovarian menstrual cyclicity in women with polycystic ovary syndrome. *Fertil Steril* 2005; 84(6):1755–1757.

18. Lydic, ML, M McNurlan, S Bembo, et al. Chromium picolinate improves insulin sensitivity in obese subjects with polycystic ovary syndrome. *Fertil Steril* 2006; 86(1):243–246.

19. Nestler, JE, et al. Ovulatory and metabolic effects of D-chiro-inositol in the polycystic ovary syndrome. *N Engl J Med* 1999; 340(17):1314–1320.

21   Thyroid Disease

1. A Major Women's Health Issue. American Autoimmune Related Diseases Association, Inc., 2001. Available at www.aarda.org/women_health_art.html.

2. Graves' Disease. The Thyroid Foundation of Canada, April 23, 2007. Available at www.thyroid.ca/Guides/HG06.html.

3. Yoshiuchi, K, et al. Stressful life events and smoking were associated with Graves' disease in women, but not in men. *Psychosom Med* 1998; 60(2):182–185.

4. Hypothyroidism. The Thyroid Foundation of Canada, April 23, 2007. Available at www.thyroid.ca/Guides/HG03.html.

5. Faughnan, M, et al. Screening for thyroid disease at the menopausal clinic. *Clin Invest Med* 1995; 18(1):11–18.

6. Duntas, LH. Oxidants, antioxidants in physical exercise and relation to thyroid function. *Horm Metab Red* 2005; 37(9):572–576.

7. Guerra, LN, C Rios de Molina Mdel, EA Miler, et al. Antioxidants and methimazole in the treatment of Graves' disease: Effect on urinary malondialdehyde levels. *Clin Chim Acta* 2005; 352(1–2):115–120.

8. Bianchi, G, et al. Oxidative stress and antioxidant metabolites in patients with hyperthyroidism: Effect of treatment. *Horm Metab Res* 1999; 31(11):620–624.

9. Costantini, F, et al. Effect of thyroid function on LDL oxidation. *Artherioscler Thromb Vasc Biol* 1998; 18(5):732–737.

10. Goswami, UC, and S Choudhury. The status of retinoids in women suffering from hyper- and hypothyroidism: Interrelationship between vitamin A, beta-carotene and thyroid hormones. *Int J Vitam Nutr Res* 1999; 69(2): 132–135.

11. Mano, T, et al. Vitamin E and coenzyme Q10 concentrations in the thyroid of patients with various thyroid disorders. *Am J Med Sci* 1998; 315(4):230–232.

12. Seven, A, et al. Biochemical evaluation of oxidative stress in propylthiouricil treated hyperthyroid patients: Effect of vitamin C supplementation. *Clin Chem Lab Met* 1998; 36(10):767–770.

13. Vcra, VB, F Skreb, I Cepelak, et al. Supplementation with antioxidants in the treatment of Graves' disease: The effect on glutathione peroxidase activity and concentration of selenium. *Clin Chim Acta* 2004; 341(1–2):55–63.

14. Bacic-Vcra V, F Skreb, I Cepelak, et al. The effect of antioxidant supplementation on superoxide dismultase activity, Cu and Zn levels, and total antioxidant status in erythrocytes of patients with Graves' disease. *Clin Chem Lab Med* 2005; 43(4):383–388.

15. Uzzan, B, et al. Effects on bone mass of long term treatment with thyroid hormones: A meta-analysis. *J Clin Endocrinol Metab* 1996; 81(12):4278–4289.

16. Yamashita, H, et al. Seasonal changes in calcium homeostasis affect the incidence of postoperative tetany in patients with Graves' disease. *Surgery* 2000; 127(4):377–382.

17. Solomon, BL, et al. Remission rates with antithyroid drug therapy: Continuing influence of iodine intake? *Ann Intern Med* 1987; 107(4):510–512.

18. Rodondi, N, D Aujesky, E Vittinghoff, et al. Subclinical hypothyroidism and the risk of coronary heart disease: A meta-analysis. *Am J Med* 2006; 119(7):541–551.

19. Pearce, EN. Hypothyroidism and dyslipidemia: Modern concepts and approaches. *Curr Cardiol Rep* 2004; 6(6):451–456.

20. Pucci, E, et al. Thyroid and lipid metabolism. *Int J Obes Relat Metab Disord* 2000; (Suppl 2):S109–S112.

21. Vierhapper, H, et al. Low-density lipoprotein cholesterol in subclinical hypothyroidism. *Thyroid* 2000; 10(11):981–984.

22. Hak, AE, et al. Subclinical hypothyroidism is an independent risk factor for atherosclerosis and myocardial infarction in elderly women: The Rotterdam Study. *Ann Intern Med* 2000; 132(4):270–278.

23. Bindels, AJ, et al. The prevalence of subclinical hypothyroidism at different total plasma cholesterol levels in middle aged men and women: A need for case-finding? *Clin Endocrinol* 1999; 50(2):217–220.

24. Becerra, A, et al. Lipoprotein(a) and other lipoproteins in hypothyroid patients before and after thyroid replacement therapy. *Clin Nutr* 1999; 18(5):319–322.

25. Teas, J, LE Braverman, MS Kurzer, et al. Seaweed and soy: Companion foods in Asian cusine and their effects on thyroid function in American women. *J Med Food* 2007; 10(1):90–100.

26. Bruce, B, M Messina, and GA Spiller. Isoflavone supplements do not affect thyroid function in iodine-replete postmenopausal women. *J Med Food* 2003; 6(4):309–316.

27. Messina, M, and G Redmond. Effects of soy protein and soybean isoflavones on thyroid function in healthy adults and hypothyroid patients: A review of the relevant literature. *Thyroid* 2006; 16(3):249–258.

28. Ozmen, B, D Ozmen, Z Parlidar, et al. Impact of renal function or folate status on altered plasma homocysteine levels in hypothyroidism. *Endocrin J* 2006; 53(10):119–124.

29. Diekman, MJ, NM van der Put, HJ Blom, et al. Determinants of changes in plasma homocysteine in hyperthyroidism and hypothyroidism. *Clin Endocrinol* (Oxford) 2001; 54(2): 197–204.

30. Nedrebo, BG, et al. Plasma total homocysteine levels in hyperthyroid and hypothyroid patients. *Metabolism* 1998; 47(1):89–93.

31. Tajiri, J, et al. Studies of hypothyroidism in patients with high iodine intake. *J Clin Endocrinol Metab* 1986; 63(2):412–417.

32. Olivieri, O, et al. Low selenium status in the elderly influences thyroid hormones. *Clin Sci* (Colch) 1995; 89(6):637–642.

33. Rayman, MP, AJ Thompson, B Bekaert, et al. Randomized controlled trial of the effect of selenium supplementation on thyroid function in the elderly in the United Kingdon. *Am J Clin Nutr* 2008; 87(2):370–378.

34. Negro, R, G Greco, T Mangieri, et al. The influence of selenium supplementation on postpartum thyroid status in pregnant women with thyroid peroxidase autoantibodies. *J Clin Endocrinol Metab* 2007; 92(4):1263–1268.

35. Gartner, R, BC Gasnier, JW Dietrich, et al. Selenium supplementation in patients with autoimmune thyroidosis decreases thyroid peroxidase antibodies concentrations. *J Clin Endocrinol Metab* 2002; 87(4):1687–1691.

36. Shakir, KM, et al. Ferrous sulfate-induced increase in requirement for thyroxine in a patient with primary hypothyroidism. *South Med J* 1997; 90(6):637–639.

37. Campbell, NR, et al. Ferrous sulfate reduces thyroxine efficacy in patients with hypothyroidism. *Ann Intern Med* 1992; 117(12): 1010–1013.

Part 7: Pelvic and Urinary Tract Health

22 Cervical Dysplasia

1. HPV and Cervical Cancer. The Canadian Cancer Society, August 21, 2008. Available at www.cancer.ca/Canada-wide/Prevention/ Other%20risk%20factors/Human%20 papillomavirus%20HPV/HPV%20and%20 cervical%20cancer.aspx?sc_lang=en.

2. Nagata, C, et al. Serum retinal level and risk of cervical cancer in cases with cervical dysplasia. *Cancer Invest* 1999; 17(4):253–258.

3. Romney, SL, et al. Effects of beta-carotene and other factors on outcome of cervical dysplasia and human papillomavirus infection. *Gynecol Oncol* 1997; 65(3):483–492.

4. Mackerras, D, et al. Randomized double-blind trial of beta-carotene and vitamin C in women with minor cervical abnormalities. *Br J Cancer* 1999; 79(9–10):1448–1453.

5. Keefe, KA, MJ Schell, C Brewer, et al. A randomized, double blind, Phase III trial using oral beta-carotene supplementation for women with high-grade cervical intraepithelial neoplasia. *Cancer Epidemiol Biomarkers Prev* 2001; 10(10):1029–1035.

6. Kantesky, PA, et al. Dietary intake and blood levels of lycopene: Association with cervical dysplasia among non-Hispanic, black women. *Nutr Cancer* 1998; 31(1):31–40.

7. Basu, J, et al. Plasma ascorbic acid and beta-carotene levels in women evaluated for HPV infection, smoking, and cervix dysplasia. *Cancer Detec Prev* 1991; 15(3):165–170.

8. Goodman, MT, et al. The association of plasma micronutrients with the risk of cervical dysplasia in Hawaii. *Cancer Epidemiol Biomarkers Prev* 1998; 7(6):537–544.

9. Whitehead, N, et al. Megaloblastic changes in the cervical epithelium: Association with oral contraceptive therapy. *JAMA* 1973; 226: 1421–1424.

10. McPherson, RS. Nutritional factors and the risk of cervical dysplasia. Proceedings and abstracts of papers presented at the 22nd annual meeting of the Society for Epidemiological Research, June 14–16, 1989, Birmingham, AL. *Am J Epidemiol* 1989; 130(4):830. [Abstract]

11. Piyathilake, CJ, M Macaluso, I Brill, et al. Lower red blood cell folate enhances HPV-16-associated risk of cervical intraepithelial neoplasia. *Nutrition* 2007; 23(3):203–210.

12. Butterworth, C, et al. Improvement in cervical dysplasia associated with folic acid therapy in

users of oral contraceptives. *Am J Clin Nutr* 1982; 35:73–82.

13. Childers, JM, et al. Chemoprevention of cervical cancer with folic acid: A phase III Southwest Oncology Group Intergroup Study. *Cancer Epidemiol Biomarkers Prev* 1995; 4:155–159.

23   Endometriosis

1. Endometriosis. MedicineNet Inc., 2009. Available at www.medicinenet.com/ endometriosis/article.htm2.

2. Sesti, F, A Pietropolli, T Capozzolo, et al. Hormonal suppression treatment or dietary therapy versus placebo in the control of painful symptoms after conservative surgery for endometriosis stage III–IV: A randomized comparative trial. *Fertil Steril* 2007; 88(6): 1541–1547.

3. Wu, MY, et al. Increase in the production of interleukin-6, interleukin-10, and interleukin-12 by lipoploysaccharide-stimulated peritoneal macrophages from women with endometriosis. *Am J Reprod Immunol* 1999; 41(1):106–111.

4. Karck, U, et al. PGE2 and PGF2 alpha release by human peritoneal macrophages in endometriosis. *Prostaglandins* 1996; 51(1): 49–60.

5. Nabekura, H, et al. Fallopian tube prostaglandin production with and without endometriosis. *Int J Fertil Menopausal Stud* 1994; 39(1):57–63.

6. Koike, H, et al. Eicosanoids production in endometriosis. *Prostaglandins Leukot Essent Fatty Acids* 1992; 45(4):331–317.

7. Koike, H, et al. Correlation between dysmenorrheic severity and prostaglandin production in women with endometriosis. *Prostaglandins Leukot Essent Fatty Acids* 1992; 46(2): 133–137.

8. Benedetto, C. Eicosanoids in primary dysmenorrhea, endometriosis and menstrual migraine. *Gynecol Endocrinol* 1989; 3(1):71–94.

9. Parazzini, F, F Chiaffarino, M Surace, et al. Selected food intake and risk of endometriosis. *Hum Reprod* 2004; 19(8):1755–1759.

10. Ibid.

11. Mojzis, J, L Varinska, G Mojzisova, et al. Antiangiogenic effects of flavonoids and chalcones. *Pharmacol Res* 2008; 57(4): 259–265.

12. Mathias, JR, et al. Relation of endometriosis and neuromuscular disease of the gastrointestinal tract: New insights. *Fertil Steril* 1998; 70(1):81–88.

13. Grodstein, F, et al. Relation of female infertility to consumption of caffeinated beverages. *Am J Epidemiol* 1993; 137(12):1353–1360.

14. Grodstein, F, et al. Infertility in women and moderate alcohol use. *Am J Public Health* 1994; 84(9):1429–1432.

15. Murphy, AA, et al. Endometriosis: A disease of oxidative stress? *Semin Reprod Endocrinol* 1998; 16(4):263–273.

16. Dawood, MY. Hormonal therapies for endometriosis: Implications for bone metabolism. *Acta Obstet Gynecol Scand* 1994; 159(Suppl):22–34.

17. Harel, Z, FM Biro, RK Kottenhahn, and SL Rosenthal. Supplementation with omega-3 polyunsaturated fatty acids in the management of dysmenorrhea in adolescents. *Am J Obstet Gynecol* 1996; 174(4):1335–1338.

18. Sesti, F, A Pietropolli, T Capozzolo, et al. Hormonal suppression treatment or dietary therapy versus placebo in the control of painful symptoms after conservative surgery for endometriosis stage III–IV: A randomized comparative trial. *Fertil Steril* 2007; 88(6): 1541–1547.

24   Interstitial Cystitis (IC)

1. Pelikan, Z, et al. The role of allergy in interstitial cystitis. *Ned Tijdschr Geneeskd* 1999; 143(25):1289–1292. [Dutch]

2. Whitmore, K, et al. Survey of the effect of Prelief on food-related exacerbation of interstitial cystitis symptoms. Philadelphia, 1998–1999, unpublished. Available at www.akpharma.com/Icrews/food_survey.htm.

3. Whitmore, K, et al. The therapeutic effects of Prelief in interstitial cystitis. Philadelphia, 2000, unpublished. Available at www. akpharma.com/Icrews/food_survey.htm.

4. Smith, SD, et al. Urinary nitric oxide synthase activity and cyclic GMP levels are decreased with interstitial cystitis and increased with urinary tract infections. *J Urol* 1996; 155(4):1432–1435.

5. Cartledge, JJ, et al. A randomized double-blind placebo-controlled crossover trial of the efficacy of L-arginine in the treatment of interstitial cystitis. *BJU Int* 2000; 85(4):421–426.

6. Smith, SD, et al. Improvement in interstitial cystitis symptom scores during treatment with oral L-arginine. *J Urol* 1997; 158(3 Pt 1):703–708.

7. Korting, GE, et al. A randomized double-blind trial of oral L-arginine for treatment of interstitial cystitis. *J Urol* 1999; 161(2):558–565.

8. Wheeler, MA, et al. Effect of long term oral L-arginine on the nitric oxide synthase pathway in the urine from patients with interstitial cystitis. *J Urol* 1997; 158(6):2045–2050.

25 Urinary Tract Infections (UTIs)

1. Avorn, J, M Manone, JH Gurwitz, et al. Reduction of bacteriuria and pyuria after ingestion of cranberry juice. *JAMA* 1994; 27(10)1:751–754.

2. Wing, DA, PJ Rumney, CW Preslicka, and JH Chung. Daily cranberry juice for the prevention of asymptomatic bacteriuria in pregnancy: A randomized, controlled pilot study. *J Urol* 2008; 180(4):1367–1372.

3. Kontiokari, T, et al. Randomised trial of cranberry-lingonberry juice and Lactobacillus GG drink for the prevention of urinary tract infections in women. *Br Med J* 2001; 322(7302):1571.

4. Avron, J, et al. Reduction of bacteriuria and pyuria after ingestion of cranberry juice. *JAMA* 1994; 271:751–754.

5. Kyo, E, et al. Immunomodulatory effects of aged garlic extract. *J Nutr* 2001; 131(Suppl 3): 1075S–1079S.

6. Amagase, H, et al. Intake of garlic and its bioactive components. *J Nutr* 2001; 131(Suppl 3):955S–962S.

7. Salman, H, et al. Effect of a garlic derivative (alliin) on peripheral blood cell immune responses. *Int J Immunopharmacol* 1999; 21(9):589–597.

8. Reid, G. Potential preventative strategies and therapies in urinary tract infection. *World J Urol* 1999; 17(6):359–363.

9. Velraeds, MM, et al. Inhibition of initial adhesion of uropathogenic Enterococcus faecalis by biosurfactants from Lactobacillus isolates. *Appl Environ Micorbiol* 1996; 62(6):1958–1963.

10. Hawthorn, LA, and G Reid. Exclusion of uropathogen adhesion to polymer surfaces by Lactobacillus acidophilus. *J Biomed Mater Res* 1990; 24(1):39–46.

11. Reid, G, et al. Is there a role for lactobacilli in prevention of urogenital and intestinal functions? *Clin Microbiol Rev* 1990; 3(4): 335–344.

12. Falagas, ME, GI Betsi, T Tokas, and S Athanasiou. Probiotics for prevention of recurrent urinary tract infections in women: A review of the evidence from microbiological and clinical studies. *Drugs* 2006; 66(9):1253–1261.

26 Ovarian Cancer

1. Leitzmann, MF, C Koebnick, KN Danforth, et al. Body mass index and risk of ovarian cancer. *Cancer* 2009; 115(4):812–822.

2. Rodriguez, C, EE Calle, D Fakhrabadi-Shokoohi, et al. Body mass index, height, and the risk of ovarian cancer mortality in a prospective cohort of postmenopausal women. *Cancer Epidemiol Biomarkers Prev* 2002; 11(9):822–828.

3. Schouten, LJ, C Rivera, DJ Hunter, et al. Height, body mass index, and ovarian cancer: A pooled analysis of 12 cohort studies. *Cancer Epidemiol Biomarkers Prev* 2008; 17(4): 902–912.

4. Mulholland, HG, LJ Murray, CR Cardwell, and MM Cantwell. Dietary glycaemic index, glycaemic load and endometrial and ovarian cancer risk: A systematic review and meta-analysis. *Br J Cancer* 2008; 99(3):434–441.

5. Larsson, SC, L Bergkvist, and A Wolk. Milk and lactose intakes and ovarian cancer risk in the Swedish Mammography Cohort. *Am J Clin Nutr* 2004; 80(5):1353–1357.

6. Fairfield, KM, DJ Hunter, GA Colditz, et al. A prospective study of dietary lactose and ovarian cancer. *Int J Cancer* 2004; 110(2):271–277.

7. Larsson, SC, A Orsini, and A Wolk. Milk, milk products and lactose intake and ovarian cancer risk: A meta-analysis of epidemiological studies. *Int J Cancer* 2006; 118(2):431–441.

8. Gates, MA, AF Vitonis, SS Tworoger, et al. Flavonoid intake and ovarian cancer risk in a population-based case-control study. *Int J Cancer* 2009; 124(8):1918–1925.

9. Rossi, M, E Negri, P Lagiou, et al. Flavonoids and ovarian cancer risk: A case-control study in Italy. *Int J Cancer* 2008; 123(4):895–898.

10. Gates, MA, SS Tworoger, JL Hecht, et al. A prospective study of dietary flavonoids intake and incidence of epithelial ovarian cancer. *Int J Cancer* 2007; 121(10):2225–2232.

11. Navarro Silvera, SA, M Jain, GR Howe, et al. Dietary folate consumption and risk of ovarian cancer: A prospective cohort study. *Eur J Cancer Prev* 2006; 15(6):511–515.

12. Larsson, SC, E Giovannucci, and A Wolk. Dietary folate intake and incidence of ovarian cancer: The Swedish Mammography study. *J Natl Cancer Inst* 2004; 96(5):396–402.

Index